Hepatocellular Carcinoma - Challenges and Opportunities of a Multidisciplinary Approach

Edited by Georgios Tsoulfas

Published in London, United Kingdom

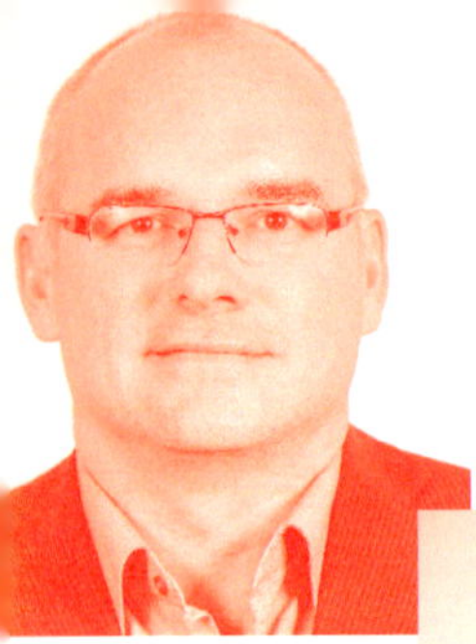

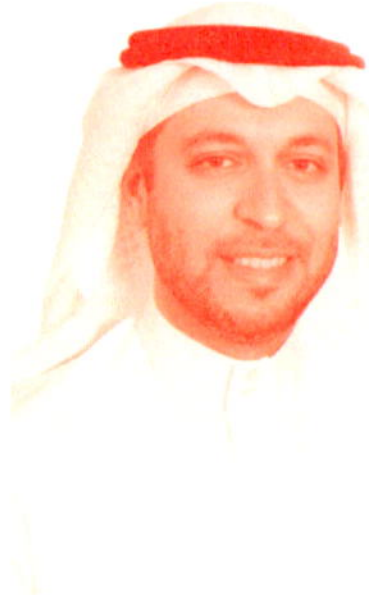

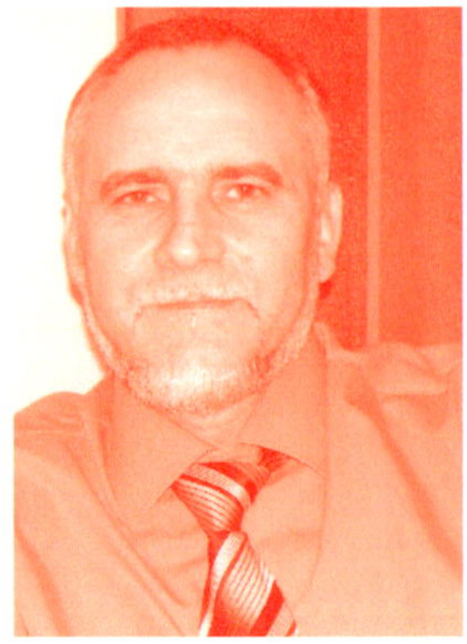

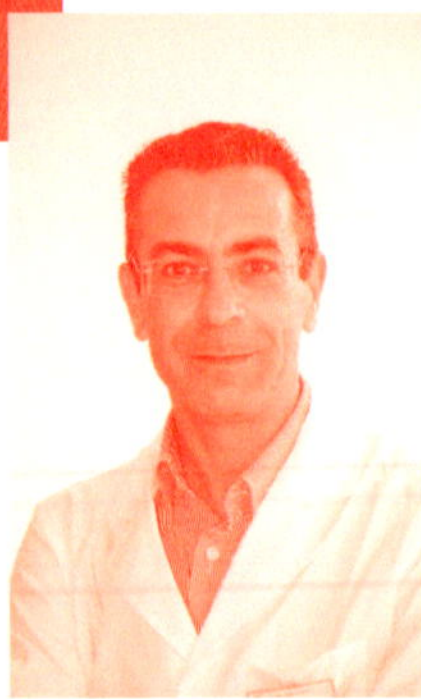

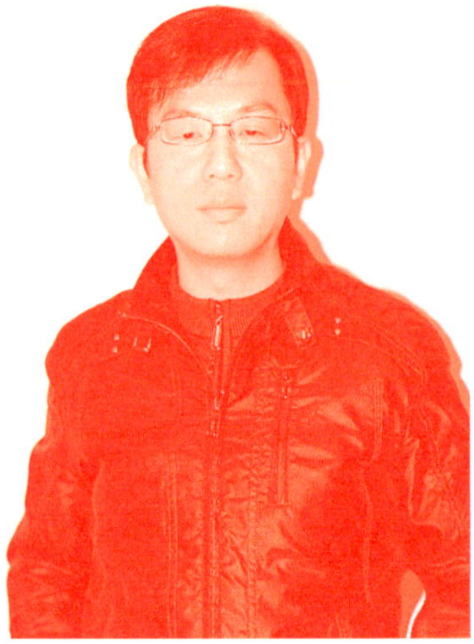

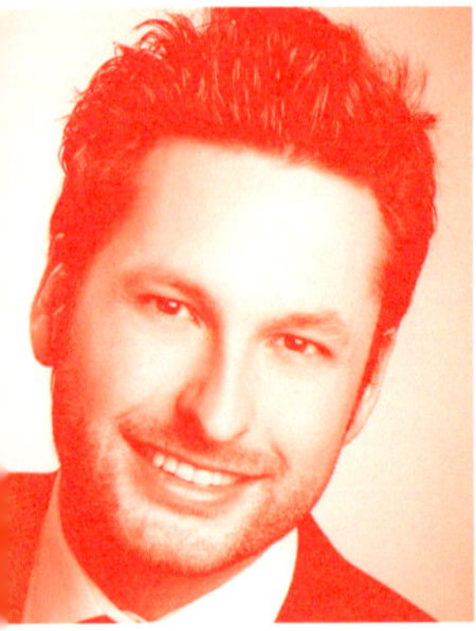

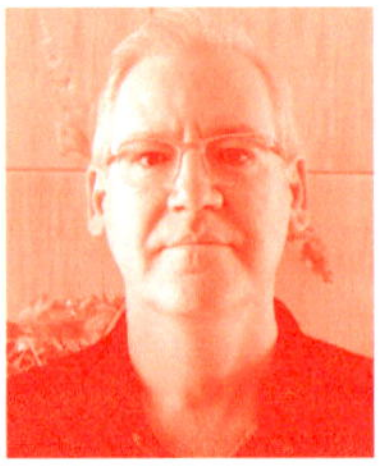

IntechOpen

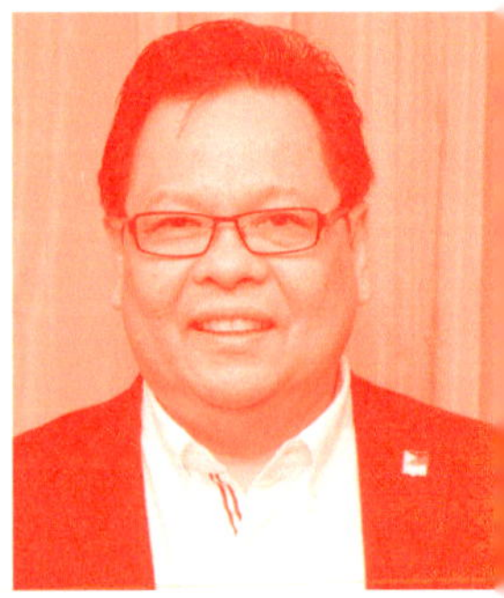

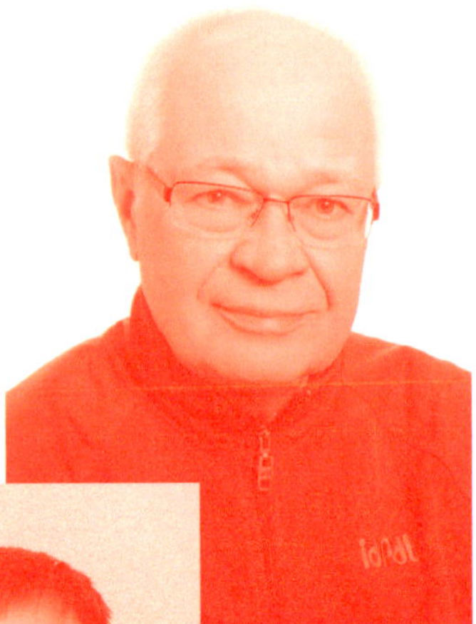

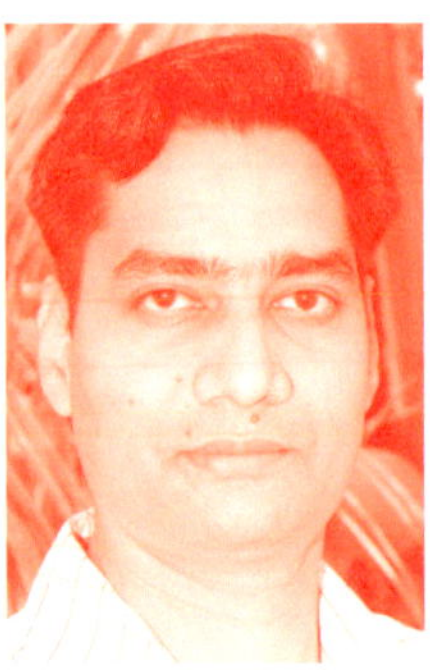

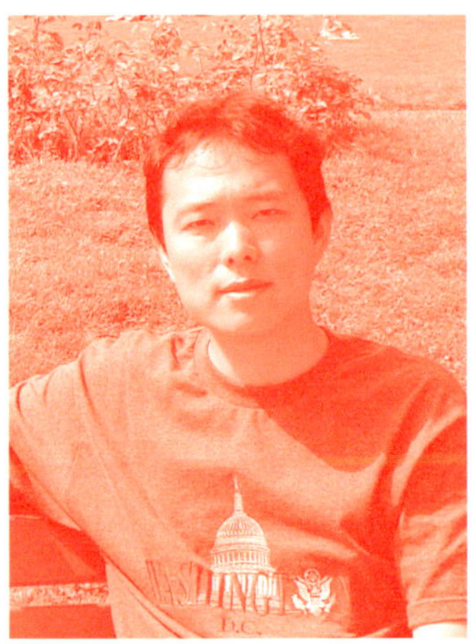

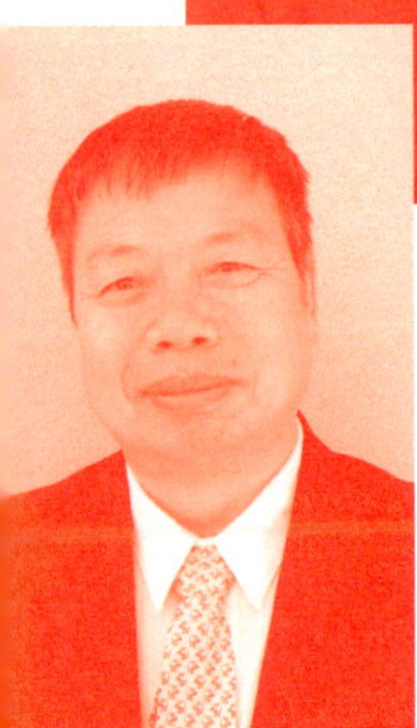

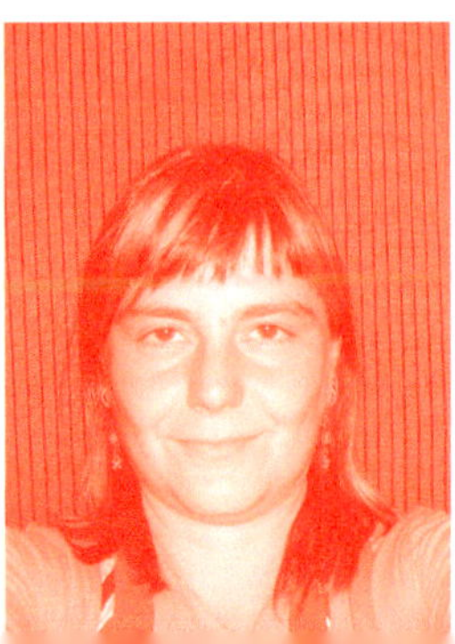

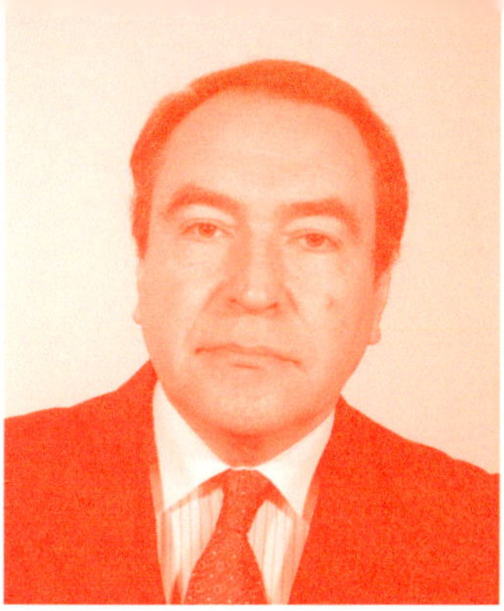
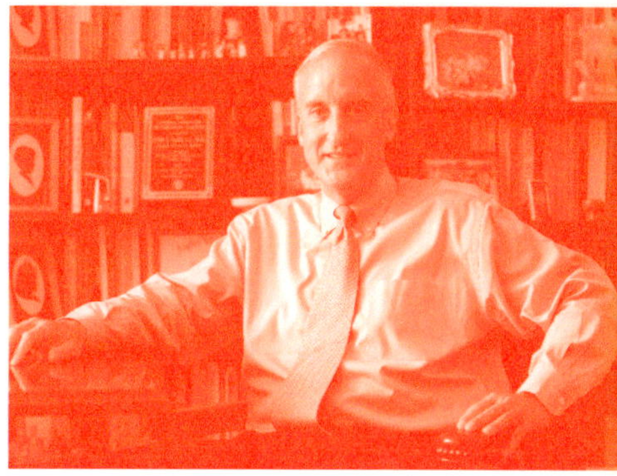
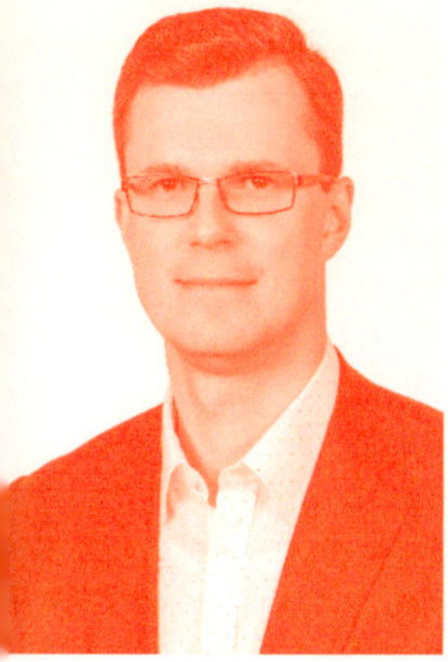
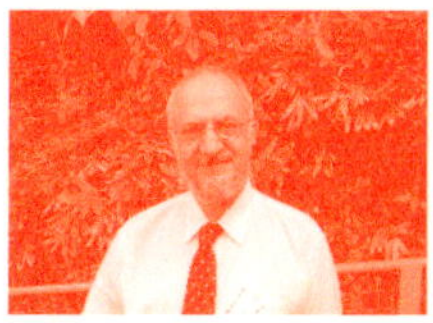
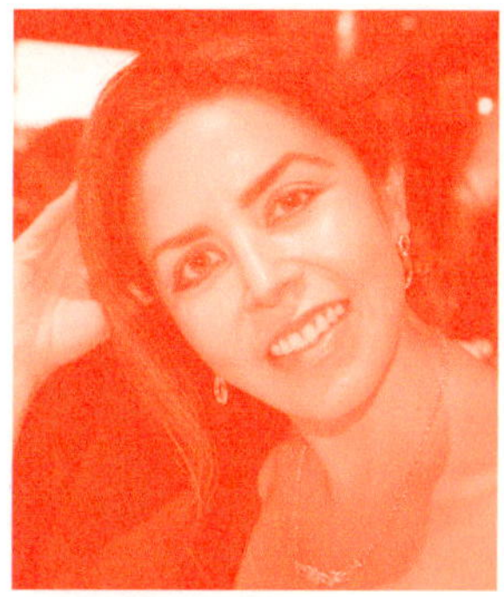

Supporting open minds since 2005

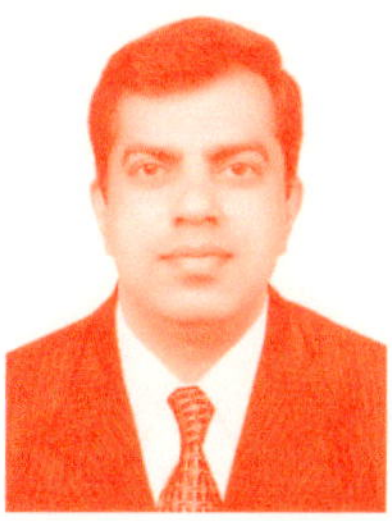
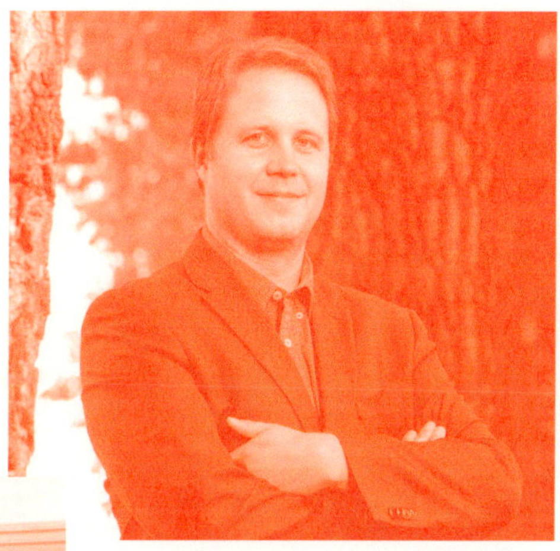
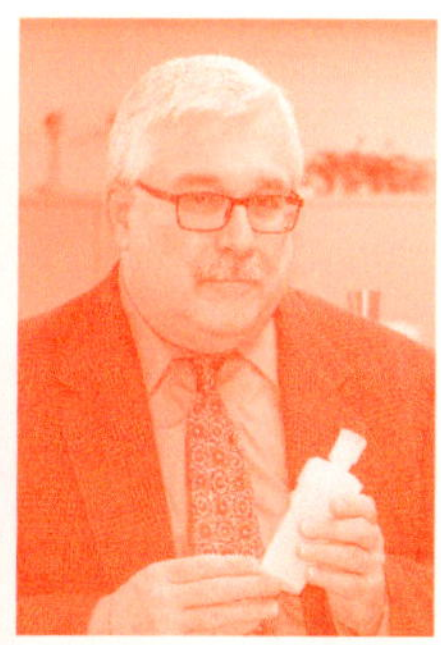
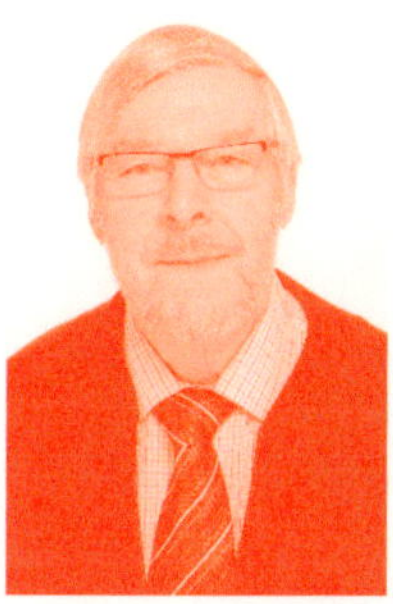
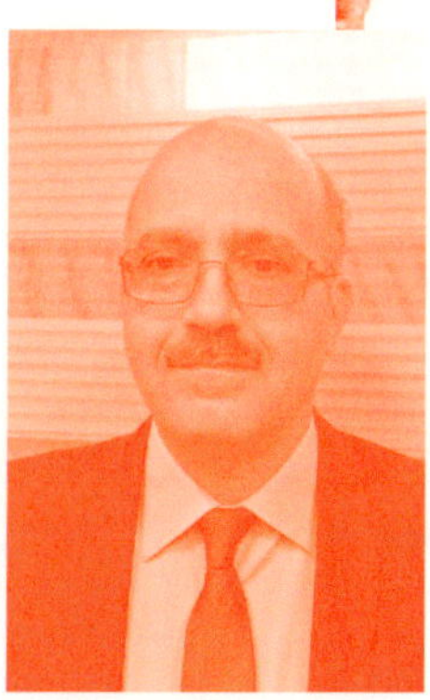
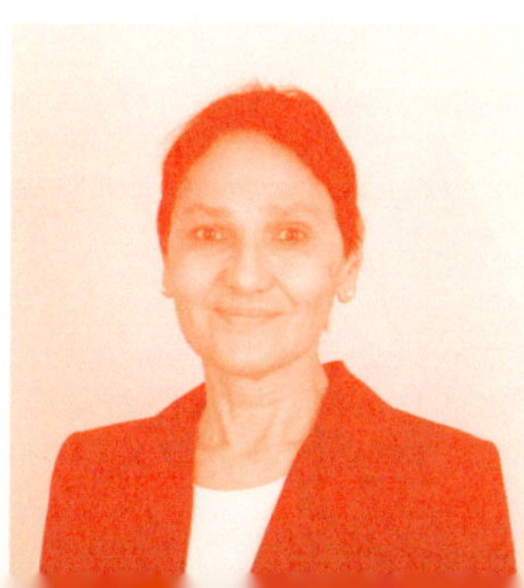
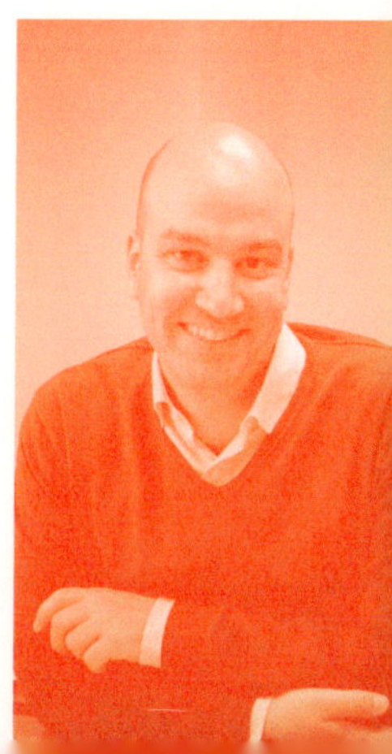

Hepatocellular Carcinoma - Challenges and Opportunities of a Multidisciplinary Approach
http://dx.doi.org/10.5772/intechopen.94813
Edited by Georgios Tsoulfas

Contributors
Cchanchai Charonpongsuntorn, Haichao Zhao, Changzhou Chen, Jiefeng He, Muntaser S. Ahmad, Osama Makhamrah, Mohammad Hjouj, Wei Zhang, Mahmoud Aryan, Ellery Altshuler, Xia Qian, Ioannis Hatzaras, Nikolaos Arkadopoulos, Melina Vlami, Guangwen Cao, Wenbin Liu, Aditya Kale, Alexandros Giakoustidis, Apostolos Koffas, Dimitrios Giakoustidis, Vasileios N. Papadopoulos, Lekshmi Kalinathan, Deepika Sivasankaran, Amritha Sennappa Sudharsan, Janet Reshma Jeyasingh, Hareni Marimuthu, Emine Turkmen Samdanci, Evangelos Felekouras, Spyridon Davakis, Michail Vailas, Alexandros Kozadinos, Panagiotis Sakarellos, Anastasia Karampa, Dimitrios Korkolis, Georgios Glantzounis, Alexandros Papalampros, Hoang Van Tong, Pham Van Dung, Nguyen Thi Mong Diep, Nguyen Linh Toan

First published in London, United Kingdom, 2022 by IntechOpen
IntechOpen is the global imprint of INTECHOPEN LIMITED, registered in England and Wales, registration number: 11086078, 5 Princes Gate Court, London, SW7 2QJ, United Kingdom
Printed in Croatia

British Library Cataloguing-in-Publication Data
A catalogue record for this book is available from the British Library

Additional hard and PDF copies can be obtained from orders@intechopen.com

Hepatocellular Carcinoma - Challenges and Opportunities of a Multidisciplinary Approach
Edited by Georgios Tsoulfas
p. cm.
Print ISBN 978-1-83969-110-2
Online ISBN 978-1-83969-111-9
eBook (PDF) ISBN 978-1-83969-112-6

For EU product safety concerns:
IN TECH d.o.o., Prolaz Marije Krucifikse Kozulić 3, 51000 Rijeka, Croatia, info@intechopen.com or visit our website at intechopen.com.

Meet the editor

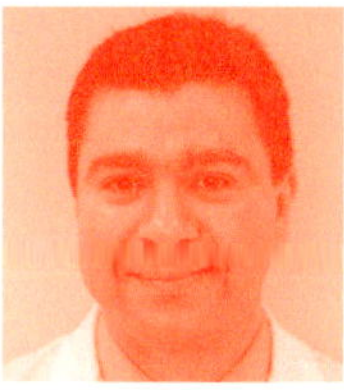

Dr. Georgios Tsoulfas received his medical degree from Brown University School of Medicine, Rhode Island, and completed his general surgery residency at the University of Iowa Hospitals and Clinics, as well as a transplant research fellowship at the Starzl Transplant Institute, University of Pittsburgh. He then completed a two-year transplantation surgery fellowship at Massachusetts General Hospital, Harvard Medical School, and then joined the Division of Solid Organ Transplantation and Hepatobiliary Surgery at the University of Rochester Medical Center, New York, as Assistant Professor of Surgery. He has currently moved back to Greece, where he is a Professor of Transplantation Surgery and Chief of the Department of Transplantation Surgery at the Aristotle University School of Medicine. He has published more than 140 papers in peer-reviewed journals and PubMed, as well as 35 book chapters. He is a reviewer for more than forty international journals and serves on the editorial boards of several others.

Contents

Preface

The combination of the high global prevalence of hepatocellular carcinoma (HCC), the complex nature of hepatic anatomy and physiology, and the continuously increasing wealth of information and techniques regarding its management, make HCC one of the most interesting and challenging areas in surgery. As such, it is also an area where a multidisciplinary approach is a necessity, especially given the combined medical and surgical issues that these patients face. The role of the surgeon is critical in the sense that decisions must be made regarding the different strategies and techniques and which one is best for the specific patient at the specific stage of the disease.

This book provides an overview of the main challenges and opportunities involved in the multidisciplinary management of HCC, whether they have to do with epidemiology, molecular diagnosis, staging, the role of immunotherapy or, of course, the great variety of surgical techniques and technologies involved in the therapy. Its value lies in the fact that the authors present us with their distilled wisdom, which is the result of substantial experience and daily involvement in this most difficult field of medicine and surgery.

Overall, this book is a useful resource for any physician, whether they are in training or in practice, treating patients with hepatic diseases.

Georgios Tsoulfas, MD, Ph.D., FICS, FACS
Professor of Transplantation Surgery,
Chief, Department of Transplantation Surgery,
Aristotle University School of Medicine,
Thessaloniki, Greece

Section 1

Epidemiology and Etiology of Hepatocellular Carcinoma

Chapter 1

Hepatitis B Virus (HBV) - Induced Hepatocarcinogenesis, a Founding Framework of Cancer Evolution and Development (*Cancer Evo-Dev*)

Wenbin Liu and Guangwen Cao

Abstract

In this chapter, we present the founding framework of a novel theory termed as Cancer Evolution-Development (*Cancer Evo-Dev*), based on the current understanding of hepatitis B virus (HBV) induced hepatocarcinogenesis. The interactions of genetic predispositions and HBV infection is responsible for the maintenance of chronic non-resolving inflammation. Under the inflammatory microenvironment, pro-inflammatory factors trans-activate the expression of cytidine deaminases and suppress the expression of uracil DNA glycosylase. The imbalance between the mutagenic forces and mutation-correcting forces facilitates the generations of somatic mutations, viral mutations, and viral integrations into the host genomes. The majority of cells with genomic mutations and mutated viruses are eliminated in survival competition. Only a small percentage of the mutated cells adapted to the hostile environment can survive, retro-differentiate, and function as cancer-initiating cells, representing a process of "mutation-selection-adaptation". *Cancer Evo-Dev* lays the theoretical foundation for understanding the mechanisms by which chronic infection of HBV promotes hepatocarcinogenesis. This theory also plays an important role in specific prophylaxis, prediction, early diagnosis, and targeted treatment of cancers.

Keywords: Hepatocarcinogenesis, hepatitis B virus, inflammation, mutation, evolution

1. Introduction

Chronic infection of hepatitis B virus (HBV) is a major cause of hepatocellular carcinoma (HCC). Although the strong etiologic relationship between HBV infection and HCC has been supported by substantial evidence, the underlying mechanism is still elusive. There are more than nine thousand studies investigating HBV-induced hepatocarcinogenesis, which yield 143 genes function in 137 pathways [1]. Most of the studies are one-sided investigations, only a few trying to provide a theoretical hypothesis and to promote the system-level understanding of HBV-induced HCC (HBV-HCC). In past decades, continuous attempts have been made to investigate carcinogenesis from an evolutionary point of view. In 1976, Dr. Nowell first proposed that most neoplasms originate from a single cell. Malignant cells are more genetically unstable than normal cells [2]. In 2006, it was pointed out that cancer clone genetic diversification and sub-clonal selection occurs within the microenvironment, which is similar to the process of Darwinian natural selection [3]. This viewpoint was put forward mainly based on morphological evidence and only a limited number of gene mutations and related signaling pathways were discussed. The widespread application of new generation sequencing promotes the investigation of genetic diversification and clonal selection within tissue ecosystems. It was found that the number of mutations in cancer range from 10 to hundreds of thousands. The majority of mutations are "passengers" and a small part are "drivers" [4]. Cancer cells acquire a variety of critical phenotypes via driver mutations, which compound to enhance the capabilities of self-renewal, migration, and invasion. The mutational spectra in cancers can reflect the characteristics of the mutational process, including the error-prone repair and genotoxic exposure [5]. Interestingly, the cytidine deaminase induced mutation is dominant in most cancers [6]. Cytidine deaminase is upregulated during inflammation and defense against many viruses, including HBV. Epidemiological and experimental evidence identified the co-evolution of HBV and cancer cells during chronic inflammation. In turn, the mutant cells and viruses also affect the inflammatory microenvironment [7]. Thus, there is a similarity between the process of carcinogenesis and Darwinian evolution. Furthermore, the investigation of cancer evolution can draw upon the understanding of developmental processes. Development is referred to the process that a fertilized egg develops into an individual. In humans, the fertilized diploid cell differentiates into various functional and/or structural cells to form different organs and tissues within 40 weeks. This process resembles the process of long-term organic evolution morphologically, from single cell creatures to multicellular creatures, and from aquatic creatures to terrestrial mammals. Some evolutionarily conserved molecules, like Hedgehog, HOX, and Myc are essential for the developmental process, suggesting evolution and development have similar inherent mechanisms [8–11]. The integration of evolution and developmental biology was termed *Evo-Devo* [12, 13]. In this chapter, we present a scientific theory of Cancer Evolution-Development (*Cancer Evo-Dev*) based on the current understanding of HBV-HCC [14]. This theoretical hypothesis can provide an evolutionary insight of profiling HCC risk and developing more reasonable predictive and prognostic strategies.

2. Framework of *Cancer Evo-Dev*

The synergetic effects of genetic predisposition and environmental factors contribute to the imbalance of the immune system, resulting in the activation and maintenance of non-resolving inflammation, that functions as the microenvironment for the *Cancer Evo-Dev*. Activated inflammatory signaling pathways can trans-activate the expression of nucleic acid editing enzymes, such as the human apolipoprotein B mRNA-editing enzyme catalytic polypeptides (APOBECs) family, thus promoting viral and somatic mutations. Viral mutants facilitate the malignant transformation of normal cells. Most mutant cells are eliminated under the selective pressure of the inflammatory microenvironment, while a small proportion of mutated cells survive. These survived mutant clones evolve to tumor-initiating cells by altering the original cell signal patterns, promoting epithelial-mesenchymal transition (EMT), or reprogramming the metabolic patterns, etc. Some established cancer markers, such as α-fetoprotein (AFP) and carcinoembryonic antigen (CEA), are usually expressed at the embryonic stage, silenced after birth, and re-expressed in cancer patients. These pieces of evidence imply that the process of *Cancer Evo-Dev* can be characterized as "backward evolution" and "retro-differentiation".

3. Chronic inflammation is indispensable for HBV-HCC evolution

As a defense mechanism responding to exogenous infection and injury, acute inflammation is beneficial to humans. However, chronic inflammation, also termed non-resolving inflammation is essential for carcinogenesis. The weak immunity, HBV mutation, and HBV genotype contribute to the chronicity of inflammation. During the development of HBV-induced HCC evolution, non-resolving inflammation is evident. By relieving hepatic inflammation, antiviral therapy can significantly lower the risks of HCC occurrence and postoperative recurrence [15, 16]. Interestingly, the risk of HCC is still significantly higher in the complete responder group of oral-administered antiviral therapy, compared with the subjects with inactive chronic hepatitis B (CHB) [17]. The active inflammation on chronic infection background also indicated postoperative recurrence [18, 19]. The close association between chronic inflammation and the risk of HCC can be explained from the perspective of *Cancer Evo-Dev*. Cancer evolution is based on two conditions: the continuous acquisition of somatic mutations and natural selection acting on the resultant phenotypic diversity [20]. These two conditions were fulfilled by HBV infection-induced chronic inflammation, that induces mutagenic factors such as APOBECs and provides selection pressure.

3.1 Chronicity of HBV infection and hepatic inflammation

The oncogenic capability of HBV is closely related to its capacity to induce and maintain chronic inflammation. The chronicity of HBV infection is dependent on 3 aspects: infection occasion, HBV genotypes, and genetic predisposition of the key immune molecules. HBV infection in early childhood is generally believed to be one of the major causes of chronic HBV infection in adulthood. The perinatal infection occurred in 8.7% and 84.2% of infants born to hepatitis B e-antigen (HBeAg)-positive mothers who did and did not receive immunoprophylaxis, respectively. The infection rates were 0.4% and 6.7% for infants born to HBeAg-negative mothers and HBeAg-positive mothers, respectively. Furthermore, the chronicity of HBV infection acquired perinatally was 28.2% and 64.5% for infants born to HBeAg-negative mothers and HBeAg-positive mothers, respectively [21]. This vulnerability of infants may due to the immaturity of the immune system. Although perinatal HBV infection is an important cause of chronic HBV infection, the chronic transformation of acute hepatitis B is the predominant cause of chronic HBV infection in adults. In China, 8.5% of patients with acute hepatitis B develop into chronic HBV infection 6 months after acute infection [22]. The HBV genotype and genetic predisposition of immune molecules contribute to this transformation.

According to sequence divergence of 8% in the whole viral genome, HBV can be classified into eight genotypes (A to H) [23]. Variant genotypes are distributed unevenly around the world, and the predominant one in mainland China is genotype C (68.3%), followed by genotype B (25.5%) [24]. Under selection pressure from the inflammatory microenvironment, the fates of different HBV genotypes are distinct. Genotype B HBV is prone to causing acute infection, whereas genotype C HBV is associated with chronic infection and contributes independently to the development of HCC [22, 25, 26].

The genetic predisposition of immune molecules is the third major cause of chronic HBV infection. The single nucleotide polymorphisms (SNPs) in the loci encoding human leukocyte antigen class II (HLA-II) are significantly associated with vaccine response as well as the risk of CHB, HBV-induced liver cirrhosis, and HBV-HCC [27–32]. Interestingly, the allele frequencies of SNPs affecting the expression of HLA-DP and HLA-DQ are variant in different human races. The polymorphic genotypes that are more frequent in the Han Chinese than in European populations are significantly associated with the increased risk of chronicity of HBV infection as well as the immune selection of HBV mutations related to end-stage liver diseases [21]. These data suggest that the Han Chinese are inherently more apt to progress into chronic infection once exposed to HBV infection than Europeans. This might be partly responsible for the fact that chronic HBV infection, HBV-induced liver cirrhosis, and HBV-HCC are more frequent in Chinese than in European populations. The genetic polymorphisms of HLA-II may facilitate the progression of CHB into HCC through predisposing immune imbalance and maintain HBV infection. Due to the chronicity of inflammation, the mutagenic force that serves as antiviral immunity is prone to injury the human genome, thus induce *Cancer Evo-Dev.*

3.2 HBV promote the generation of inflammatory mutations

The APOBECs are powerful endogenous mutagenic factors that can catalyze irreversible cytidine and deoxycytidine deamination to convert bases from cytosine to uracil, creating a cytosine-to-uracil mismatch in minus-strand and reverse-transcript G-to-A (guanosine-to-adenosine) transitions in plus-stranded DNA. APOBEC3s play important roles in the innate immune system [7]. Mutagenesis mediated by APOBEC3s can increase the viral mutation load to a level that exceeds the threshold for viral viability. Accordingly, APOBEC3s can similarly increase the number of somatic mutations to a threshold that exceeds the host's repair ability and starts the *Cancer Evo-Dev*. Three mechanisms prevent the induction of somatic mutations by the APOBEC3s family. First, APOBEC3s rarely express in normal tissues, and short-term activation of APOBEC3s is beneficial for eliminating pathogens. Second, the cytidine deaminase activity of APOBEC3s is applied almost exclusively to single-stranded nucleotides, in which mutagenesis is 200–300 times more efficient than it is in double-stranded DNA. Third, the uracil-induced mutagenesis of APOBEC3s is counteracted by uracil–DNA glycosylase (UNG), that plays an important role in the base-excision repair mechanism [7, 33]. However, genetic susceptibility, viral mutations, and an unbalanced immune system interact with each other to prevent the absolute elimination of HBV, resulting in chronic inflammation accompanied with APOBEC3s expression. During the HBV-induced malignant transformation, inflammatory signaling pathways including interleukin 6 (IL-6)/signal transducer and activator of transcription 3 (STAT3) and tumor necrosis factor α (TNF-α)/ nuclear factor kappa B (NF-κB) are activated, which up-regulate the expression of APOBEC3s [7]. Among the members of APOBEC3s, APOBEC3B was identified as the major subtype responsible for the APOBEC-signature somatic mutations in multiple cancers [34]. The mutagenic effect of inflammatory factors on the HBV genome depends on the degree of the damage to the APOBEC3B–UNG balance. IL-6 can increase the expression of APOBEC3B and decrease the expression of UNG. The functional polymorphisms located in the *APOBEC3B* promoter (rs2267401-G) and *UNG* enhancer (rs3890995-C) predispose the IL-6 induced APOBEC3B-UNG imbalance and increase the risk of HCC [35].

3.3 HBV affects the selection pressure of the inflammatory microenvironment

In an inflammatory microenvironment, continuous necrosis and proliferation can help to accumulate somatic mutations, and tumor-initiating cell clones with strong viability are selected. HBV replication directly reflects the selective stress and influences the evolution of HCC. It has been revealed by various studies that HBV DNA load increases the risk of HCC in CHB patients [25, 36]. A high level of HBV DNA load either in serum or liver tissue predicts poor postoperative prognosis in HCC [37]. Meanwhile, HBV in turn affecting the selective pressure of the inflammatory microenvironment. The innate immune and adaptive immune against HBV are both participate in the selection of malignant cells. During the chronic infection of HBV, APOBEC3B is stimulated and reduces the occupancy of H3K27me3 on the promoter of CC-chemokine ligand 2 (CCL2). By this mechanism, APOBEC3B upregulates the CCL2 to enhance the recruitment of tumor-associated macrophages (TAMs) and myeloid-derived suppressor cells (MDSCs). TAMs and MDSCs suppress the function of $CD8^{+}$T cells and are associated with a poor prognosis of HCC [38]. HBV can transmit into natural killer (NK) cells through exosomes, thereby inducing the disfunction of NK cells, which promotes the HCC evolution [39, 40]. HBV also induced the exhaustion of HBV-specific $CD8^{+}$ T cells through impairing the mitochondrial functions, including electron transport, membrane transport, and the transcription of mitochondrial DNA [41]. The glucose metabolism of T cells is reprogramed by HBV, which leads to increased lactate production and decreased migration of T cells [42]. During chronic infection, HBV promotes the recruitment of regulatory T cells (Tregs) through activating the growth factor-beta (TGF-β)/ miR-34a/ CC-motif chemokine ligand 22 (CCL22) axis [43]. The increased Tregs suppress HCC antigen-specific immune responses and HBV antigen-specific immune response at the same time [44]. Thus, the HBV that survives the survival competition can in turn affect the inflammatory microenvironment.

4. Roles of HBV mutation during the process of HCC evolution

During HBV-induced hepatocarcinogenesis, viruses also experience the process of evolution. Viral evolution serves as a valuable clue to investigate the mechanism underlying the HBV-HCC [45]. The generation and accumulation of HBV mutations abide by the Darwinian model: mutation-selection–adaptation. In the inflammatory microenvironment, most HBV mutants are eliminated by the antiviral immune response. Only a tiny fraction of mutant viruses that facilitate the regeneration of hepatocytes can survive and gradually develop into the HCC-promoting clones.

4.1 The generation of HBV mutation

Two major mechanisms are responsible for the generation of HBV mutation. The first pattern is the replicative errors. During viral replication, the partially double-stranded HBV DNA is generated from an intermediate RNA through the reverse transcription activity of the viral polymerase. Due to lack of proofreading capacity, the HBV genome has a higher mutation rate than other DNA viruses, which is in the range of 1.5×10^{-5} to 5×10^{-5} nucleotide substitutions per site per year, which can increase after HBeAg seroconversion [46]. The second viral mutation pattern is induced by host cytidine deaminases [7]. The APOBEC family has a dual effect on HBV: reduction of HBV and induction of HBV mutations [47]. The expression levels of APOBEC3s are positively correlated with the quasispecies complexity of HBV [48]. The genetic polymorphisms predisposing the IL-6 induced APOBEC3B-UNG imbalance significantly promote the generation of HCC related HBV mutations [35]. Although many HBV genome fragments, including the Enhancer II (EnhII) / basal core promoter (BCP)/ precore region and the S region, are generally sensitive to editing by members of APOBEC3 [49–53], the sequence encoding HBV X protein (HBx) is more vulnerable. APOBEC3 prefers the HBx region as its editing target and generates carboxylic acid–terminal truncated HBx (Ct-HBx). Although most HBV mutations are random, the directional evolution of HBV occurs under the selective pressures of chronic inflammation. In the immune tolerance phase of chronic infection, the immune pressure is weak, and most of the individual viruses are wild-type. Immune pressure increases with the progression of chronic inflammation, which facilitates the gradual occurrence of viral mutations, especially in HBeAg-negative individuals [54, 55]. HCC-related HBV mutations are selected by the immune microenvironment before the occurrence of HCC and can be used as predictive markers. Single-nucleotide polymorphisms of the inflammatory signaling pathway genes, including STAT3, NF-κB, HLA-DP, and HLA-DQ have been demonstrated to maintain the chronic infection and to facilitate the selection of HCC-related HBV mutations that contribute to the risk of liver cancer [32, 56, 57]. However, those viral mutants that affect the pre-cancer hepatocytes are less infectious to normal liver cells, which leads to a process of "dead-end" evolution.

4.2 The "dead-end" evolution of HBV

Hepatitis B virus belongs to the Hepadnaviridae family and is evolutionarily conservative in the long-term evolution of species [58]. However, the evolution of the HBV genome is evident in infected individuals during chronic infection. Previous research by our group established the wild-type HBV sequences of HBV subgenotypes B2 and C2, based on the whole HBV genome sequenced using 1000 asymptomatic carriers of the HBV surface antigen from community-based epidemiologic surveys. Based on the wild-type HBV sequences, HCC-related mutations and their development patterns were subsequently identified. We also observed that HBV mutations posing a significant HCC risk are located mainly within the BCP and preS regions [59–61]. During the HBV-induced carcinogenic "trilogy" (chronic hepatitis, liver cirrhosis, HCC), the species and frequencies of those mutations often accumulate consecutively and can be used to predict the occurrence and development of liver cirrhosis and HCC [15, 32, 56, 62]. Retrospective and prospective cohort studies have both identified a combination of HBV mutations (C1653T, A1762T/G1764A, and T1753V) that have significant predictive value [32, 63, 64]. Among them, the A1762T/G1764A mutation usually appears in the early stage; other mutations, including T1753V, C1653T, preS deletion, are evident only in a late stage of the evolution [65]. Reaction to chronic HBV infection (characterized by the immune response–induced hepatocyte injury and release of transaminase) is usually accompanied by HBeAg seroconversion and an increase in HBV mutations, indicating the selective effect of immune cells on viral mutants. The deficiency of $CD8^+$ T cell epitopes is one of the main features of HBV mutations. The mutant virus with a low density of $CD8^+$ T cells epitopes can evade immune eradication [66, 67]. The proportion of mutant preS/S region is higher in patients with occult HBV infection than in CHB patients [67, 68]. Therefore, CD^+8 T cell is essential for the immune selection of HCC-related HBV mutants.

Hepatitis B virus acquired during infancy or early childhood, or at the early infection stage in adults, is usually the wild type [15, 32, 56]. During the chronic inflammation process, especially after an HBeAg shift from HBeAg-positive to HBeAg-negative, mutant HBV subgroups gradually increase. Although the HCC-related HBV mutants are present in fetal cord blood, neonatal infection is usually caused by wild-type HBV rather than by mutant subgroups. At 1–15 years in HBV-infected children, the frequencies of HCC-related mutations increase with increasing age. However, compared with their mothers, who have been exposed to chronic infection for at least about 25 years, the children have fewer HCC-related HBV mutations [65]. The foregoing results are based on analyses of serum HBV. In individuals with chronic HBV infection, most all HBV is synthesized in hepatocytes and released into the circulation at a pace of up to 10^{11} viral particles daily [69]. The immune microenvironment of circulation, tumor tissue, and tumor-adjacent liver tissue are all necessary for the HBV evolution [48]. Interestingly, HBV evolves more advanced in the sera than in the tumors of HCC patients. The evolutionary similarity between the sera-derived HBV strains and adjacent tissue-derived ones is significantly stronger than that between sera-derived HBV strains and tumor-derived ones [48]. Although tumor-adjacent tissues are pathologically categorized as "normal," they are typical precancerous lesions and have already entered the middle stage of the cancer evolutionary process. The HCCs that relapse more than 2 years after resection are considered to be recurrent HCC and not a result of the initial HCC cell diffusion into remnant liver tissue [18]. The species and frequencies of certain HBV mutations in adjacent tissues are distinct in the different populations. Together with immune markers and expression levels of inflammatory genes, they can therefore be used to predict prognosis in HCC patients receiving curative surgery. For example, HBV mutations in the EnhII/BCP/PreC region, such as A1762T/G1764A, can serve as predictive markers for survival and recurrence [18], indicating that HBV evolution in adjacent tissues continues until the patient dies. Antiviral therapy can block HBV evolution in adjacent tissues by easing inflammation and notably prolongs survival in HCC patients [15].

Taken together, the Hepadnaviridae family members are highly conservative across species [65]. Wild-type HBV has the advantage of infecting hepatocytes, facilitating viral spread from one individual to another, and contributing to the maintenance of its viral species. The HCC-related mutants can cause malignant transformation but have lost the advantage of person-to-person infection. Those mutants are therefore usually eliminated at the death of the carriers, which is termed "dead-end" evolution.

4.3 High-risk HBV mutations promote the *Cancer Evo-Dev*

During hepatocarcinogenesis, high-risk HBV mutations are selected by the immune microenvironment. Because of overlapping open reading frames, HBV mutations altering the genes necessary for viral replication are unlikely transferred into their progeny viruses. Natural selection ensures only the fittest survive to pass their genes on to the next generation. Thus, the random natural mutations are therefore constrained to special regions of the HBV genome, especially in the fragment of HBx gene and large envelope protein gene fragment (preS1/preS2/S). These HBV mutations that survive the selective pressure can promote the evolution of HCC, which is supported by many pieces of evidence from epidemiology studies and mechanism studies.

Previous longitudinal studies, especially cohort studies, support that combo HBV mutations including A1762T/G1764A, C1653T, and T1753V in HBx gene in sera can predict the occurrence of HCC [64, 70]. The mutations in the HBV preS fragment, including the preS deletion, accumulate during the process of inflammation-HCC transformation, which is significantly associated with increased risk of HCC [62, 71, 72]. Epidemiological evidence identified the interaction effect between HBV mutations and genetic polymorphisms of immune molecules. For the population with the infection of genotype B HBV, the SNPs of HLA-DP, including rs3077 (T allele), rs2281388 (T allele), rs3135021 (G allele), and rs9277535 (G allele) can promote the HBV persistence and are associated with a higher prevalence of HBV mutation increasing HCC risk. Moreover, the effects of HBV mutations on HCC risk are selectively significant in subjects with these HLA-DP SNPs that promote HBV persistence [32]. For the population with the infection of genotype C HBV, the HLA-DQ SNP, rs9275319 (GG genotype), is significantly associated with an increased prevalence of preS1 start codon mutation, an HCC-risk mutation [63]. The SNPs of STAT3 SNPs appear to promote HCC evolution in the host with HBV mutations [56]. The interaction effect of STAT3 rs1053004 with T1674C/G and the interaction effect of STAT3 rs4796793 with preS2 start codon mutation are both significantly associated with an increased HCC risk. The T allele of rs223406 impairs the promoter activity of NFKBIA, a key molecule of the NF-κB signaling pathway. The interaction of rs223406 T allele with A1762T/G1764A is significantly associated with an increased risk of HCC [57]. The genetic polymorphisms predisposing the imbalance of APOBEC3B and UNG increase the risk of HCC through through facilitate the generation of APOBEC3B-signature HBV mutations. Furthermore, the positive rate of APOBEC-signature HBV mutations consecutively increased from asymptomatic HBsAg carrier (ASC) to HCC in HBV-infected subjects [35]. This line of evidence highlights the important role of HBV mutation in the process of HCC evolution.

Experimental evidence also confirms that HBV mutation can endow the hepatocytes with a survival advantage. The HBx with A1762T/G1764A–based combo mutations can upregulate the expression of S-phase kinase-associated protein 2 (SKP2) by activating E2F1, a transcription factor, downregulate cell cycle inhibitors, and facilitate the ubiquitin-mediated proteasomal degradation of p21, thereby enhancing the proliferation of HCC cells [73, 74]. Moreover, HBx with A1762T/G1764A–based combo mutations also enhance the cell migration through activating the Wnt/β-catenin signaling pathway [75]. Ct-HBx mutation can promote cell metastasis and invasiveness by activating the C-Jun/matrix metalloproteinase protein 10 signaling pathway [15, 76]. The HBx gene with K130M/V131I mutations enhances HCC evolution by activating the arachidonic acid metabolism and the hypoxia-inducible factor-1a [77, 78]. Besides the mutated HBx gene, the mutated preS1, preS2, and S regions also notably facilitate carcinogenesis [18, 61]. The preS2 region with F141L can significantly downregulate the expression of the p53 pathway and upregulate the expression of cyclin-dependent kinase 4 and cyclin A, thereby promoting proliferation and colony-forming rates [79]. The accumulation of mutant envelop protein in the endoplasmic reticulum (ER) leads to the activation of ER stress signaling pathway [80]. ER stress promotes HCC evolution through generating reactive oxygen species (ROS), inducing oxidative DNA damage, and ultimately increasing genomic instability [81, 82]. Although HBV mutation plays important role in hepatocarcinogenesis, somatic mutation of the human genome is the direct cause of cell evolution.

5. Roles of somatic mutation during the process of HCC evolution

The spontaneous rate of somatic mutations is not high enough to trigger the evolution process. HBV participates in the alteration of the host genome, both directly and indirectly. First, HBV can cause somatic mutations by directly integrating into the human genome. Second, mutant HBV contributes to the maintenance of non-resolving inflammation, that induces long-term up-regulation of APOBECs [7]. Somatic mutations can be classified according to their effects on *Cancer Evo-Dev*. A small proportion of the mutations can lead to advantageous phenotypes that are positively selected during the evolution process and thus are called "driver" mutations. The remaining mutations are "passengers" that contribute very little to carcinogenesis [4]. Due to survival competition and the positive selection of the inflammatory microenvironment, driver mutations accumulate sufficiently to promote malignant transformation. The distribution, combination, and dynamic patterns of driver mutations reflex the pressure of microenvironmental selection and growth advantage of cell subsets. As HCC has many etiological causes and experiences a long evolutionary process, the somatic mutation spectrum is most heterogeneous [6, 83]. The driver somatic mutations affect multiple functions, like signaling pathways, EMT, and energy metabolism.

5.1 Somatic mutations alter "stem-ness" signaling pathways

Based on the investigations of whole-exome sequencing, it is found that the somatic mutation in HCC evolution mainly altering six cancer related pathways: signaling pathway related with telomere maintenance, Wnt/b-catenin pathway, P53 and cell cycle pathway, oxidative stress pathway, epigenome modifiers, RAS/RAF/ mitogen-activated protein kinase pathway, and PI3K/AKT/mTOR pathways [84]. Among them, the somatic mutation related to telomeres pathway is most frequent. Telomerase is activated in more than 90% HCC patients. Somatic mutation within the promoter of telomerase reverse transcriptase (*TERT*) is the major cause with the prevalence ranging from 54–60%. The second cause is the HBV integration in the *TERT* promoter, which is observed in 10–15% of HCC patients. Interestingly, the mutation of catenin beta 1 (*CTNNB1*) is more frequent in hepatitis C virus induced HCC, indicated a different way of *Cancer Evo-Dev* [85, 86]. The frequencies of mutation in other hot genes range from 5–20%. Although the spectrums and frequencies of altered genes vary greatly among individuals, they are usually clustered to pathways or functional groups that are closely related to stem-ness and embryonic characteristics. In this regard, global mutation rates of functionally related genes are added together to define the mutation rate of a given signaling pathway. Mutation rates of Wnt/β-catenin, p53/cell cycle control, JAK/STAT, and PI3k/mTOR pathways range from 12–72%. Similar outstanding outcomes are also observed in functional gene groups of chromatin remodeling and telomere maintenance. Therefore, it is promising to use combo somatic mutations as predictive and prognostic biomarkers just like gene signatures [19].

5.2 Somatic mutations affect HCC evolution through regulating EMT

APOBECs can promote gene demethylation and remove epigenetic memory to stabilize the pluripotent state in embryonic stem cells through deaminating 5-methylcytosine (5mC) or 5-hydroxymethylcytosine (5hmC) [87, 88]. EMT is a landmark event of *Cancer Evo-Dev*, which is driven by transcription factors, like ZEB1, ZEB2, SNAI1, and SNAI2. AID, a member of the APOBECs family, is upregulated by inflammatory signals and induces demethylation of the promoters of ZEB1, ZEB2, SNAI1, and SNAI2. Silencing AID leads to increased methylation of CpG island proximal to the promoters of these EMT regulators, thus inhibits EMT and invasion of cells [89]. AID-induced, CpG methylation-dependent mutagenesis is proven to be a common feature of cancer evolution [90]. Therefore, it is reasonable to postulate that re-expression of embryonic factors in cancers might result from epigenetic reprogramming caused by APOBECs family, that is upregulated by proinflammatory factors.

5.3 Somatic mutations reprogram energy metabolism

To support the rapid growth of malignant cells, tumor tissues prefer to use glycolysis for energy production, even in the presence of oxygen. Glucose is more easily to be metabolized to lactate in tumor tissues than in normal tissues. This pattern of energy metabolism was identified in 1920 and was termed as Warburg effect [91]. Warburg effect in TAMs promotes vascular network formation, augments extravasation of tumor cells out of blood vessels, and induces higher levels of EMT at inflammatory foci within the tumor [92]. In the microenvironment with both hypoxia and hypoglycemia, stem cell-, angiogenic-, and EMT-biomarkers, as well as glycoprotein-P content and invasiveness of cancer cells are enhanced [93]. Thus, we believe that the Warburg effect promotes the evolutionary process of cancer under both hypoxia and hypoglycemia conditions. The Warburg effect can provide essential energy for cell survival in a hostile microenvironment, furthermore, glycolysis generates the raw material for DNA synthesis of progeny cells. HBV infection and somatic mutation are both the possible origin of Warburg phenotype. In HBV-HCC, the major pattern of single nucleotide variants in mitochondrial DNA (mtDNA) is C > T, that is the character of APOBEC induced mutation. This kind of mutation mainly occurs in the D-loop region of mtDNA and promotes the proliferation, invasion, and metastasis of HCC cells [94]. Pyruvate kinase M2 (PKM2), an alternatively spliced variant of the pyruvate kinase gene that is preferentially expressed during embryonic development and in cancer cells, alters the final rate-limiting step of glycolysis, resulting in the cancer-specific Warburg effect [95]. Besides the Warburg effect, HCC cells also enhance other patterns of energy metabolism during evolution. For example, the inactivating mutation of ribosomal S6 kinase 2 (RSK2) can support cholesterol metabolism in HCC [96].

5.4 HBV integration

HBV integration is a kind of somatic mutation that is specific to the HBV-induced *Cancer Evo-Dev.* Although the HCC in an individual can be monoclonal, HBV integration is common in most clones, indicating it is the early driver event for HCC evolution [83]. The HBV integration can be detected in 85–90% of HBV-HCC patients [97]. Moreover, the prevalence of HBV integration is 60–75% in HCCs from patients with occult HBV infection, indicating the HBV integration contributes to the occult HBV infection induced HCC [98, 99]. Approximately five thousand HBV integration events have been reported and more than half of them locate in the intergenic regions. Only the HBV integration events within thirteen genes are repeated in diverse studies [1]. *TERT*, mixed-lineage leukemia 4 (*MLL4*), fibronectin 1 (*FN1*), cyclin E1 (*CCNE1*), and cyclin A2(*CCNA2*) are the top five most frequently integrated genes [85, 100–105]. The X and core genes of HBV are the regions that most frequently insert into the human genome [103, 105]. Cis-activation of host genes is an important mechanism by which HBV integration promotes HCC evolution. The highest frequency of HBV integration is observed in the promoter region of *TERT* [85, 100–105]. The HBV integration within the *TERT* promoter leads to an increased mRNA level of *TERT*, that is significantly associated with a poor prognosis of HCC [103, 105]. MLL4 is the second most frequently integrated gene and the HBV integration mainly locate in the introns and exons [85, 105]. Since *MLL* gene family has methyltransferase activity, the HBV integration within *MLL4* may promote HCC evolution in an epigenetic way. As the third most frequently integrated gene, *FN1* is reported to create a microenvironment promoting metastasis of lung cancer [106]. Most HBV integration events within *FN1* are detected in the adjacent tissues of HCC, indicating these mutations may contribute to the microenvironment of the early stage of HCC evolution [85, 101]. HBV integration is associated with an increased expression of *CCNE1*, that is reported to promote hepatic inflammation and hepatocarcinogenesis [107]. The HBV-*CCNA2* chimeric transcript encodes a chimeric protein promoting cell cycle progression [108]. Besides affecting the expression or function of coding genes, HBV integration within the region of long interspersed nuclear elements (LINEs) can generate HBx-LINE1 chimeric transcript acting as long non-coding RNA (lncRNA). This lncRNA increases the activity of the Wnt pathway through decrease the level of miR-122 [104]. The DNA fragment with HBV integration can be used as a circulating biomarker of HCC recurrence. The HBV-host chimera DNA can be detected in more than 90% of HCC patients before surgery. After the surgery, HBV-host chimera DNA can still be detected in 20% of HCC patients, which may come from the mutant hepatocytes at the early stage of evolution and are significantly associated with HCC recurrence [109]. Thus, most HBV integration occurs randomly. The integration mutations that endow the hepatocytes with survival advantage will have the opportunity of accumulation.

As mentioned above, hepatocarcinogenesis involves the co-evolution of HBV and transformed cells. The interaction between somatic mutation and HBV mutation occurs during this process. The deletion, duplication, and translocation are observed near the insertion site of integrated HBV fragments [84]. The frequency of HBV mutation is positive associated with the level of HBV integration. The prevalence of HBx mutation is significantly higher in patients with HBV integration in *TERT* promoter (35%) than in patients without these integration events (19.8%) [83]. There are studies reporting the selective expression of mutant HBx and preS2 genes in the tumor tissues from patients with occult HBV infection [110]. These pieces of evidence support that the integration and selection of mutant HBV fragments play important roles in the HCC evolution.

6. Conclusion

Based on studies of HBV-induced hepatocarcinogenesis (a typical evolutionary process), we put forward the theory of *Cancer Evo-Dev*. Under conditions of genetic predisposition, exogenous factors such as viral infection can induce chronic inflammation. The elimination of chronic infection can relieve inflammation, reducing the incidence of cancer and subsequently extending effective survival. As the theory describes, tumor-initiating cells obtain survival advantage during the evolutionary process of mutation-selection–adaptation by activating a "stem-ness" pathway and simultaneously causing evolutionary heterogeneity. Critical molecules in a functional subnetwork that maintains and promotes the *Cancer Evo-Dev* process can be demonstrated using systems biology approaches. The development of high-efficiency inhibitors that will target these critical molecules and block corresponding signal pathways could be a powerful treatment strategy in advanced cancers. The theory of *Cancer Evo-Dev* will serve three purposes: first, the early prevention that reduces the cancer incidence and delays its onset; second, targeted therapy that reduces morbidity and mortality rates. Therefore, this theory can contribute to the realization of "P4 pattern" medicine (predictive, preventive, personalized, and participatory).

Acknowledgements

This work was supported by grant 2015CB554006 from the National Key Basic Research Program of China, grants 91529305, 81520108021, and 81673250, and 81521091 from the National Natural Science Foundation of China.

Conflict of interest

The authors declare no conflict of interest.

Author details

Wenbin Liu and Guangwen Cao*
Department of Epidemiology, Second Military Medical University, Shanghai, China

*Address all correspondence to: gcao@smmu.edu.cn

References

[1] Lee WY, Bachtiar M, Choo CCS, Lee CG. Comprehensive review of Hepatitis B Virus-associated hepatocellular carcinoma research through text mining and big data analytics. Biol Rev Camb Philos Soc. 2019;94(2):353-367. DOI: 10.1111/brv.12457

[2] Nowell PC. The clonal evolution of tumor cell populations. Science. 1976;194(4260):23-28. DOI: 10.1126/science.959840

[3] Merlo LM, Pepper JW, Reid BJ, Maley CC. Cancer as an evolutionary and ecological process. Nat Rev Cancer. 2006;6(12):924-935. DOI: 10.1038/nrc2013

[4] Greaves M, Maley CC. Clonal evolution in cancer. Nature. 2012;481(7381):306-313. DOI: 10.1038/nature10762

[5] Stratton MR. Exploring the genomes of cancer cells: progress and promise. Science. 2011;331(6024):1553-1558. DOI: 10.1126/science.1204040

[6] Alexandrov LB, Nik-Zainal S, Wedge DC, Aparicio SA, Behjati S, Biankin AV, et al. Signatures of mutational processes in human cancer. Nature. 2013;500(7463):415-421. DOI: 10.1038/nature12477

[7] Deng Y, Du Y, Zhang Q, Han X, Cao G. Human cytidine deaminases facilitate hepatitis B virus evolution and link inflammation and hepatocellular carcinoma. Cancer letters. 2014; 343(2):161-171. DOI: 10.1016/j.canlet.2013.09.041

[8] Wang S, Zhang J, Jiao W, Li J, Xun X, Sun Y, et al. Scallop genome provides insights into evolution of bilaterian karyotype and development. Nat Ecol Evol. 2017;1(5):120. DOI: 10.1038/s41559-017-0120

[9] Deschamps J, Duboule D. Embryonic timing, axial stem cells, chromatin dynamics, and the Hox clock. Genes Dev. 2017;31(14):1406-1416. DOI: 10.1101/gad.303123.117

[10] Lettice LA, Devenney P, De Angelis C, Hill RE. The Conserved Sonic Hedgehog Limb Enhancer Consists of Discrete Functional Elements that Regulate Precise Spatial Expression. Cell Rep. 2017;20(6):1396-1408. DOI: 10.1016/j.celrep.2017.07.037

[11] Zhong C, Zhou YK, Yang SS, Zhao JF, Zhu XL, Chen HH, et al. Developmental expression of the N-myc downstream regulated gene (Ndrg) family during Xenopus tropicalis embryogenesis. Int J Dev Biol. 2015;59(10-12):511-517. DOI: 10.1387/ijdb.150178xh

[12] Raff RA. Evo-devo: the evolution of a new discipline. Nat Rev Genet. 2000;1(1):74-79. DOI: 10.1038/35049594

[13] Carroll SB. Evo-devo and an expanding evolutionary synthesis: a genetic theory of morphological evolution. Cell. 2008;134(1):25-36. DOI: 10.1016/j.cell.2008.06.030

[14] Cao GW. Cancer Evo-Dev, a novel hypothesis derived from studies on hepatitis B virus-induced carcinogenesis. Hepatoma Res. 2017;3:241-259. DOI: 10.20517/2394-5079.2017.45

[15] Yin J, Li N, Han Y, Xue J, Deng Y, Shi J, et al. Effect of antiviral treatment with nucleotide/nucleoside analogs on postoperative prognosis of hepatitis B virus-related hepatocellular carcinoma: a two-stage longitudinal clinical study. J Clin Oncol. 2013;31(29):3647-3655. DOI: 10.1200/JCO.2012.48.5896

[16] Chen LP, Zhao J, Du Y, Han YF, Su T, Zhang HW, et al. Antiviral treatment to prevent chronic hepatitis B or C-related hepatocellular carcinoma. World J Virol.

2012;1(6):174-183. DOI: 10.5501/wjv.v1.i6.174

[17] Cho JY, Paik YH, Sohn W, Cho HC, Gwak GY, Choi MS, et al. Patients with chronic hepatitis B treated with oral antiviral therapy retain a higher risk for HCC compared with patients with inactive stage disease. Gut. 2014; 63(12):1943-1950. DOI: 10.1136/gutjnl-2013-306409

[18] Chen L, Zhang Q, Chang W, Du Y, Zhang H, Cao G. Viral and host inflammation-related factors that can predict the prognosis of hepatocellular carcinoma. European journal of cancer. 2012;48(13):1977-1987. DOI: 10.1016/j.ejca.2012.01.015

[19] Liu WB, Yang F, Shao DY, Cao GW. Novel predictive and prognostic strategies of hepatitis B virus related hepatocellular carcinoma. Hepatoma Res. 2016;2:331-340. DOI: 10.20517/2394-5079.2016.38

[20] Gatenby RA, Gillies RJ, Brown JS. Of cancer and cave fish. Nat Rev Cancer. 2011;11(4):237-238. DOI: 10.1038/nrc3036

[21] Li Z, Hou X, Cao G. Is mother-to-infant transmission the most important factor for persistent HBV infection? Emerg Microbes Infect. 2015;4(5):e30. DOI: 10.1038/emi.2015.30

[22] Zhang HW, Yin JH, Li YT, Li CZ, Ren H, Gu CY, et al. Risk factors for acute hepatitis B and its progression to chronic hepatitis in Shanghai, China. Gut. 2008;57(12):1713-1720. DOI: 10.1136/gut.2008.157149

[23] Norder H, Courouce AM, Coursaget P, Echevarria JM, Lee SD, Mushahwar IK, et al. Genetic diversity of hepatitis B virus strains derived worldwide: genotypes, subgenotypes, and HBsAg subtypes. Intervirology. 2004;47(6):289-309. DOI: 10.1159/000080872

[24] Yin J, Zhang H, He Y, Xie J, Liu S, Chang W, et al. Distribution and hepatocellular carcinoma-related viral properties of hepatitis B virus genotypes in Mainland China: a community-based study. Cancer epidemiology, biomarkers & prevention : a publication of the American Association for Cancer Research, cosponsored by the American Society of Preventive Oncology. 2010; 19(3):777-786. DOI: 10.1158/1055-9965.EPI-09-1001

[25] Chan HL, Tse CH, Mo F, Koh J, Wong VW, Wong GL, et al. High viral load and hepatitis B virus subgenotype ce are associated with increased risk of hepatocellular carcinoma. J Clin Oncol. 2008;26(2):177-182. DOI: 10.1200/JCO.2007.13.2043

[26] Chan HL, Hui AY, Wong ML, Tse AM, Hung LC, Wong VW, et al. Genotype C hepatitis B virus infection is associated with an increased risk of hepatocellular carcinoma. Gut. 2004; 53(10):1494-1498. DOI: 10.1136/gut.2003.033324

[27] Kamatani Y, Wattanapokayakit S, Ochi H, Kawaguchi T, Takahashi A, Hosono N, et al. A genome-wide association study identifies variants in the HLA-DP locus associated with chronic hepatitis B in Asians. Nat Genet. 2009;41(5):591-595. DOI: 10.1038/ng.348

[28] Guo X, Zhang Y, Li J, Ma J, Wei Z, Tan W, et al. Strong influence of human leukocyte antigen (HLA)-DP gene variants on development of persistent chronic hepatitis B virus carriers in the Han Chinese population. Hepatology. 2011;53(2):422-428. DOI: 10.1002/hep.24048

[29] Hu Z, Liu Y, Zhai X, Dai J, Jin G, Wang L, et al. New loci associated with chronic hepatitis B virus infection in Han Chinese. Nat Genet. 2013;45(12):1499-1503. DOI: 10.1038/ng.2809

[30] Png E, Thalamuthu A, Ong RT, Snippe H, Boland GJ, Seielstad M. A genome-wide association study of

hepatitis B vaccine response in an Indonesian population reveals multiple independent risk variants in the HLA region. Hum Mol Genet. 2011;20(19): 3893-3898. DOI: 10.1093/hmg/ddr302

[31] Jiang DK, Sun J, Cao G, Liu Y, Lin D, Gao YZ, et al. Genetic variants in STAT4 and HLA-DQ genes confer risk of hepatitis B virus-related hepatocellular carcinoma. Nat Genet. 2013;45(1):72-75. DOI: 10.1038/ng.2483

[32] Zhang Q, Yin J, Zhang Y, Deng Y, Ji X, Du Y, et al. HLA-DP polymorphisms affect the outcomes of chronic hepatitis B virus infections, possibly through interacting with viral mutations. J Virol. 2013;87(22):12176-12186. DOI: 10.1128/JVI.02073-13

[33] Siriwardena SU, Chen K, Bhagwat AS. Functions and Malfunctions of Mammalian DNA-Cytosine Deaminases. Chem Rev. 2016;116(20):12688-12710. DOI: 10.1021/acs.chemrev.6b00296

[34] Kuong KJ, Loeb LA. APOBEC3B mutagenesis in cancer. Nat Genet. 2013;45(9):964-965. DOI: 10.1038/ng.2736

[35] Liu W, Wu J, Yang F, Ma L, Ni C, Hou X, et al. Genetic Polymorphisms Predisposing the Interleukin 6-Induced APOBEC3B-UNG Imbalance Increase HCC Risk via Promoting the Generation of APOBEC-Signature HBV Mutations. Clin Cancer Res. 2019;25(18):5525-5536. DOI: 10.1158/1078-0432.CCR-18-3083

[36] Yang HI, Yuen MF, Chan HL, Han KH, Chen PJ, Kim DY, et al. Risk estimation for hepatocellular carcinoma in chronic hepatitis B (REACH-B): development and validation of a predictive score. Lancet Oncol. 2011;12(6):568-574. DOI: 10.1016/S1470-2045(11)70077-8

[37] Yeh CT, So M, Ng J, Yang HW, Chang ML, Lai MW, et al. Hepatitis B virus-DNA level and basal core promoter A1762T/G1764A mutation in liver tissue independently predict postoperative survival in hepatocellular carcinoma. Hepatology. 2010;52(6):1922-1933. DOI: 10.1002/hep.23898

[38] Wang D, Li X, Li J, Lu Y, Zhao S, Tang X, et al. APOBEC3B interaction with PRC2 modulates microenvironment to promote HCC progression. Gut. 2019;68(10):1846-1857. DOI: 10.1136/gutjnl-2018-317601

[39] Yang Y, Han Q, Hou Z, Zhang C, Tian Z, Zhang J. Exosomes mediate hepatitis B virus (HBV) transmission and NK-cell dysfunction. Cell Mol Immunol. 2017;14(5):465-475. DOI: 10.1038/cmi.2016.24

[40] Zhang QF, Yin WW, Xia Y, Yi YY, He QF, Wang X, et al. Liver-infiltrating CD11b(−)CD27(−) NK subsets account for NK-cell dysfunction in patients with hepatocellular carcinoma and are associated with tumor progression. Cell Mol Immunol. 2017;14(10):819-829. DOI: 10.1038/cmi.2016.28

[41] Fisicaro P, Barili V, Montanini B, Acerbi G, Ferracin M, Guerrieri F, et al. Targeting mitochondrial dysfunction can restore antiviral activity of exhausted HBV-specific CD8 T cells in chronic hepatitis B. Nat Med. 2017;23(3):327-336. DOI: 10.1038/nm.4275

[42] Masson JJ, Billings HW, Palmer CS. Metabolic reprogramming during hepatitis B disease progression offers novel diagnostic and therapeutic opportunities. Antivir Chem Chemother. 2017;25(2):53-57. DOI: 10.1177/2040206617701372

[43] Yang P, Li QJ, Feng Y, Zhang Y, Markowitz GJ, Ning S, et al. TGF-beta-miR-34a-CCL22 signaling-induced Treg cell recruitment promotes venous metastases of HBV-positive hepatocellular carcinoma. Cancer Cell. 2012;22(3):291-303. DOI: 10.1016/j.ccr.2012.07.023

[44] Zhang HH, Mei MH, Fei R, Liu F, Wang JH, Liao WJ, et al. Regulatory T cells in chronic hepatitis B patients affect the immunopathogenesis of hepatocellular carcinoma by suppressing the anti-tumour immune responses. J Viral Hepat. 2010;17 Suppl 1:34-43. DOI: 10.1111/j.1365-2893.2010.01269.x

[45] Yang F, Ma LT, Cao GW. Hepatocellular carcinoma: co - evolution of hepatocytes and hepatitis B virus. Zhonghua Gan Zang Bing Za Zhi. 2017;25(5):321-324. DOI: 10.3760/cma.j.issn.1007-3418.2017.05.001

[46] Orito E, Mizokami M, Ina Y, Moriyama EN, Kameshima N, Yamamoto M, et al. Host-independent evolution and a genetic classification of the hepadnavirus family based on nucleotide sequences. Proc Natl Acad Sci U S A. 1989;86(18):7059-7062. DOI: 10.1073/pnas.86.18.7059

[47] Noguchi C, Imamura M, Tsuge M, Hiraga N, Mori N, Miki D, et al. G-to-A hypermutation in hepatitis B virus (HBV) and clinical course of patients with chronic HBV infection. J Infect Dis. 2009;199(11):1599-1607. DOI: 10.1086/598951

[48] Yin J, Chen X, Li N, Han X, Liu W, Pu R, et al. Compartmentalized evolution of hepatitis B virus contributes differently to the prognosis of hepatocellular carcinoma. Carcinogenesis. 2021;42(3):461-470. DOI: 10.1093/carcin/bgaa127

[49] Vartanian JP, Henry M, Marchio A, Suspene R, Aynaud MM, Guetard D, et al. Massive APOBEC3 editing of hepatitis B viral DNA in cirrhosis. PLoS Pathog. 2010;6(5):e1000928. DOI: 10.1371/journal.ppat.1000928

[50] Suspene R, Guetard D, Henry M, Sommer P, Wain-Hobson S, Vartanian JP. Extensive editing of both hepatitis B virus DNA strands by APOBEC3 cytidine deaminases in vitro and in vivo. Proc Natl Acad Sci U S A. 2005;102(23):8321-8326. DOI: 10.1073/pnas.0408223102

[51] Beggel B, Munk C, Daumer M, Hauck K, Haussinger D, Lengauer T, et al. Full genome ultra-deep pyrosequencing associates G-to-A hypermutation of the hepatitis B virus genome with the natural progression of hepatitis B. J Viral Hepat. 2013;20(12):882-889. DOI: 10.1111/jvh.12110

[52] Kock J, Blum HE. Hypermutation of hepatitis B virus genomes by APOBEC3G, APOBEC3C and APOBEC3H. J Gen Virol. 2008;89(Pt 5): 1184-1191. DOI: 10.1099/vir.0.83507-0

[53] Reuman EC, Margeridon-Thermet S, Caudill HB, Liu T, Borroto-Esoda K, Svarovskaia ES, et al. A classification model for G-to-A hypermutation in hepatitis B virus ultra-deep pyrosequencing reads. Bioinformatics. 2010;26(23):2929-2932. DOI: 10.1093/bioinformatics/btq570

[54] Han YF, Zhao J, Ma LY, Yin JH, Chang WJ, Zhang HW, et al. Factors predicting occurrence and prognosis of hepatitis-B-virus-related hepatocellular carcinoma. World J Gastroenterol. 2011;17(38):4258-4270. DOI: 10.3748/wjg.v17.i38.4258

[55] Hannoun C, Horal P, Lindh M. Long-term mutation rates in the hepatitis B virus genome. J Gen Virol. 2000;81(Pt 1):75-83. DOI: 10.1099/0022-1317-81-1-75

[56] Xie J, Zhang Y, Zhang Q, Han Y, Yin J, Pu R, et al. Interaction of signal transducer and activator of transcription 3 polymorphisms with hepatitis B virus mutations in hepatocellular carcinoma. Hepatology. 2013;57(6):2369-2377. DOI: 10.1002/hep.26303

[57] Zhang Q, Ji XW, Hou XM, Lu FM, Du Y, Yin JH, et al. Effect of functional nuclear factor-kappaB genetic polymorphisms on hepatitis B virus

persistence and their interactions with viral mutations on the risk of hepatocellular carcinoma. Ann Oncol. 2014;25(12):2413-2419. DOI: 10.1093/annonc/mdu451

[58] Schaefer S. Hepatitis B virus taxonomy and hepatitis B virus genotypes. World J Gastroenterol. 2007; 13(1):14-21. DOI: 10.3748/wjg.v13.i1.14

[59] Yin J, Xie J, Liu S, Zhang H, Han L, Lu W, et al. Association between the various mutations in viral core promoter region to different stages of hepatitis B, ranging of asymptomatic carrier state to hepatocellular carcinoma. Am J Gastroenterol. 2011;106(1):81-92. DOI: 10.1038/ajg.2010.399

[60] Yin J, Xie J, Zhang H, Shen Q, Han L, Lu W, et al. Significant association of different preS mutations with hepatitis B-related cirrhosis or hepatocellular carcinoma. J gastroenterol. 2010;45(10): 1063-1071. DOI: 10.1007/s00535-010-0253-1

[61] Liu S, Xie J, Yin J, Zhang H, Zhang Q, Pu R, et al. A matched case-control study of hepatitis B virus mutations in the preS and core promoter regions associated independently with hepatocellular carcinoma. J Med Virol. 2011;83(1):45-53. DOI: 10.1002/jmv.21829

[62] Liu S, Zhang H, Gu C, Yin J, He Y, Xie J, et al. Associations between hepatitis B virus mutations and the risk of hepatocellular carcinoma: a meta-analysis. J Natl Cancer Inst. 2009; 101(15):1066-1082. DOI: 10.1093/jnci/djp180

[63] Ji X, Zhang Q, Li B, Du Y, Yin J, Liu W, et al. Impacts of human leukocyte antigen DQ genetic polymorphisms and their interactions with hepatitis B virus mutations on the risks of viral persistence, liver cirrhosis, and hepatocellular carcinoma. Infect Genet Evol. 2014;28:201-209. DOI: 10.1016/j.meegid.2014.09.032

[64] Yin J, Wang J, Pu R, Xin H, Li Z, Han X, et al. Hepatitis B Virus Combo Mutations Improve the Prediction and Active Prophylaxis of Hepatocellular Carcinoma: A Clinic-Based Cohort Study. Cancer Prev Res. 2015;8(10):978-988. DOI: 10.1158/1940-6207.CAPR-15-0160

[65] Li Z, Xie Z, Ni H, Zhang Q, Lu W, Yin J, et al. Mother-to-child transmission of hepatitis B virus: evolution of hepatocellular carcinoma-related viral mutations in the post-immunization era. J Clin Virol. 2014;61(1):47-54. DOI: 10.1016/j.jcv.2014.06.010

[66] Maman Y, Blancher A, Benichou J, Yablonka A, Efroni S, Louzoun Y. Immune-induced evolutionary selection focused on a single reading frame in overlapping hepatitis B virus proteins. J Virol. 2011;85(9):4558-4566. DOI: 10.1128/JVI.02142-10

[67] Chen BF. Hepatitis B virus pre-S/S variants in liver diseases. World J Gastroenterol. 2018;24(14):1507-1520. DOI: 10.3748/wjg.v24.i14.1507

[68] Huang X, Ma C, Zhang Q, Shi Q, Huang T, Liu C, et al. Impact of "a" determinant mutations on detection of hepatitis B surface antigen (HBsAg) in HBV strains from Chinese patients with occult hepatitis B. Journal of medical virology. 2017;89(10):1796-1803. DOI: 10.1002/jmv.24859

[69] Nowak MA, Bonhoeffer S, Hill AM, Boehme R, Thomas HC, McDade H. Viral dynamics in hepatitis B virus infection. Proc Natl Acad Sci U S A. 1996;93(9): 4398-4402. DOI: 10.1073/pnas.93.9.4398

[70] Sung FY, Lan CY, Huang CJ, Lin CL, Liu CJ, Chen PJ, et al. Progressive accumulation of mutations in the hepatitis B virus genome and its impact on time to diagnosis of hepatocellular carcinoma. Hepatology. 2016;64(3):720-731. DOI: 10.1002/hep.28654

[71] Chen CH, Hung CH, Lee CM, Hu TH, Wang JH, Wang JC, et al. Pre-S

deletion and complex mutations of hepatitis B virus related to advanced liver disease in HBeAg-negative patients. Gastroenterology. 2007;133(5):1466-1474. DOI: 10.1053/j.gastro.2007.09.002

[72] Liu WC, Wu IC, Lee YC, Lin CP, Cheng JH, Lin YJ, et al. Hepatocellular carcinoma-associated single-nucleotide variants and deletions identified by the use of genome-wide high-throughput analysis of hepatitis B virus. J Pathol. 2017;243(2):176-192. DOI: 10.1002/path.4938

[73] Huang Y, Tong S, Tai AW, Hussain M, Lok AS. Hepatitis B virus core promoter mutations contribute to hepatocarcinogenesis by deregulating SKP2 and its target, p21. Gastroenterology. 2011;141(4):1412-1421, 1421 e1411-1415. DOI: 10.1053/j.gastro.2011.06.048

[74] Huang Y, Tai AW, Tong S, Lok AS. HBV core promoter mutations promote cellular proliferation through E2F1-mediated upregulation of S-phase kinase-associated protein 2 transcription. J Hepatol. 2013;58(6):1068-1073. DOI: 10.1016/j.jhep.2013.01.014

[75] Chen Z, Tang J, Cai X, Huang Y, Gao Q, Liang L, et al. HBx mutations promote hepatoma cell migration through the Wnt/beta-catenin signaling pathway. Cancer Sci. 2016;107(10):1380-1389. DOI: 10.1111/cas.13014

[76] Sze KM, Chu GK, Lee JM, Ng IO. C-terminal truncated hepatitis B virus x protein is associated with metastasis and enhances invasiveness by C-Jun/matrix metalloproteinase protein 10 activation in hepatocellular carcinoma. Hepatology. 2013;57(1):131-139. DOI: 10.1002/hep.25979

[77] Chiu AP, Tschida BR, Sham TT, Lo LH, Moriarity BS, Li XX, et al. HBx-K130M/V131I Promotes Liver Cancer in Transgenic Mice via AKT/FOXO1 Signaling Pathway and Arachidonic Acid Metabolism. Mol Cancer Res. 2019;17(7):1582-1593. DOI: 10.1158/1541-7786.MCR-18-1127

[78] Liu LP, Hu BG, Ye C, Ho RL, Chen GG, Lai PB. HBx mutants differentially affect the activation of hypoxia-inducible factor-1alpha in hepatocellular carcinoma. Br J Cancer. 2014;110(4):1066-1073. DOI: 10.1038/bjc.2013.787

[79] Huang J, Deng Q, Wang Q, Li KY, Dai JH, Li N, et al. Exome sequencing of hepatitis B virus-associated hepatocellular carcinoma. Nat Genet. 2012;44(10):1117-1121. DOI: 10.1038/ng.2391

[80] Pollicino T, Cacciola I, Saffioti F, Raimondo G. Hepatitis B virus PreS/S gene variants: pathobiology and clinical implications. J Hepatol. 2014;61(2):408-417. DOI: 10.1016/j.jhep.2014.04.041

[81] Hsieh YH, Su IJ, Wang HC, Chang WW, Lei HY, Lai MD, et al. Pre-S mutant surface antigens in chronic hepatitis B virus infection induce oxidative stress and DNA damage. Carcinogenesis. 2004;25(10):2023-2032. DOI: 10.1093/carcin/bgh207

[82] Wang LH, Huang W, Lai MD, Su IJ. Aberrant cyclin A expression and centrosome overduplication induced by hepatitis B virus pre-S2 mutants and its implication in hepatocarcinogenesis. Carcinogenesis. 2012;33(2):466-472. DOI: 10.1093/carcin/bgr296

[83] Cui X, Wei W, Wang C, Qi Y, Qin X, Huang L, et al. Studies on the correlation between mutation and integration of HBV in hepatocellular carcinoma. Biosci Rep. 2020;40(8). DOI: 10.1042/BSR20201988

[84] Levrero M, Zucman-Rossi J. Mechanisms of HBV-induced hepatocellular carcinoma. J Hepatol. 2016;64(1):S84-S101. DOI: 10.1016/j.jhep.2016.02.021

[85] Sung WK, Zheng H, Li S, Chen R, Liu X, Li Y, et al. Genome-wide survey of recurrent HBV integration in hepatocellular carcinoma. Nat Genet. 2012; 44(7):765-769. DOI: 10.1038/ng.2295

[86] Totoki Y, Tatsuno K, Covington KR, Ueda H, Creighton CJ, Kato M, et al. Trans-ancestry mutational landscape of hepatocellular carcinoma genomes. Nat Genet. 2014;46(12):1267-1273. DOI: 10.1038/ng.3126

[87] Nabel CS, Jia H, Ye Y, Shen L, Goldschmidt HL, Stivers JT, et al. AID/APOBEC deaminases disfavor modified cytosines implicated in DNA demethylation. Nat Chem Biol. 2012;8(9):751-758. DOI: 10.1038/nchembio.1042

[88] Kumar R, DiMenna L, Schrode N, Liu TC, Franck P, Munoz-Descalzo S, et al. AID stabilizes stem-cell phenotype by removing epigenetic memory of pluripotency genes. Nature. 2013; 500(7460):89-92. DOI: 10.1038/nature12299

[89] Munoz DP, Lee EL, Takayama S, Coppe JP, Heo SJ, Boffelli D, et al. Activation-induced cytidine deaminase (AID) is necessary for the epithelial-mesenchymal transition in mammary epithelial cells. Proc Natl Acad Sci U S A. 2013;110(32):E2977-E2986. DOI: 10.1073/pnas.1301021110

[90] Rogozin IB, Lada AG, Goncearenco A, Green MR, De S, Nudelman G, et al. Activation induced deaminase mutational signature overlaps with CpG methylation sites in follicular lymphoma and other cancers. Sci Rep. 2016;6:38133. DOI: 10.1038/srep38133

[91] Koppenol WH, Bounds PL, Dang CV. Otto Warburg's contributions to current concepts of cancer metabolism. Nat Rev Cancer. 2011;11(5):325-337. DOI: 10.1038/nrc3038

[92] Penny HL, Sieow JL, Adriani G, Yeap WH, See Chi Ee P, San Luis B, et al. Warburg metabolism in tumor-conditioned macrophages promotes metastasis in human pancreatic ductal adenocarcinoma. Oncoimmunology. 2016;5(8):e1191731. DOI: 10.1080/2162402X.2016.1191731

[93] Marin-Hernandez A, Gallardo-Perez JC, Hernandez-Resendiz I, Del Mazo-Monsalvo I, Robledo-Cadena DX, Moreno-Sanchez R, et al. Hypoglycemia Enhances Epithelial-Mesenchymal Transition and Invasiveness, and Restrains the Warburg Phenotype, in Hypoxic HeLa Cell Cultures and Microspheroids. J Cell Physiol. 2017;232(6):1346-1359. DOI: 10.1002/jcp.25617

[94] Yin C, Li DY, Guo X, Cao HY, Chen YB, Zhou F, et al. NGS-based profiling reveals a critical contributing role of somatic D-loop mtDNA mutations in HBV-related hepatocarcinogenesis. Ann Oncol. 2019;30(6):953-962. DOI: 10.1093/annonc/mdz105

[95] Garcia-Heredia JM, Carnero A. Decoding Warburg's hypothesis: tumor-related mutations in the mitochondrial respiratory chain. Oncotarget. 2015;6(39):41582-41599. DOI: 10.18632/oncotarget.6057

[96] Chan LK, Ho DW, Kam CS, Chiu EY, Lo IL, Yau DT, et al. RSK2-inactivating mutations potentiate MAPK signaling and support cholesterol metabolism in hepatocellular carcinoma. J Hepatol. 2021;74(2):360-371. DOI: 10.1016/j.jhep.2020.08.036

[97] Pollicino T, Saitta C, Raimondo G. Hepatocellular carcinoma: the point of view of the hepatitis B virus. Carcinogenesis. 2011;32(8):1122-1132. DOI: 10.1093/carcin/bgr108

[98] Saitta C, Tripodi G, Barbera A, Bertuccio A, Smedile A, Ciancio A, et al. Hepatitis B virus (HBV) DNA integration in patients with occult HBV infection and hepatocellular carcinoma.

Liver Int. 2015;35(10):2311-2317. DOI: 10.1111/liv.12807

[99] Wong DK, Cheng SCY, Mak LL, To EW, Lo RC, Cheung TT, et al. Among Patients with Undetectable Hepatitis B Surface Antigen and Hepatocellular Carcinoma, a High Proportion Has Integration of HBV DNA into Hepatocyte DNA and No Cirrhosis. Clin Gastroenterol Hepatol. 2020;18(2):449-456. DOI: 10.1016/j.cgh.2019.06.029

[100] Bonilla Guerrero R, Roberts LR. The role of hepatitis B virus integrations in the pathogenesis of human hepatocellular carcinoma. J Hepatol. 2005;42(5):760-777. DOI: 10.1016/j.jhep.2005.02.005

[101] Ding D, Lou X, Hua D, Yu W, Li L, Wang J, et al. Recurrent targeted genes of hepatitis B virus in the liver cancer genomes identified by a next-generation sequencing-based approach. PLoS Genet. 2012;8(12):e1003065. DOI: 10.1371/journal.pgen.1003065

[102] Jiang Z, Jhunjhunwala S, Liu J, Haverty PM, Kennemer MI, Guan Y, et al. The effects of hepatitis B virus integration into the genomes of hepatocellular carcinoma patients. Genome Res. 2012;22(4):593-601. DOI: 10.1101/gr.133926.111

[103] Toh ST, Jin Y, Liu L, Wang J, Babrzadeh F, Gharizadeh B, et al. Deep sequencing of the hepatitis B virus in hepatocellular carcinoma patients reveals enriched integration events, structural alterations and sequence variations. Carcinogenesis. 2013;34(4):787-798. DOI: 10.1093/carcin/bgs406

[104] Lau CC, Sun T, Ching AK, He M, Li JW, Wong AM, et al. Viral-human chimeric transcript predisposes risk to liver cancer development and progression. Cancer Cell. 2014;25(3):335-349. DOI: 10.1016/j.ccr.2014.01.030

[105] Zhao LH, Liu X, Yan HX, Li WY, Zeng X, Yang Y, et al. Genomic and oncogenic preference of HBV integration in hepatocellular carcinoma. Nat Commun. 2016;7:12992. DOI: 10.1038/ncomms12992

[106] Liu J, Cao L, Meng J, Li Y, Deng P, Pan P, et al. The fibrotic microenvironment promotes the metastatic seeding of tumor cells into the lungs via mediating the ZEB1-AS1/miR-200b-3p/ZEB1 signaling. Cell Cycle. 2020;19(20):2701-2719. DOI: 10.1080/15384101.2020.1826236

[107] Ehedego H, Mohs A, Jansen B, Hiththetiya K, Sicinski P, Liedtke C, et al. Loss of Cyclin E1 attenuates hepatitis and hepatocarcinogenesis in a mouse model of chronic liver injury. Oncogene. 2018;37(25):3329-3339. DOI: 10.1038/s41388-018-0181-8

[108] Chiu YT, Wong JK, Choi SW, Sze KM, Ho DW, Chan LK, et al. Novel pre-mRNA splicing of intronically integrated HBV generates oncogenic chimera in hepatocellular carcinoma. J Hepatol. 2016;64(6):1256-1264. DOI: 10.1016/j.jhep.2016.02.005

[109] Li CL, Ho MC, Lin YY, Tzeng ST, Chen YJ, Pai HY, et al. Cell-Free Virus-Host Chimera DNA From Hepatitis B Virus Integration Sites as a Circulating Biomarker of Hepatocellular Cancer. Hepatology. 2020;72(6):2063-2076. DOI: 10.1002/hep.31230

[110] Hatazawa Y, Yano Y, Okada R, Tanahashi T, Hayashi H, Hirano H, et al. Quasispecies variant of pre-S/S gene in HBV-related hepatocellular carcinoma with HBs antigen positive and occult infection. Infect Agent Cancer. 2018;13:7. DOI: 10.1186/s13027-018-0179-4

Chapter 2

Histopathological Features of the Steatohepatitic Variant of Hepatocellular Carcinoma and Its Relationship with Fatty Liver Disease

Emine Turkmen Samdanci

Abstract

Hepatocellular carcinoma (HCC) is the most common primary malignant tumor of the liver in adults. Steatohepatitic HCC (SH-HCC) is a recently described, rarer variant of HCC and is associated with nonalcoholic fatty liver disease (NAFLD). The relationship between fatty liver disease and/or steatohepatitis and SH-HCC is now known. This subtype can be confused with lipid-containing nodules (such as cirrhotic nodules, regenerative nodules, focal nodular hyperplasia) clinically, radiologically and histopathologically. Here, the histopathological features of SH-HCC, its relationship with fatty liver disease and briefly its clinical features will be discussed. In addition, histopathological features of this specific variant, immunohistochemical staining of the tumor and diagnostic difficulties in tru-cut biopsies will also be discussed. Actually, I think this article will raise clinicopathological awareness about this rare variant.

Keywords: Hepatocellular carcinoma, steatohepatitic HCC, steatohepatitis, NASH, alcoholic steatohepatitis, IHC

1. Introduction

Hepatocellular carcinoma (HCC) is the most common primary malignant tumor of the liver in adults, the fifth most common cancer in the world and also the third most common cancer of cancer-related deaths [1]. It is the malignancy of hepatocytes with varying degrees of differentiation [2]. The most common cause of death in patients with HCC is cirrhosis. Despite all the unknowns, heptocarcinogenesis is a multistep process, and chronic inflammation plays the major role [2–6].

2. Epidemiology and etiology

HCC has a multifactorial etiology, and its incidence and prevalence varies by country [7]. Although the incidence of HCC is different in different geographies, the incidence increases with age [8]. It is more common in men than in women (male:female ratio; ranging between 2:1 and 4:1 in various countries). Cirrhosis, viral hepatitis, alcohol, aflatoxin, metabolic diseases, metabolic syndrome characterized by fatty liver are the main causes of HCC etiology. Although the activation of the WNT/B-catenin pathway is one of the main events in HCC, the effects of viral antigens on the nucleus, mutations, and DNA instability constitute the pathogenesis of HCC [9]. There are also molecular studies showing that activation of the JAK/STAT pathway also contributes to the development of SH-HCC [1, 10].

2.1 Cirrhosis

Most patients with HCC have underlying liver cirrhosis. Cirrhosis is therefore considered a major risk factor for HCC [8, 11, 12]. Although macronodular cirrhosis is considered as a higher risk for HCC than micronodular cirrhosis, cirrhotic liver can create HCC for any reason [13]. Cirrhosis also has a geographical distribution, the etiology of cirrhosis is chronic viral hepatitis in Asian countries, and nonviral causes in European and American countries [14]. Despite this known association between cirrhosis and HCC, HCC also develops from the noncirrhotic liver [15–17].

2.2 Viral hepatitis (hepatitis B and hepatitis C)

Most HCCs develop from the background of chronic viral hepatitis, including hepatitis B and Hepatitis C [18–21]. Viral hepatitis-related HCCs are more common in countries where hepatitis B and hepatitis C are more prevalent, such as Asia and Africa. Viral-related HCC appears to be decreasing in countries where clinical follow-up increases, and whom include hepatitis B vaccine in regular vaccination programme. Integration of hepatitis B virus into the host hepatocyte genome is thought to initiate hepatocarcinogenesis. In the etiology of HCC, hepatitis C is as important as hepatitis B [22–24]. Being men and older, having coinfection (such as HBV, HIV), alcohol use, diabetes, and fatty liver constitute a high risk for HCC formation. Even the development of HCC in liver coinfected with hepatitis C and hepatitis B viruses, is higher than in those infected with other viruses [13]. It is thought that ongoing liver damage and accompanying regeneration caused by the immune response and direct cytopathic effect in hepatitis C infection induce malignant transformation [25, 26].

2.3 Aflatoxin

Consumption of foods contaminated with aflatoxins produced by fungi can lead to the formation of HCC [8, 27, 28]. Aflatoxin B1, one of the toxin types, is thought to be mainly responsible for HCC formation [8]. It contributes to the formation of HCC by making mutations (Guanin and Thymine mutations) in DNA via cytochrome p450. Aflatoxin exposure is thought to affect patients with chronic HCV hepatitis more [8, 29, 30].

2.4 Alcohol

The relationship between alcohol use and HCC is both by direct effect and being a cofactor in viral infections [31, 32]. Reactive oxygen radicals, that occur while alcohol is metabolized to acetaldehyde, initiate hepatocarcinogenesis by causing damage and transformation in DNA. HCC development in alcoholic cirrhosis is in the form of DNA instability caused by DNA hypomethylation [33–36].

2.5 Metabolic diseases

HCC can develop in some of the livers with metabolic diseases. However, the development of HCC is more common with hereditary hemochromatosis, tyrosinemia and α1-antiripsin deficiency [37–41]. In these diseases, the direct toxic effect of accumulations (such as iron), mutation (p53 mutation), immunological abnormalities and DNA damage by lipid peroxidation initiate the development of HCC [8, 42, 43].

2.6 Metabolic syndrome and fatty liver disease

Metabolic syndrome is a mortal endocrinopathy that is accompanied by systemic disorders such as abdominal obesity that begins with insulin resistance, diabetes, dyslipidemia, hypertension and coronary artery disease. This situation has led to an increase in HCC formation, which has the characteristics of metabolic syndrome [44–47]. The risk of HCC increases 2–3 times in patients with diabetes [37, 48, 49]. The increase in metabolic syndrome in developed countries also brought an increase in nonalcholic fatty liver disease (NAFLD) [50–55].

In obese patients, the decrease in the release of fatty acids from adipose tissue, tumor necrosis factor-α and adiponectin causes insulin resistance and thus chronic hyperinsulinemia. Insulin and insulin growth factor-1 (IGF-1) contribute to hepatocarcinogenesis by preventing apoptosis and increasing cellular proliferation with the signals they send to insulin receptors and IGF-1 receptors [8].

Since steatohepatitic HCC (SH-HCC) will be mentioned here, NAFLD, steatohepatitis and their associated HCC formation mechanism are explained in a little more detail.

There are many studies on the incidence and prevalence of HCC in NAFLD cases, with rates varying between 3 and 35% [51, 56, 57]. Steatohepatitis varies between 3 and 5%. In some cohort studies, the rate of development of HCC (1-year cumulative incidence) was reported as 2–5% in patients with NAFLD compared to hepatitis C cases. The 5-year incidence was reported as 11% [51, 58]. In another study, the annual cumulative rate was 2–6%. In a retrospective study, NAFLD was detected in 21.2% of HCC cases. In fact, 23% of NAFLD patients without histopathologically and radiologically significant cirrhosis developed HCC [59]. In a different study, HCC develops in 5% of patients with cirrhosis secondary to NAFLD [53]. In cohort studies with large case series, both steatosis and steatohepatitis in nontumoral liver were found to be statistically significant with HCC. Moreover, a close relationship between the steatohepatitic variant of HCC (SH-HCC), which has been recently defined, and NAFLD has been described and demonstrated [22, 53, 58, 60]. Although its relationship with fatty liver diseases has been clarified, there are studies showing that SH-HCC can also develop in viral hepatitis [16, 61].

3. Clinical features

The clinical manifestations of HCC are quite ambiguous and are related to the tumor and underlying chronic liver disease [1]. Usually, patients show signs in advanced stages and even miss the chance of treatment. Patients may present with upper abdominal pain, hepatomegaly, splenomegaly, weight loss, jaundice or decompensated liver finding such as ascites [1, 8]. HCC most commonly spreads intrahepaticly via the portal vein [1]. While HCC spreads with intrahepatic portal vein branches, the main portal vein and hepatic vein involvement can also be seen.

Invasion of the bile duct causes liver decompensation, resulting in rapid ascites accumulation, obstructive jaundice, variceal hemorrhages, and hepatic encephalopathy [8]. Although extrahepatic dissemination is rare, it can metastasize to the lung, lymph nodes, bone, and adrenal gland in advanced disease [1]. Paraneoplastic syndrome findings such as hypoglycemia, hypercholesterolemia, hyperkalemia, gynecomastia, carcinoid syndrome, hypertrophic pulmonary osteoarthropathy, osteopetrosis, hypertension, hyperthyroidism, porphyria cutanea tarda can be seen [8]. Median suvival in patients with clinical findings who have the chance for curative treatment is around 1–3 months, and survival over 1 year is also unusual. Today, thanks to definitive treatments and advanced surgeries, patients at risk of developing HCC are followed more closely and the tumor is diagnosed at an early stage [8, 28]. Radiologic imaging methods (ultrasound, computed tomography, magnetic resonance imaging, angiography) are used for the diagnosis of liver masses and HCC [8, 17, 62, 63].

4. Pathological features

HCC is a highly heterogeneous tumor. Heterogeneity is both molecular and morphological [64, 65]. Understanding the heterogeneity is important for the diagnosis, treatment and follow-up of the disease [64].

HCCs below 2 cm are called small HCC (s-HCC) and early HCC (e-HCC) [1, 64, 66]. These tumors are divided into two as prominent nodular or indistinct nodules [64]. Early-HCC is in the form of nodules with indistinct borders and usually develops from a dysplastic nodule background. They are well differentiated, develop from the background of fibrosis-cirrhosis, and are radiologically hypovascular and rarely vascular invasion (5%) [1, 64]. Small-HCC has a prominent pseudocapsule, is well-moderately differentiated, radiologically hypervascular, and invades more frequently (40%) [1, 64]. Pedinculated HCC has a growth pattern protruding from the capsular surface [67]. Diffuse HCC is in the form of proliferation of small tumor nodules and resembles cirrhotic nodules (cirrhotomimetic) [64]. SH-HCC is more solid than other HCC subtypes and has more golden-yellow color due to the lipid contains. When the macroscopic specimen is carefully examined, fibrotic bands that divide the tumor into lobules can be seen. The tumor usually tends to be well-circumscribed or nodular and may range in diameter from 0.5 cm to 11 cm [68]. The prognosis of SH-HCC is similar to that of classical HCC [40, 57, 69, 70]. Although nontumoral liver can be cirrhotic or noncirrhotic, it is usually yellowish-brown in color suggestive of fatty liver (**Figure 1**).

After these macroscopic definitions and macroscopic heterogeneity, it is necessary to mention microscopic heterogeneity. This heterogeneity is also reflected in the histopathological subtyping of HCC [71]. In the 5th edition of WHO classification of the tumors of the digestive system (2019), the subtypes of HCC are as follows; fibrolamellar, scirrhus, cear cell type, steatohepatitic, macrotrabecular massive, chromophobe, neutrophil-rich, lympocyte-rich [1]. More on SH-HCC will be mentioned here. SH-HCC is a newly identified subtype of HCC. It accounts for approximately 5–20% of all HCCs [1]. It is characterized by steatohepatitic features such as steatosis in tumor cells, balloon degeneration, inflammation, Mallory-Denk bodies and pericellular fibrosis [58, 72]. Tumor is usually related to MetS and steatohepatitis is detected in the background [22, 39, 57, 61, 69, 72]. Some studies have shown that steatosis and interstitial fibrosis are the main findings for SH-HCC [22, 40]. However, the minimum amount of steatosis in the steatohepatitic area in some tumors

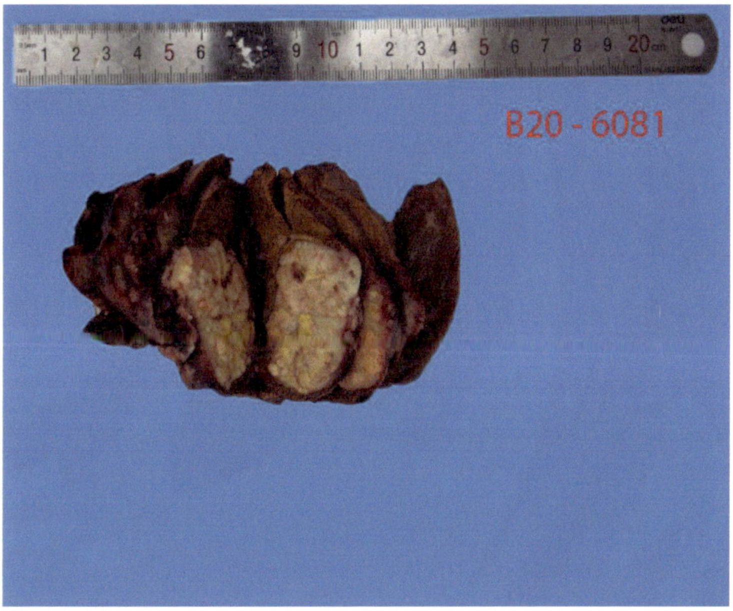

Figure 1.
Tumor with nodular border is seen in the brown-yellow noncirrhotic liver. The tumor is lobulated by fibrotic bands and has yellow areas.

that are histomorphologically SH-HCC, the presence of only steatosis in some cases, the presence of steatotic areas or cells in HCC are confusing points in the diagnosis of SH-HCC. Despite all this confusion, the steatohepatitic area in HCC is diagnostic for SH-HCC. For the histopathological diagnosis of SH-HCC, the cut-off for steatohepatitic features was described more than 5% of the tumor before but later moved to 50% [10, 39, 64, 72]. Hepatocellular carcinoma morphologically has 4 histological growth patterns: trabecular, solid (compact), pseudoaglandular (pseudoacinar), and macrotrabecular (trabecular thickness consisting of more than 10 cells) [1]. When SH-HCC is examined microscopically, a steatotic tumor is seen, separated from the generally steatotic liver (cirrhotic or non-cirrhotic) by a nodular or infiltrative margin. Large fat droplets are detected in tumor cells. Mallory-Denk bodies are detected in most tumors. Thin connective tissue growth (pericellular fibrosis), trabecular fibrosis, and randomly distributed collagen bundles surrounding tumor cells can be easily selected. Trabecular fibrosis, including randomly distributed collagen bundles in the tumor, and fibrosis surrounding tumor cells (pericellular) can be easily distinguished. Inflammation in the tumor is also remarkable. The inflammation is lymphocyte predominant with sparse plasma cells. More prominent neutrophil and lymphocyte infiltrations can be detected around tumor cells which contains Mallory-Denk bodies. The nuclei of tumor cells have atypia. This atypia is mild in well-differentiated tumors and quite pronounced in poorly differentiated tumors. They may even have bizarre nuclei suggested of sarcomas or pleomorphic carcinomas. However, mitotic activity is very low. Again, as in classical HCC and other subtypes, the tumor does not contain portal tracts and unpaired arteries can be seen (**Figures 2–4**) [1, 10, 45, 68, 72, 73]. The differentiation of SH-HCC is the same as that of classical HCC and is graded as well differentiated (Grade1: Tumor cells resemble mature hepatocytes with minimal to mild atypia), moderately differentiated (Grade 2: Distinctly malignant and histomorphology strongly suggests hepatocellolar differentiation) and poorly differentiated (Grade 3: Clearly malignant, but histomorphology strongly suggests spectrum of

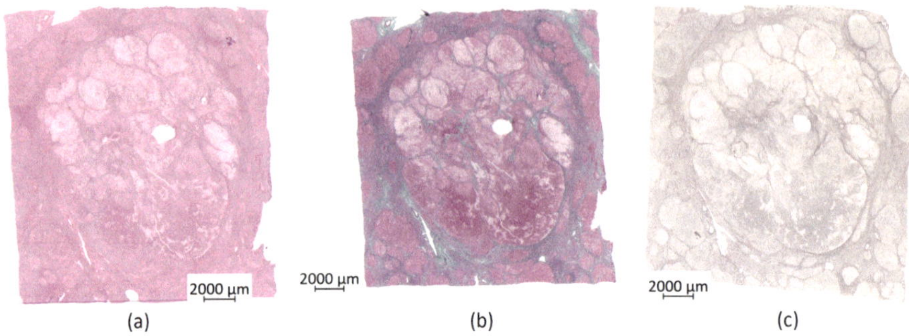

Figure 2.
The tumor (pale area) is located in the center of the figure, surrounded by cirrhotic nodules (a, Hematoxylin and Eosin-H&E). Masson's trichrome (b) and reticulin (c) stains, both the tumor and its surrounding micronodular cirrhotic background are more prominent.

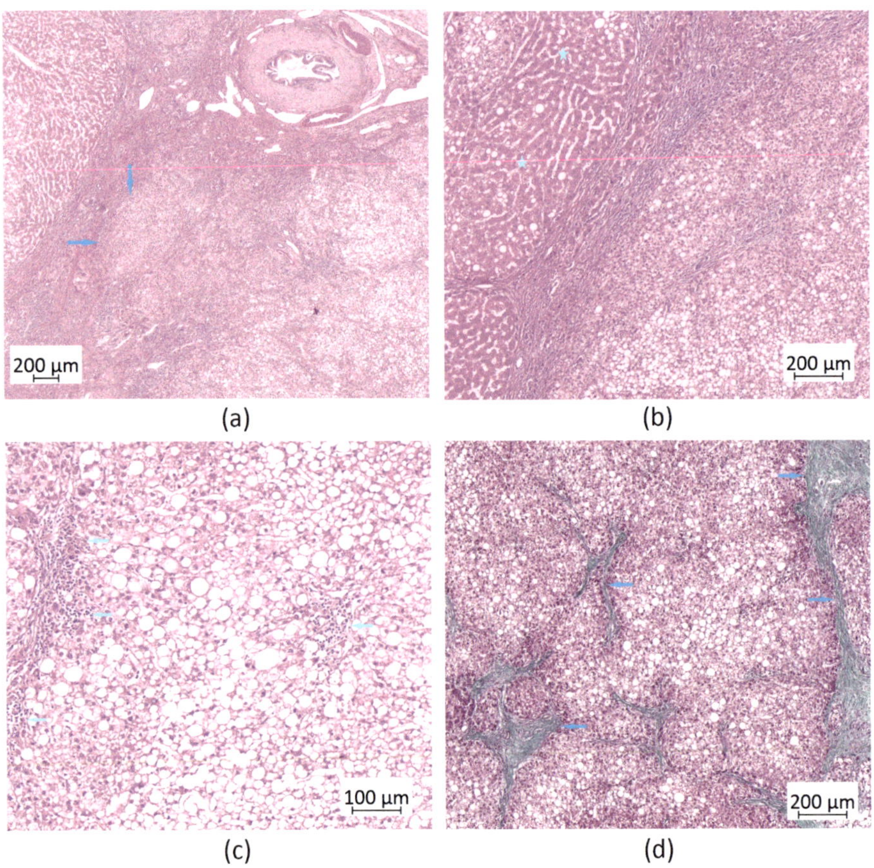

Figure 3.
The parenchymal invasion area of steatohepatitic HCC is seen (arrows) (a), the tumor is seen adjacent to the fatty cirrhotic nodule (stars) (b), presence of large lipid droplets and chronic inflammation (arrows) (c), Masson's trichrome stain shows thick fibrous septa (arrows) (d).

poorly differentiated carcinomas) [1]. Most SH-HCCs are moderately differentiated and have a trabecular pattern and a pseudoglandular pattern [52].

Immunohistochemical antibodies are helpful and supportive in the diagnosis of HCC [74]. Although heppar-1, glypican-3, glutamine synthetase, arginase, heat shock protein-70 (HSP-70), β-catenin and sinusoidal staining with CD34, canalicular staining pattern with polyclonal carcinoma embryogenic antigen (pCEA) and CD10 antibodies are used in the diagnosis of HCC, immune studies for SH-HCC are limited (**Figure 5**) [22, 68, 72, 75].

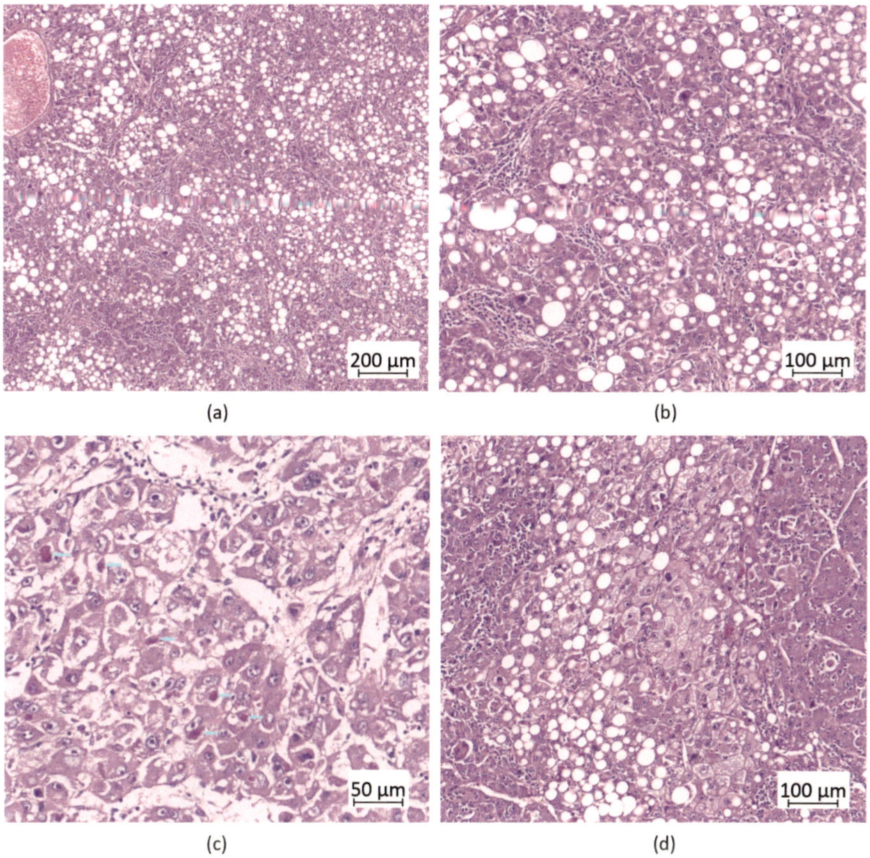

Figure 4.
Dense inflammation and fibrosis (a), pleomorphism (b), Mallory-Denk bodies (arrows) (c), and ballooning (cells with pale cytoplasm) (d) are seen in different areas of the tumor.

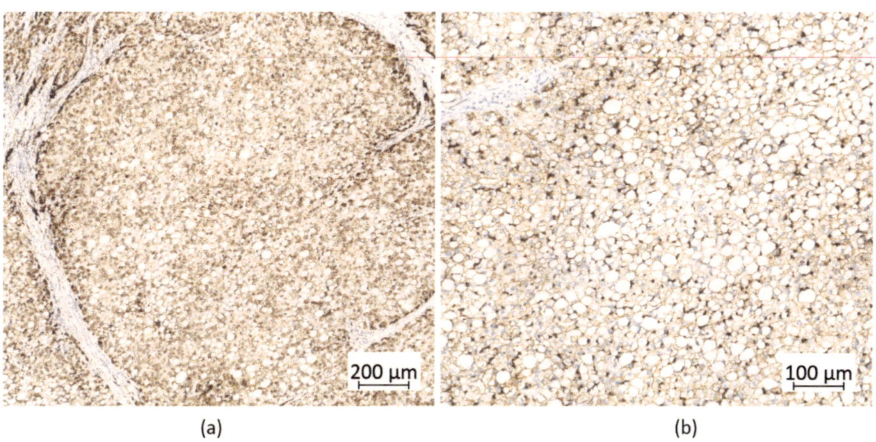

Figure 5.
Glutamine synthetase shows positive cytoplasmic staining (a), CD10 antibody shows positive canalicular staining (b).

The histopathological diagnosis of SH-HCC is usually easy in cases with explant and resection. However, tru-cut biopsies, which represent a small part of the tumor, may have diagnostic difficulties. These diagnostic difficulties are due to both the heterogeneity of the tumor and its similar morphological appearance to NAFLD with advanced fibrosis. A tru-cut biopsy from focal nodular hyperplasia (FNH) with fatty changes sometimes can be confused with a diagnosis of nodular and well differentiated SH-HCC. This difference between the diagnosis in the tru-cut biopsy and the resection material should not be interpreted as a misdiagnosis. Before interpreting it as an erroneous diagnosis, it should be remembered that this diagnostic difference is due to the heterogeneous and fat-containing nature of the tumor. Pathologists should remember that bile duct proliferation, presence of central scar (histologically and radiologically), and thick-walled abnormal vascular structures in the fibrous septa are more common in FNH when examining this tru-cut biopsy. Since fibrosis can be seen in both SH-HCC and FNH, it may not clarify the differential diagnosis. Non-invasive border and immunohistochemical staining (sinusoidal CD34 staining, glypican-3 positivity and diffuse glutamine synthetase staining) may be helpful in the differential diagnosis of steatohepatitis [8, 11, 68, 72]. Differentiation from classical HCC can be made by evaluating morphological and immune markers together [68]. In spite of all this, it would be appropriate to consult a pathologist experienced in liver pathology in cases where tumor specification could not be made.

The relationship between NAFLD, NASH, and HCC (especially SH-HCC) is now known. Adequate tumor sampling should be performed in resection materials, explants, particularly when identifying subtypes of large-diameter HCCs. It should be noted that classical HCC and other subtypes, including SH-HCC, have a heterogeneous histomorphology. While patients with metabolic syndrome, insulin resistance, obesity, fatty liver and steatohepatitis are followed up, careful radiological examination should be performed for SH-HCC that may develop from this background. In other words, the terminology of "neoplastic steatogenesis" should be kept in mind.

Author details

Emine Turkmen Samdanci
Pathology Department, School of Medicine, Inonu University, Malatya, Turkey

*Address all correspondence to: esamdanci@gmail.com

References

[1] WHO Classification of Tumours Editorial Board. Digestive System Tumours. Lyon (France): International Agency for Research on Cancer; 2019. (WHO classification of tumours series, 5th ed.;vol.1).

[2] Calderaro J, Couchy G, Imbeaud S, Amaddeo G, Letouzé E, Blanc JF, Laurent C, Hajji Y, Azoulay D, Bioulac-Sage P, Nault JC, Zucman-Rossi J.J Histological subtypes of hepatocellular carcinoma are related to gene mutations and molecular tumour classification. Hepatol. 2017 Oct;67(4):727-738.

[3] Schirmacher P, Rogler CE, Dienes HP. Current pathogenetic and molecular concepts in viral liver carcinogenesis. Virchows Arch B Cell Pathol Incl Mol Pathol. 1993;63(2):71-89.

[4] Popper H, Thung SN, McMahon BJ, Lanier AP, Hawkins I, Alberts SR. Evolution of hepatocellular carcinoma associated with chronic hepatitis B virus infection in Alaskan Eskimos Arch Pathol Lab Med. 1988 May;112(5):498-504.

[5] El-Serag HB. Hepatocellular carcinoma. N Engl J Med 2011;365:1118-1127.

[6] Forner A, Llovet JM, Bruix J. Hepatocellular carcinoma. Lancet 2012;379:1245-1255.

[7] Di Bisceglie AM, Carithers RL Jr, Gores GJ. Hepatocellular carcinoma. Hepatology. 1998 Oct;28(4):1161-5. doi: 10.1002/hep.510280436.

[8] Goodman ZD, Terracciano LM, Wee A. Tumours and tumour-like lesions of the liver. In: MacSween's Pathology of the Liver 6th Edition,Churchill Livinstone, 2012. 761-851.

[9] Van Treeck BJ, Mounajjed T, Moreira RK, Orujov M, Allende DS, Bellizzi AM, Lagana SM, Davila JI, Jessen E, Graham RP. Transcriptomic and Proteomic Analysis of Steatohepatitic Hepatocellular Carcinoma Reveals Novel Distinct Biologic Features. Am J Clin Pathol. 2021 Jan 4;155(1):87-96. doi: 10.1093/ajcp/aqaa114.

[10] Vij M, Calderaro J. Pathologic and molecular features of hepatocellular carcinoma: An update World J Hepatol. 2021 Apr 27;13(4):393-410. doi: 10.4254/wjh.v13.i4.393.

[11] Lefkowitch JH. In: Scheuer's Liver Biopsy Interpretation. 9th Edition. Elsevier. 2016.193-250

[12] Calderaro J, Ziol M, Paradis V, Zucman-Rossi J. Molecular and histological correlations in liver cancer.J Hepatol. 2019 Sep;71(3):616-630. doi: 10.1016/j.jhep.2019.06.001. Epub 2019 Jun 10.

[13] Fattovich G, Stroffolini T, Zagni I, Donato F. Hepatocellular carcinoma in cirrhosis: incidence and risk factors. Gastroenterology. 2004 Nov;127(5 Suppl 1):S35-50. doi: 10.1053/j.gastro.2004.09.014.

[14] Nzeako UC, Goodman ZD, Ishak KG. Hepatocellular carcinoma in cirrhotic and noncirrhotic livers. A clinico-histopathologic study of 804 North American patients.Am J Clin Pathol. 1996 Jan;105(1):65-75. doi: 10.1093/ajcp/105.1.65.

[15] Leung C, Yeoh SW, Patrick D, et al. Characteristics of hepatocellular carcinoma in cirrhotic and non-cirrhotic non-alcoholic fatty liver disease. World J Gastroenterol. 2015;21:1189-1196.

[16] Aykutlu U, Argon A, Orman M, Ulukaya S, Zeytunlu M, Karasu Z,

Günşar F, Nart D, Akarca U, Yilmaz F. Steatotic and Steatohepatitic Hepatocellular Carcinomas: Features in a Series With Predominantly Viral Etiology.Am J Surg Pathol. 2021 Apr 8. doi: 10.1097/PAS.0000000000001714. Online ahead of print.

[17] Gupta N, Rastogi A, Bihari C. Steatohepatitic hepatocellular carcinoma-a case report with literature review. Indian J Surg Oncol. 2014 Jun;5(2):161-3. doi: 10.1007/s13193-014-0297-4. Epub 2014 Feb 27.

[18] Perz JF, Armstrong GL, Farrington LA, Hutin YJ, Bell BP. The contributions of hepatitis B virus and hepatitis C virus infections to cirrhosis and primary liver cancer worldwide. J Hepatol. 2006 Oct;45(4):529-38. doi: 10.1016/j.jhep.2006.05.013. Epub 2006 Jun 23.

[19] Hayashi PH, Di Bisceglie AM. The progression of hepatitis B- and C-infections to chronic liver disease and hepatocellular carcinoma: epidemiology and pathogenesis. Med Clin North Am. 2005 Mar;89(2):371-89. doi: 10.1016/j.mcna.2004.08.014.

[20] Sun CA, Wu DM, Lin CC, Lu SN, You SL, Wang LY, Wu MH, Chen CJIncidence and cofactors of hepatitis C virus-related hepatocellular carcinoma: a prospective study of 12,008 men in Taiwan. Am J Epidemiol. 2003 Apr 15;157(8):674-82. doi: 10.1093/aje/kwg041.

[21] Tan A, Yeh SH, Liu CH, Claudia C, Chen PJ. Viral hepatocarcinogenesis: from infection to cancer Liver Int . 2008 Feb;28(2):175-88. doi: 10.1111/j.1478-3231.2007.01652.x.

[22] Ando S, Shibahara J, Hayashi A, Fukayama M. β-catenin alteration is rare in hepatocellular carcinoma with steatohepatitic features: immunohistochemical and mutational study. Virchows Arch. 2015 Nov;467(5):535-42. doi: 10.1007/s00428-015-1836-2. Epub 2015 Aug 27.

[23] Tornillo L, Carafa V, Richter J, Sauter G, Moch H, Minola E, Gambacorta M, Bianchi L, Vecchione R, Terracciano LM. Marked genetic similarities between hepatitis B virus-positive and hepatitis C virus-positive hepatocellular carcinomas. J Pathol. . 2000 Nov;192(3):307-12. doi: 10.1002/1096-9896(2000)9999:9999<::AID-PATH706>3.0.CO;2-O.

[24] Di Bisceglie AM, Lyra AC, Schwartz M, Reddy RK, Martin P, Gores G, Lok AS, Hussain KB, Gish R, Van Thiel DH, Younossi Z, Tong M, Hassanein T, Balart L, Fleckenstein J, Flamm S, Blei A, Befeler AS; Hepatitis C-related hepatocellular carcinoma in the United States: influence of ethnic status.Liver Cancer Network.Am J Gastroenterol. 2003 Sep;98(9):2060-3. doi: 10.1111/j.1572-0241.2003.t01-1-07641.x.

[25] Liang TJ, Heller T. Pathogenesis of hepatitis C-associated hepatocellular carcinoma. Gastroenterology. 2004 Nov;127(5 Suppl 1):S62-71. doi: 10.1053/j.gastro.2004.09.017.

[26] Block TM, Mehta AS, Fimmel CJ, Jordan R. Molecular viral oncology of hepatocellular carcinoma. Oncogene. 2003 Aug 11;22(33):5093-107. doi: 10.1038/sj.onc.1206557.

[27] Qian GS, Ross RK, Yu MC, Yuan JM, Gao YT, Henderson BE, Wogan GN, Groopman JD. A follow-up study of urinary markers of aflatoxin exposure and liver cancer risk in Shanghai, People's Republic of China.Cancer Epidemiol Biomarkers Prev. 1994 Jan-Feb;3(1):3-10.

[28] Llovet JM, Zucman-Rossi J, Pikarsky E, Sangro B, Schwartz M, Sherman M, Gores G. Hepatocellular carcinoma. Nat Rev Dis Primers. 2016

Apr 14;2:16018. doi: 10.1038/nrdp.2016.18.

[29] Chen CH, Wang MH, Wang JH, Hung CH, Hu TH, Lee SC, Tung HD, Lee CM, Changchien CS, Chen PF, Hsu MC, Lu SN. Aflatoxin exposure and hepatitis C virus in advanced liver disease in a hepatitis C virus endemic area in Taiwan. Am J Trop Med Hyg. 2007 Oct;77(4):747-52.

[30] Zhang W, He H, Zang M, Wu Q, Zhao H, Lu LL, Ma P, Zheng H, Wang N, Zhang Y, He S, Chen X, Wu Z, Wang X, Cai J, Liu Z, Sun Z, Zeng YX, Qu C, Jiao YGenetic Features of Aflatoxin-Associated Hepatocellular Carcinoma. Gastroenterology. 2017 Jul;153(1):249-262.e2. doi: 10.1053/j.gastro.2017.03.024. Epub 2017 Mar 29

[31] Davila JA, Morgan RO, Shaib Y, McGlynn KA, El-Serag HB. Hepatitis C infection and the increasing incidence of hepatocellular carcinoma: a population-based study. Gastroenterology. 2004 Nov;127(5):1372-80. doi: 10.1053/j.gastro.2004.07.020.

[32] Ganne-Carrié N, Nahon P. Hepatocellular carcinoma in the setting of alcohol-related liver disease. J Hepatol. 2019 Feb;70(2):284-293. doi: 10.1016/j.jhep.2018.10.008.

[33] Morgan TR, Mandayam S, Jamal MM. Alcohol and hepatocellular carcinoma. Gastroenterology. 2004 Nov;127(5 Suppl 1):S87-96. doi: 10.1053/j.gastro.2004.09.020.

[34] Stickel F, Schuppan D, Hahn EG, Seitz HK. Cocarcinogenic effects of alcohol in hepatocarcinogenesis. Gut. 2002 Jul;51(1):132-9. doi: 10.1136/gut.51.1.132.

[35] Lieber CS. Alcohol and the liver: 1994 update. Gastroenterology. 1994 Apr;106(4):1085-105. doi: 10.1016/0016-5085(94)90772-2.

[36] Ceni E, Mello T, Galli A. Pathogenesis of alcoholic liver disease: role of oxidative metabolism. World J Gastroenterol. 2014 Dec 21;20(47):17756-72. doi: 10.3748/wjg.v20.i47.17756.

[37] Nair S, Mason A, Eason J, Loss G, Perrillo RP. Is obesity an independent risk factor for hepatocellular carcinoma in cirrhosis? Hepatology. 2002 Jul;36(1):150-5. doi: 10.1053/jhep.2002.33713.

[38] Kowdley KV. Iron, hemochromatosis, and hepatocellular carcinoma. Gastroenterology. 2004 Nov;127(5 Suppl 1):S79-86. doi: 10.1016/j.gastro.2004.09.019.

[39] Salomao M, Remotti H, Vaughan R, Siegel AB, Lefkowitch JH, Moreira RK. The steatohepatitic variant of hepatocellular carcinoma and its association with underlying steatohepatitis. Hum Pathol. 2012; 43 (5):737±46. Epub 2011/10/25. doi: 10.1016/j.humpath.2011.07.005 PMID: 22018903

[40] Jafri W, Kamran M. Hepatocellular Carcinoma in Asia: A Challenging Situation. Euroasian J Hepatogastroenterol. 2019 Jan-Jun;9(1):27-33. doi: 10.5005/jp-journals-10018-1292.

[41] Sotiropoulos GC, Molmenti EP, Lang H, Beckebaum S, Kaiser GM, Brokalaki EI, Frilling A, Malagó M, Neuhauser M, Broelsch CE. Surgery for hepatocellular carcinoma arising in hereditary hemochromatosis. Eur Surg Res. 2006;38(4):371-6. doi: 10.1159/000094532. Epub 2006 Jul 11

[42] Vautier G, Bomford AB, Portmann BC, Metivier E, Williams R, Ryder SD. p53 mutations in british patients with hepatocellular carcinoma: clustering in genetic hemochromatosis. Gastroenterology. 1999 Jul;117(1):154-60. doi: 10.1016/s0016-5085(99)70562-7.

[43] Dragani TA. Risk of HCC: genetic heterogeneity and complex genetics. J Hepatol. 2010 Feb;52(2):252-7. doi: 10.1016/j.jhep.2009.11.015. Epub 2009 Nov 24.

[44] Siegel AB, Zhu AX. Metabolic syndrome and hepatocellular carcinoma: two growing epidemics with a potential link.Cancer. 2009 Dec 15;115(24):5651-61. doi: 10.1002/cncr.24687.

[45] Takahashi Y, Fukusato T. . Histopathology of nonalcoholic fatty liver disease/nonalcoholic steatohepatitis. World J Gastroenterol. 2014 Nov 14;20(42):15539-48. doi: 10.3748/wjg.v20.i42.15539.

[46] Anstee QM, Reeves HL, Kotsiliti E, Govaere O, Heikenwalder M. From NASH to HCC: current concepts and future challenges. Nat Rev Gastroenterol Hepatol. 2019 Jul;16(7):411-428. doi: 10.1038/s41575-019-0145-7.

[47] McGlynn KA, Petrick JL, El-Serag HB. Epidemiaology of Hepatocellular Carcinoma. Hepatology. 2021 Jan;73 Suppl 1(Suppl 1):4-13. doi: 10.1002/hep.31288. Epub 2020 Nov 24.

[48] Caldwell SH, Crespo DM, Kang HS, Al-Osaimi AM. Obesity and hepatocellular carcinoma. Gastroenterology. 2004 Nov;127(5 Suppl 1):S97-103. doi: 10.1053/j.gastro.2004.09.021.

[49] Calle EE, Rodriguez C, Walker-Thurmond K, Thun MJ. Overweight, obesity, and mortality from cancer in a prospectively studied cohort of U.S. adults. N Engl J Med. 2003 Apr 24;348(17):1625-38. doi: 10.1056/NEJMoa021423.

[50] Younossi ZM, Koenig AB, Abdelatif D, et al. Global epidemiology of nonalcoholic fatty liver disease-meta-analytic assessment of prevalence, incidence, and outcomes. Hepatology 2016;64:73e84.

[51] Degasperi E, Colombo M. Distinctive features of hepatocellular carcinoma in non-alcoholic fatty liver disease. Lancet Gastroenterol Hepatol 2016;1:156e64.

[52] Jain D, Nayak NC, Kumaran V, Saigal S. Steatohepatitic hepatocellular carcinoma, a morphologic indicator of associated metabolic risk factors: a study from India.Arch Pathol Lab Med. 2013 Jul;137(7):961-6. doi: 10.5858/arpa.2012-0048-OA.

[53] Alexander J, Torbenson M, Wu TT, Yeh MM. Non-alcoholic fatty liver disease contributes to hepatocarcinogenesis in non-cirrhotic liver: a clinical and pathological study.J Gastroenterol Hepatol. 2013 May;28(5):848-54. doi: 10.1111/jgh.12116.

[54] Zhang X. NAFLD Related-HCC: The Relationship with Metabolic Disorders. Adv Exp Med Biol. 2018;1061:55-62. doi: 10.1007/978-981-10-8684-7_5.

[55] Michelotti GA, Machado MV, Diehl AM.Nat Rev NAFLD, NASH and liver cancer.Gastroenterol Hepatol. 2013 Nov;10(11):656-65. doi: 10.1038/nrgastro.2013.183. Epub 2013 Oct 1.

[56] Vernon G, Baranova A, Younossi ZM. Systematic review: the epidemiology and natural history of non-alcoholic fatty liver disease and non-alcoholic steatohepatitis in adults. Aliment Pharmacol Ther 2011; 34: 274-85.

[57] Shibahara J, Ando S, Sakamoto Y, Kokudo N, Fukayama M. Hepatocellular carcinoma with steatohepatitic features: a clinicopathological study of Japanese patients.Histopathology. 2014 Jun;64(7):951-62. doi: 10.1111/his.12343. Epub 2014 Feb 5.

[58] Yeh MM, Liu Y, Torbenson M. Steatohepatitic variant of hepatocellular carcinoma in the absence of metabolic

syndrome or background steatosis: a clinical, pathological, and genetic study. Hum Pathol. 2015 Nov;46(11):1769-75. doi: 10.1016/j.humpath.2015.07.018. Epub 2015 Aug 4

[59] Dyson J, Jacques B, Chattopadyhay D, et al. Hepatocellular cancer:the impact of obesity, type 2 diabetes and a multidisciplinary team.J Hepatol 2014; 60: 110-17.

[60] Baffy G, Brunt EM, Caldwell SH (2012) Hepatocellular carcinoma in non-alcoholic fatty liver disease: an emerging menace. J Hepatol 56:1384-1391. doi:10.1016/j.jhep.2011.10.027

[61] Lee JS, Yoo JE, Kim H, Rhee H, Koh MJ, Nahm JH, Choi JS, Lee KH, Park YN. Tumor stroma with senescence-associated secretory phenotype in steatohepatitic hepatocellular carcinoma. PLoS One. 2017 Mar 8;12(3):e0171922. doi: 10.1371/journal.pone.0171922. eCollection 2017.

[62] Ikeda K, Saitoh S, Koida I, Tsubota A, Arase Y, Chayama K, Kumada H. Imaging diagnosis of small hepatocellular carcinoma.Hepatology. 1994 Jul;20(1 Pt 1):82-7. doi: 10.1016/0270-9139(94)90137-6.

[63] Inui S, Kondo H, Tanahashi Y, Fukukura Y, Sano K, Morisaka H, Saito K, Kondo F, Fukusato T, Furui S, Oba H. Steatohepatitic hepatocellular carcinoma: imaging findings with clinicopathological correlation.Clin Radiol. 2021 Feb;76(2):160.e15-160.e25. doi: 10.1016/j.crad.2020.09.011. Epub 2020 Oct 10.

[64] Torbenson MS. Hepatocellular carcinoma: making sense of morphological heterogeneity, growth patterns, and subtypes. Hum Pathol. 2020 Dec 30:S0046-8177(20)30262-8. doi: 10.1016/j.humpath.2020.12.009. Online ahead of print.

[65] Torbenson M, Washington K. Pathology of liver disease: advances in the last 50years. Hum Pathol 2020 Jan;95:78e98.

[66] Kojiro M. Pathology of hepatocellular carcinoma. India: Replika Presss Pvt. Ltd.; 2006. p. 174.

[67] Yeh CN, Lee WC, Jeng LB, Chen MF. Pedunculated hepatocellular carcinoma: clinicopathologic study of 18 surgically resected cases. World J Surg 2002;26:1133e8.

[68] Olofson AM, Gonzalo DH, Chang M, Liu X. Steatohepatitic Variant of Hepatocellular Carcinoma: A Focused Review. Gastroenterology Res . 2018 Dec;11(6):391-396. doi: 10.14740/gr1110. Epub 2018 Dec 17.

[69] Qin J, Higashi T, Nakagawa S, Fujiwara N, Yamashita YI, Beppu T, Baba H, Kobayashi M, Kumada H, Gunasekaran G, Schiano TD, Thung SN, Fiel MI, Hoshida Y, Ward SC. Steatohepatitic Variant of Hepatocellular Carcinoma Is Associated With Both Alcoholic Steatohepatitis and Nonalcoholic Steatohepatitis: A Study of 2 Cohorts With Molecular Insights. Am J Surg Pathol. 2020 Oct;44(10):1406-1412. doi: 10.1097/PAS.0000000000001533

[70] Hoshida Y, Nijman SM, Kobayashi M, et al. Integrative transcriptome analysis reveals common molecular subclasses of human hepatocellular carcinoma. Cancer Res. 2009;69:7385-7392.

[71] Samdanci ET, Akatli AN, Soylu NK. Clinicopathological Features of Two Extremely Rare Hepatocellular Carcinoma Variants: a Brief Review of Fibrolamellar and Scirrhous Hepatocellular Carcinoma. .J Gastrointest Cancer. 2020 Dec;51(4):1187-1192. doi: 10.1007/s12029-020-00500-1.

[72] Salomao M, Yu WM, Brown Jr RS, Emond JC, Lefkowitch JH.

Steatohepatitic hepatocellular carcinoma (SH-HCC): a distinctive histological variant of HCC in hepatitis C virus-related cirrhosis with associated NAFLD/NASH. Am J Surg Pathol 2010;34:1630-6.

[73] Jabbour TE, Lagana SM, Lee H. Update on hepatocellular carcinoma: Pathologists' review World J Gastroenterol, 2019 Apr 14;25(14):1653-1665.

[74] Yasir S, Chen ZE, Said S, Wu TT, Torbenson M. Biopsies of hepatocellular carcinoma with no reticulin loss: an important diagnostic pitfall.Hum Pathol. 2021 Jan;107:20-28. doi: 10.1016/j.humpath.2020.09.015. Epub 2020 Oct 8.

[75] Taniai M, Hashimoto E, Tobari M, Kodama K, Tokushige K, Yamamoto M, Takayama T, Sugitani M, Sano K, Kondo F, Fukusato T. Clinicopathological investigation of steatohepatitic hepatocellular carcinoma: A multicenter study using immunohistochemical analysis of adenoma-related markers..Hepatol Res. 2018 Nov;48(12):947-955. doi: 10.1111/hepr.13203. Epub 2018 Oct 15.

Section 2

Diagnosis and Staging of Hepatocellular Carcinoma

Chapter 3

Multimodal Imaging of Hepatocellular Carcinoma Using Dynamic Liver Phantom

Muntaser S. Ahmad, Osama Makhamrah and Mohammad Hjouj

Abstract

Liver phantom is used at various medical levels, such as detecting hepatocellular carcinoma (HCC) in the early stages, training medical staff to deal with HCC by taking biopsies, developing new sequences on medical imaging devices, confirming the image quality, applying treatments to HCC, and others. All of the trials should be applied before entering the real human body. The phantom includes properties very similar to those of the human body, as well as the properties of liver cancer and how it is treated within the body through its biological form. Therefore, the present chapter aims to provide comprehensive information to consider when fabricating HCC-containing phantoms and the characteristics of those phantoms in proportion to multimodal medical imaging to aid in understanding the main target of dynamic phantom for HCC.

Keywords: Liver phantom, HCC, Dynamic Phantom, Multimodality Imaging, phantom characteristic

1. Introduction

Cancer is one of the most common diseases in the world and threatens human life on an unprecedented scale. Hepatocellular carcinoma (HCC) is one of the cancer types that originate in the human liver, and usually, it discovers at a late stage [1, 2]. The detection of HCC at the early stage increases the clinical efficacy of treatment by 60% compared to late detection. Several methods are used to detect HCC; alpha-fetoprotein (AFP); Ultrasound (US); computed tomography (CT); magnetic resonance imaging (MRI); and hybrid fluorodeoxyglucose positron emission tomography with FDG PET/CT [3].

The difficulties of detecting liver cancer in its early stages lie with researchers and medical practitioners. Therefore, researchers need to provide any method that will enable them to achieve this goal. Thus, the researchers turned to a tool that can be used to detect liver cancer before the actual application to the real patient. One such tool is the phantom, which mimics hepatocellular carcinoma [4, 5].

2. Diagnosis of HCC

HCC is detected in several medical methods, one of which is the use of non-invasive medical imaging technology. For HCC, the detection depends primarily on the detection of vascular perturbation of cancer. Therefore, contrast media enhancement is used in medical imaging techniques, which are relied upon to detect these disorders through the three imaging phases: late arterial phase, Porto-venous phase (PVP), and delayed phase.

The HCC is supplied by the hepatic artery, while the normal liver parenchymal cells are nourished by the portal vein. Based on this information, it is possible to distinguish between HCC and normal liver cells by contrast enhancement in both CT and MRI scans. The HCC cells show hyper-vascularity in the late arterial phase, while in the Porto-venous phase it appears less bright because it contains blood free of contrast (washout), and these features are known as classic features. These characteristics of cancer depend on the size of cancer itself, as the early stages of cancer do not have a large blood supply, in this stage are usually less than 1 cm in size, but in the advanced stages of cancer, it reaches 1-2 cm or more [6, 7].

2.1 HCC diagnosis in CT and MRI

The sensitivity of both CT and MRI to detect HCC varies according to HCC size. The sensitivity of MRI reaches 62% compared to 48% in CT for the HCC of less than 2 cm, while it reaches 95% in MRI compared with 92% in CT for HCC more than 2 cm. The major difference in both modalities lies in the detection of lesions less than 1 cm. Although MRI shows better results than CT, both have low specificity [8].

The image characteristics of both MRI and CT scans are similar in detecting liver cancer through the use of contrast enhancement. It appears as a very bright (strong signal) in the arterial phase and is less bright (lower signal) in the porto-venous phase and in the delay phase, it appears black. However, in MRI it appears hyper-intensity also on T2-weighted and diffusion-weighted images. A specific contrast agent is used in the MRI to increase the sensitivity of the examination in the detection of HCC, which is the gadolinium-ethoxybenzyl-diethylenetriamine pentaacetic acid (Gd-EOB-DTPA, Primovist, or Eovist). The reason is that only 50% of gadoxetic acid is absorbed into the liver cells and it is excreted by bile ducts and the remaining 50% is excreted by the kidneys [9].

In the arterial stage, the excessive enhancement this stage is caused by increases in the arterial supply of the nodules. While the washout appearance in the PVP and delayed phase depends on different factors such as the new drainage in the veins, the liver background enhancement, the amount of blood supply in the portal vein, the hyper-cellularity rate of a tumor, and the fundamental components of the cancer tissue. Indeed, the hemodynamic changing in the nodules through the development of carcinogenesis starts with decreasing the arterial supplies and presence of portal perfusion, after that the decreases on both arterial supplies and portal blood supplies would occur. Subsequently, the increase of arterial vascularity is developed, and the hypervascular pattern would appear [10]. **Figure 1** shows the typical features for HCC in MRI and **Figure 2** Shows a typical pattern of HCC in CT.

2.2 Contrast-enhanced ultrasound

Contrast-enhanced ultrasound (CEUS) can be used in ultrasound imaging to detect HCC. However, the possibility of error in diagnosis is high in this technique,

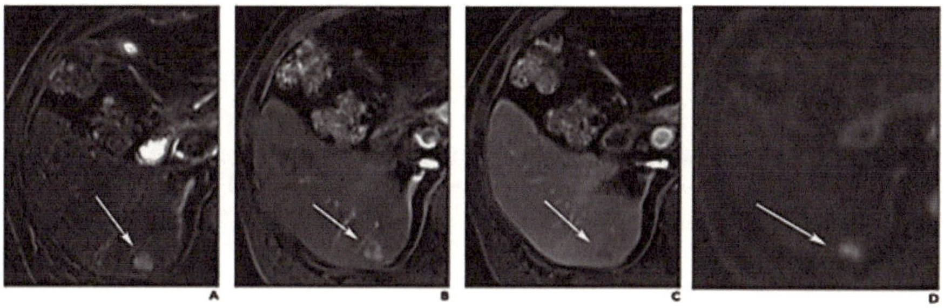

Figure 1.
Typical enhancement patterns of HCC; (A): Hyperintensity on T2 weighted image; (B): Arterial enhancement (arrow) on arterial phase image; (C): Tumor shows washout on portal venous phase image; and (D): Diffusion restriction on DWI [11].

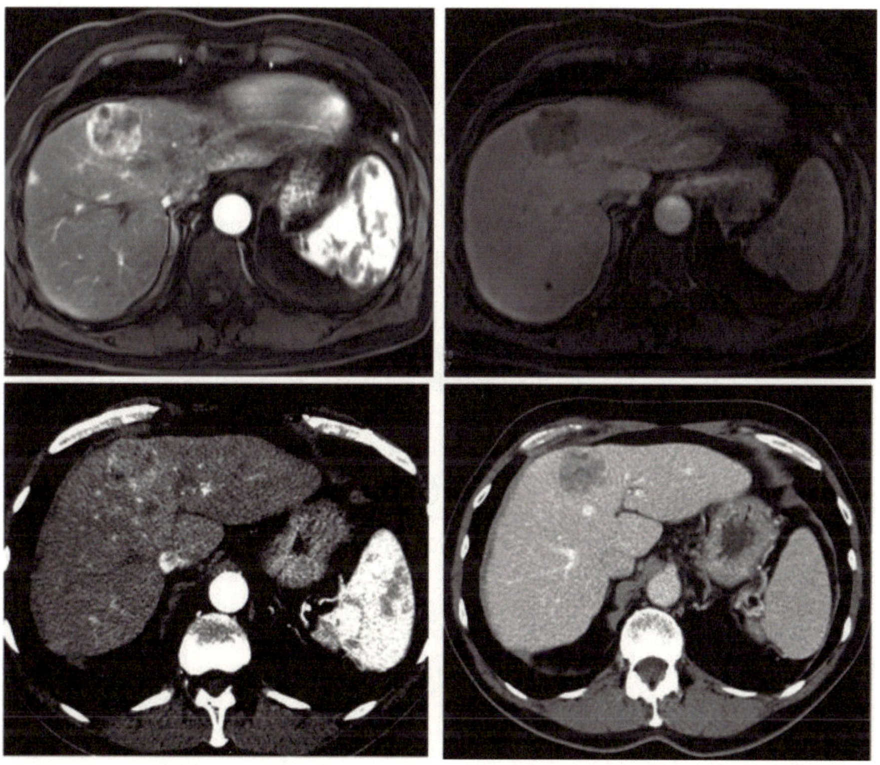

Figure 2.
Typical vascular pattern of HCC in CT: Liver lesion in the right hepatic lobe observed in a cirrhotic patient. The lesion is presenting a typical HCC vascular pattern with arterial hyperenhancement (left images) and venous wash-out (right images) visible both in magnetic resonance imaging (MRI) (upper row) and computed tomography (CT) (lower row) [12].

due to the rapid washout of the CEUS in less than 60 seconds after contrast material injection, and thus increases the risk of diagnostic error [7].

The contrast media used in CEUS such as sulfur hexafluoride and octafluoropropane combined with a phospholipid shell has a short arterial phase, so the liver exploration is not adequate to visualize the deep lesions [13]. Another problem with ultrasound is the inability to review the output image. CEUS and contrast enhanced MRI in lesions less than 2 cm can be used to improve diagnosis [14].

2.3 FDG-PET/CT

FDG PET/CT imaging is based on molecular imaging in different diagnoses of cancers. HCC is characterized by a low uptake of the FDG, and therefore the sensitivity of the examination is reduced compared with MRI and CT. Where it reaches less than 70%. In addition, normal liver cells absorb FDG significantly, and thus the sensitivity of detecting HCC than normal cells would be less [15].

3. Liver dynamic phantom component for hepatocellular carcinoma

3.1 Liver phantom

Different liver MRI phantoms are commercially available, that mimics blood vessels structures, tumor models, and real appearance [16]. However, none of them is a dynamic phantom. There are many commercial phantoms that offer 3D liver designs, but they are quite pricey. Therefore, we need to fabricate a liver phantom that is available at a lower cost. These phantoms use in multimodal medical imaging (US, CT and MR) such as CIRS model 057A [17], IOUSFAN® phantom [18], and Quality Assurance in Radiology and Medicine (QRM) GmbH supplies another version of a semi-anthropomorphic liver phantom (QRM-Abdomen Phantom, QRM GmbH, Möhrendorf, Germany) [19].

In previous studies, many chemical materials have been used to fabricate the human liver as TMMs. Most of these materials are represented on carrageenan [20], Poly Acrylic Acid (PAA), agar, PolyVinyl Alcohol (PVA) [21], polysaccharide, agarose [22], gelatin and silicone [23], polyurethane [4], commercial rigid plastics [24], and elastomeric (rubber-like) materials [25]. Shevchenko et al., (2011) [26], and Chmarra et al. (2013) [27], developed a phantom to simulate the liver using candle gel with cellulose. The simulation included the liver blood vessels in a simple form and the phantom was used for CT and US imaging. Another study conducted by Rethy et al. (2018) [4], using polyurethane to simulate the liver due to its durability. The phantom involved the simulation of the arterial and venous system of the liver with high accuracy as it was the first phantom that applying the contrast media. Phantom has been used on various medical modalities including CT, MRI, and US. All of Advantages and disadvantages of chemical materials for phantom fabrication were summarized in Appendix A.

The liver phantoms were increasingly used in clinical practices for different purposes including medical training and education, surgical and interventional planning, diagnosis and treatment planning, and research aims. Qiu et al., (2018) [25], developed a 3D phantom used as a surgical assistant for various human organs to provide an effective pre-operative planning solution. The study used rigid-plastic materials to create and develop a body that mimics the human liver. Another study conducted by Zein et al. (2013) [28], in the development of a human liver model using the PolyJet process, where simulated three liver models of three liver donors. These phantoms were used in anatomical evaluations before and during the surgical procedure. Javan and Zeman, (2018) [24] developed a 3D-printed model using polyamide material to fabricate the liver. The study was conducted for liver anatomical evaluation and to develop advanced functional interventional liver phantom. With a different purpose of the phantom, Bazrafshan et al. (2014) [29], developed a liver phantom made of acrylamide gel used in the development of tools for thermal mapping and coagulation progress which is applied in thermal tumor ablation methods such as radiofrequency ablation, and laser-induced interstitial thermotherapy.

3.2 HCC phantom

Several previous studies have included liver phantom within HCC samples. All of these studies focused on differentiating between normal liver cells and HCC by varying the density, intensity, and echogenicity for CT, MRI, and US, respectively. However, none has dealt with HCC samples in a dynamic way that simulates three phases; Arterial phase; Porto-venous phase; and Delayed phase, as in typical HCC.

Rethy et al. (2018) [4], designed a phantom similar to the human liver. This design contained HCC made of polyurethane blended with calcium carbonate. Where they used the concentration of −100 parts by weight (pbw) of polyurethane and 0.6% of Sephadex added with 5% calcium carbonate bw. Chmarra et al. (2013) [27], also designed another human liver phantom, including HCC samples which is made from agarose, with glycerol. The samples were made with 7.5 g of agarose, 30 ml of glycerol, 200 ml of distilled water, and 4 g of sephadex. The phantom was applied to various medical modalities and showed similar results to human tissue characteristics. In addition, the Javan and Zeman, (2018) [24] developed a 3D phantom of the liver containing cancer samples using polyamide material. The normal liver cells were distinguished using resin while polymer was used to simulate the internal structures which is allowed the catheters and wires for passaging. In contrast, Shevchenko et al. (2011) [26], developed a liver phantom including tumor model made from agarose-glycerol mix. The phantom was applied under CT and US imaging while it was not applied under MRI. K. Li et al., (2017) [30] conducted a study of Evaluation of the ablation margin of hepatocellular carcinoma for testing Radiofrequency ablation on the HCC which was made from carrageenan. The phantom was applied in CEUS, CT, and MRI.

3.3 Dynamic phantom

Dynamic contrast-enhanced (DCE) imaging is a method used to measure the kinetic perfusion of tumors within the body. It is also used to simulate the motion of blood circulatory inside the organ and to improve the diagnostic value, radiation treatment planning, treatment effectiveness, and monitoring [31]. This technique was used to simulate the perfusion in different tissues. However, most of the capillaries could not be imitated accurately [32]. This technique relies on the dynamic movement of contrast agent (CA) through different tissues. Therefore, the technique depends on the measurement of time-attenuation curves (TAC) for CA through the intra-arterial, intra-venous, and delay phases. The differences of CA physio-chemical properties such as solubility, viscosity, and electric charge effect on tumor pharmacokinetics [32].

The quantitative parameters such as blood flow, permeability, and blood volume control the amount of blood supply to the cancer cell. Each stage of cancer requires a different blood perfusion. Thus, it is possible to simulate the stages of cancer through DCE technique. There are several issues that need to be considered when using dynamic phantom. The phantom should be in a container that allows the transfer of contrast material from the arteries to the veins through the study samples, the substance of the sample should possess the appearance of HCC, the sample should interact with the contrast material, the sample should work to remove the contrast material without altering the sample structure, flexibility regarding changing the HCC samples without affecting the liver parenchyma structure, and the phantom should allow the pumping and disposal process of the contrast material by using an automatic injector and suction device [33, 34].

4. Phantoms properties-related modality

In order to use the phantom instead of the human tissue, different human tissue characteristics must be present in the phantom. In addition, when simulating an organ of human body, the shape, size and characteristics of the phantom must be similar to that organ. The materials used in the simulation must be non-toxic, non-degradable over time without change in properties, easy to manufacture and inexpensive. Each medical imaging modality has its own features to detect a special tissue charactarestic, the features must exist in the manufactured Phantom to mimik the human biological tissue. An explanation of these characteristics to be available in the Phantom according to medical imaging modality type.

4.1 Computed tomography

The phantom fabricated to CT device should has the same mass density (ρ_m) resulting in the same CT numbers or Hounsfield units (HU), same linear attenuation coefficient (AC), same effective atomic number (Zeff), and the same electron density (ρ_e) of the human tissue [16]. CT numbers can be calculated by the Eq. (1) [35]:

$$CTnumber(HU) = \frac{\mu_{tissue} - \mu_{water}}{\mu_{water}} * 1000 \tag{1}$$

While the linear attenuation coefficient (μ) can be calculated using the Eq. (2):

$$I_x = I_0 * e^{-\mu x} \tag{2}$$

While the effective atomic number (Zeff) can be calculated through the Eq. (3):

$$Z_{eff} = \sqrt[x]{w_1 Z_1^x + w_2 Z_2^x + w_3 Z_3^x + \ \dots \ + w_n Z_n^x} \tag{3}$$

Finally, the electron density (ρ_e) and mass density (ρ_m) are calculated using the Eq. (4):

$$\rho_e = \rho_m * NA * Z/A \tag{4}$$

Where μ_{tissue} is the linear attenuation coefficient for the tissue, μ_{water} is the linear attenuation coefficient of water, I_x is x-ray intensity after interact with human tissue, I_0 is x-ray intensity before interact with human tissue, x is the human tissue thickness, w_n is the number of atom Z_n in the compound, Z_n is the atomic number of the element, NA is the Avogadro's number, and A is the atomic mass of the element [16].

4.2 Magnetic resonance phantoms

The majority of MRI phantoms are represented in a fluid-filled model. These phantoms differ in their dimensions and forms depending on the body organ to be simulated. The phantoms are fabricated in order to achieve several purposes including evaluate image contrast, evaluate image uniformity, estimate spatial resolution, improve the signal-noise ratio (SNR), check the accuracy of slice thickness, and achieve geometric accuracy.

MRI phantom should have several characteristics compatible with MRI technology, these characteristics include tissue-specific relaxation for both; longitudinal relaxation time (T1) and transverse relaxation time (T2); variation of signal intensity with temperature changing; the mechanical properties should be fixed over an extended period [36]; and the phantom should be suitable to fit in the existing MRI coils [37]. The recovery time and decaying time depend on molecular motion in the local environment. Thus, T1 and T2 relaxation times changing with different diseases such as inflammation, hemorrhage, and any biological dysfunction. Also, the T1 and T2 relaxation times depend on tissue rigidity and viscosity. Low signal intensity on T1W and T2W appears when using phantom materials with greater viscosity and higher rigidity.

MRI phantoms have been manufactured using either aqueous solutions or polymer gels. Aqueous solutions are usually doped with paramagnetic ions like MnCl2, CuSO4, GdCl3, and NiCl2. These materials are used for testing MRI equipment because it has the property of stability. However, they are affected by motion artifacts and need a container to maintain shape [36]. Regarding gel phantoms, a lot of materials have been used in the literatures for fabricating MRI phantom including gelatin [38], gelatin-agar [39], agarose [40], agar [41], PVA [42], polysaccharide TX-150 [43], polysaccharide TX-151 [44], PAA [45], room-temperature-vulcanizing (RTV) silicone [46], and carrageenan [30, 47].

The properties of materials used to fabricate the MRI phantom are categorized into four groups including chemical properties, mechanical properties (density, pressure, elasticity, and hardness), electrical properties (conductivity and permittivity), and imaging properties (relaxation times T1 and T2). The chemical properties of the material examine using several vibrational spectroscopic techniques (VST). Different VST was used to know the chemical properties of the different samples including Fourier transform infrared spectroscopy (FTIR) [48], Near-infrared spectroscopy (NIRS), Mid-infrared Spectroscopy (MIR), Raman spectroscopy, and hyperspectral imaging (HSI) [49].

The mechanical properties of the phantom are among the most important properties that should be taken into considerations to give the best simulation of the human body organs. These properties consist of density, compressive modulus, elastic modulus, and toughness. Density depends on the quantity of mass per unit volume. The material densities should be around 1.03 ± 0.04 g/cm^3 which is closed to human tissue density [50]. The concentration of materials used in the phantom fabrication manipulates until reaches the suitable human tissue density. To confirm the stability of phantom density, several readings take overtime to monitor any density changes for phantom materials. Compressive modulus or compressibility expresses the material's ability to withstand pressure without changing the shape or size. The unit of compression strength is the pascal (Pa). Different models are used to measure the compression modulus such as the standard test method used for polymers; flexible cellular polymeric materials used for cellular [51]; and tensile strength for fused filament fabrication [52]. According to these models, the compressive strength measurements are different. Instron compression-testing machine is widely used in estimating compressive strength.

An electric is any insulated object that polarizes through applying an electric field. The most common property used in electricity is conductivity (σ) which is varied with frequency. For example, liver conductivity increases with increasing frequency [53]. Conductivity is the amount of resistance of the material or a material's ability to conduct electrical current. The signal intensity unit of electrical conductivity is siemens per meter (S/m or S.m-1) [54]. The dielectric Win DETA 5.64 from Novocontrol Technologies is used to measure the polymer dielectric properties.

4.3 Ultrasound

The phantom fabricated in the ultrasound should have the same velocity of sound or acoustic velocity, same Attenuation coefficient (AC), same acoustic impedance (Z), and same backscatter coefficient of the human tissue [55, 56]. The acoustic velocity (C_s) can be calculated by the Eq. (5):

$$C_s = \left(\frac{d_p}{d_\rho}\right)^{0.5} = \left(\frac{k_s}{\rho}\right)^{0.5} \tag{5}$$

While the Attenuation coefficient (α_s) in the ultrasound can be calculated through the Eq. (6):

$$\alpha_s = \alpha_w - \frac{1}{\Delta x}(\ln A_s - \ln A_w - 2\ln[1 - R]) \tag{6}$$

The R magnitude can be calculated by this Eq. (7):

$$R = \frac{Z_2 - Z_1}{Z_2 + Z_1} \tag{7}$$

The Backscatter coefficient (BS) is calculated by the Eq. (8):

$$BS(f,z) = \frac{S_s(f,z)}{S_R(f,z)} BS_R(f,z)A(f,z) \tag{8}$$

Where d_p is the pressure change in Pascal, $d_\rho$is the change of density in Kg.m-3, k_s is the modulus of bulk elasticity, α_w is the water attenuation coefficient, A_s is the ultrasound pulse amplitude, A_w is the water amplitude, R is the coefficient of acoustical reflection at the interface between material and water itself, Z_2 is the acoustic impedance of the material, Z_1 is the acoustic impedance of the water, S_s is the sample spectra, S_R is the phantom spectra, BS_R is the reference phantom backscatter, A is compensates function for attenuation along the propagation path, f is the frequency of ultrasonic wave, and z is the region depth of analysis [16].

4.4 Scintillation camera imaging

The following characteristics should be present on the phantom under scintillation camera imaging: same sensitivity, spatial resolution, count rate linearity, and contrast recovery of some radiopharmaceuticals such as 99mTc, 90Y, and 166Ho [57]. The Calibration factor (CF) can be calculated by the Eq. (9):

$$CF_{cps/_{Bq}} = {cps/_A} \tag{9}$$

While the sensitivity (S) or minimum detectable activity can be calculated through the Eq. (10):

$$S = \frac{4.65\sqrt{N}}{CF * t} + \frac{3}{CF * t} \tag{10}$$

Where cps is count per second of the phantom, A is the activity amount inside the phantom, N is the total background counts of the region of interest and t is the count time [16].

5. Conclusions

In summary, in order to achieve the best simulation of hepatocellular carcinoma, researchers should investigate as much as possible the characteristics of this disease and how it behaves inside the real human body. It varies from stage to stage, and therefore the simulation of HCC should be in a specific for each stage and likes to take into account the size of the cancer and the blood supply to it in each stage. Then the characteristics of the phantom should match with the characteristics of the multimodality imaging to be used for screening.

Acknowledgements

We would like to acknowledge the Universiti Sains Malaysia staff especially Dr. Nursakinah Suardi, Proff. Ahmad Shukri, and Dr. Nik Noor Ashikin Nik Ab Razak for supporting our research.

Conflict of interest

The authors declare no conflict of interest.

Appendices and nomenclature

Advantages and disadvantages of chemical materials for phantom fabrication.

Material	Material advantage	Material disadvantage	Material used in image modality
PAA gel	Elastic and easily formed • Used for multi-layered sample. • Inexpensive. • low ↓ Temperature fluctuations.	Time stability for 5 months Requires storage in sealed glass tubes	Suitable for MRI device
Carrageenan gel	Easily mold to different shapes. Inexpensive.	The relaxation time different. During hardness.	Suitable for MRI device
PAAG gel	Provides wide sites for hydrogen.	Properties affected by temperature.	Suitable for MRI device
Agar gel	Hydrophilic organic materials. Easily formed by temperature.	Properties affected by temperature. Restricted movement in free water.	Suitable for MRI, US, CT and scintillation camera imaging
Agarose gel	Independent of temperature. Used in different shape. Stable in long period	Time stability for 5 months. More complicated components than agar. Affected by bacterial infection	Suitable for MRI and CT
PVA (cryogel)	Low-cost price. Stable in long time. Easily handling.		Suitable for MRI and US
Polyurethane gel	High elastic recover. Resistance to	Complex in molecular design.	Suitable for US

Material	Material advantage	Material disadvantage	Material used in image modality
	bacterial infection Low. Low viscosity.		
Gelatine-alginate	High Stability. Store beneath water.	Complex structure. Lack of longevity.	Suitable for US and scintillation camera
Silicone polymer, RTV	Robust material. High Stability for long time. Easily formed.	Mismatching with biological tissues.	Suitable for CT
Commercial rigid plastics	High Stability in shape. High Stability for long time.	Stiffness more than normal tissue. Complex structure. Need specific device.	Suitable for CT and scintillation camera imaging.
Elastomeric (rubber-like) materials	Good flexibility. Good Elasticity	Complex structure. Need specific device.	Suitable for MRI and US

Author details

Muntaser S. Ahmad[1*], Osama Makhamrah[2] and Mohammad Hjouj[2]

1 Faculty of Applied Medical Health, Department of Medical Imaging, Palestine Ahliya University, Bethlehem, Palestine

2 Faculty of Health Professions, Medical Imaging Department, Al-Quds University, Jerusalem, Palestine

*Address all correspondence to: wmuntaser@gmail.com

References

[1] Heimbach, J. K., Kulik, L. M., Finn, R. S., Sirlin, C. B., Abecassis, M. M., Roberts, L. R., ... & Marrero, J. A. (2018). AASLD guidelines for the treatment of hepatocellular carcinoma. Hepatology, 67(1), 358-380.

[2] European Association For The Study Of The Liver. EASL clinical practice guidelines: management of hepatocellular carcinoma. Journal of hepatology. 2018 Jul 1;69(1):182-236.

[3] Ahmad, M. S., Suardi, N., Shukri, A., Mohammad, H., Oglat, A. A., Abunahel, B. M., ... & Makhamrah, O. (2019). Current status regarding tumour progression, surveillance, diagnosis, staging, and treatment of HCC: a literature review. Journal of Gastroenterology and Hepatology Research, 8(2), 2841-2852.

[4] Rethy, A., Sæternes, J. O., Halgunset, J., Mårvik, R., Hofstad, E. F., Sánchez-Margallo, J. A., & Langø, T. (2018). Anthropomorphic liver phantom with flow for multimodal image-guided liver therapy research and training. International journal of computer assisted radiology and surgery, 13(1), 61-72. DOI: 10.1007/s11548-017-1669-3.

[5] McGarry, C. K., Grattan, L. J., Ivory, A. M., Leek, F., Liney, G. P., Liu, Y., ... & Clark, C. H. (2020). Tissue mimicking materials for imaging and therapy phantoms: a review. Physics in Medicine & Biology. DOI: 10.1088/1361-6560/abbd17.

[6] Li, Y., Wang, L. H., Zhang, H. T., Wang, Y. T., Liu, S., Zhou, W. L., ... & Yang, J. Y. (2018). Disulfiram combined with copper inhibits metastasis and epithelial–mesenchymal transition in hepatocellular carcinoma through the NF-κB and TGF-β pathways. Journal of cellular and molecular medicine, 22(1), 439-451. DOI: 10.1111/jcmm.13334.

[7] Schellhaas, B., Görtz, R. S., Pfeifer, L., Kielisch, C., Neurath, M. F., & Strobel, D. (2017). Diagnostic accuracy of contrast-enhanced ultrasound for the differential diagnosis of hepatocellular carcinoma: ESCULAP versus CEUS-LI-RADS. European journal of gastroenterology & hepatology, 29(9), 1036-1044. DOI: 10.1097/MEG.0000000000000916.

[8] Ayuso, C., Rimola, J., Vilana, R., Burrel, M., Darnell, A., García-Criado, Á., ... & Brú, C. (2018). Diagnosis and staging of hepatocellular carcinoma (HCC): current guidelines. European journal of radiology, 101, 72-81. DOI: 10.1016/j.ejrad.2018.01.025.

[9] Paisant, A., Vilgrain, V., Riou, J., Oberti, F., Sutter, O., Laurent, V., ... & Aubé, C. (2020). Comparison of extracellular and hepatobiliary MR contrast agents for the diagnosis of small HCCs. Journal of hepatology, 72(5), 937-945. DOI: 10.1016/j.jhep.2019.12.011.

[10] Ippolito, D., Querques, G., Okolicsanyi, S., Franzesi, C. T., Pecorelli, A., Lombardi, S., ... & Sironi, S. (2018). Dynamic contrast enhanced perfusion CT imaging: a diagnostic biomarker tool for survival prediction of tumour response to antiangiogenetic treatment in patients with advanced HCC lesions. European journal of radiology, 106, 62-68. DOI: 10.1016/j.ejrad.2018.07.012.

[11] Choi, M. H., Choi, J. I., Lee, Y. J., Park, M. Y., Rha, S. E., & Lall, C. (2017). MRI of small hepatocellular carcinoma: typical features are less frequent below a size cutoff of 1.5 cm. American Journal of Roentgenology, 208(3), 544-551. DOI: 10.2214/AJR.16.16414.

[12] Schraml, C., Kaufmann, S., Rempp, H., Syha, R., Ketelsen, D., Notohamiprodjo, M., & Nikolaou, K.

(2015). Imaging of HCC—current state of the art. Diagnostics, 5(4), 513-545. DOI: 10.3390/diagnostics5040513.

[13] Dietrich, C. F., Nolsøe, C. P., Barr, R. G., Berzigotti, A., Burns, P. N., Cantisani, V., ... & Zheng, R. (2020). Aktualisierte Leitlinien und Empfehlungen für die gute klinische Praxis für CEUS der Leber. Ultraschall Med, 562-585. DOI: 10.1055/a-1177-0530.

[14] Huang, J. Y., Li, J. W., Lu, Q., Luo, Y., Lin, L., Shi, Y. J., ... & Lyshchik, A. (2020). Diagnostic accuracy of CEUS LI-RADS for the characterization of liver nodules 20 mm or smaller in patients at risk for hepatocellular carcinoma. Radiology, 294(2), 329-339. DOI: 10.1148/radiol.2019191086.

[15] Sabaté-Llobera, A., Mestres-Martí, J., Reynés-Llompart, G., Lladó, L., Mils, K., Serrano, T., ... & Ramos, E. (2021). 2-[18F] FDG PET/CT as a Predictor of Microvascular Invasion and a High Histological Grade in Patients with a Hepatocellular Carcinoma. Cancers, 13 (11), 2554. DOI: 10.3390/cancers13112554.

[16] Ahmad, M. S., Suardi, N., Shukri, A., Mohammad, H., Oglat, A. A., Alarab, A., & Makhamrah, O. (2020). Chemical characteristics, motivation and strategies in choice of materials used as liver phantom: a literature review. Journal of medical ultrasound, 28(1), 7. DOI: 10.4103/JMU.JMU_4_19.

[17] I. Computerized Imaging Reference Systems, "Triple modality 3D abdominal phantom, Model 057A.," Available from: http://www.Cirsinc.Com/Products/Modality/65/Triple-Modality-3D- Abdominal-Phantom/, pp. 297–300, 2017.

[18] L. Kyoto Kagaku Co., "Abdominal Intraoperative & Laparoscopic Ultrasound Phantom 'IOUSFAN,'" Available from: http://www.kyotokagaku.com/products/detail03/us-3.html., vol. 66, no. 3, pp. 373–378, 2017.

[19] QRM for quality assurance in radiology and medicine, "QRM-Liver-Phantom," Available from: http://www.qrm.de/content/products/anthropomorphic/liver_phantom.htm, vol. 88, no. 5, pp. 606–619, 2019.

[20] Lv, S., Long, Y., Su, Z., Zheng, R., Li, K., Zhou, H., ... & Xu, E. (2019). Investigating the accuracy of ultrasound-ultrasound fusion imaging for evaluating the ablation effect via special phantom-simulated liver tumors. Ultrasound in medicine & biology, 45 (11), 3067-3074. DOI: 10.1016/j.ultrasmedbio.2019.07.415.

[21] Nazem, F., Ahmadian, A., Seraj, N. D., & Giti, M. (2014). Two-stage point-based registration method between ultrasound and CT imaging of the liver based on ICP and unscented Kalman filter: a phantom study. International journal of computer assisted radiology and surgery, 9(1), 39-48. DOI: 10.1007/s11548-013-0907-6.

[22] Mitchell, M. D., Kundel, H. L., Axel, L., & Joseph, P. M. (1986). Agarose as a tissue equivalent phantom material for NMR imaging. Magnetic resonance imaging, 4(3), 263-266. DOI: 10.1016/0730-725X(86)91068-4.

[23] Kao, Y. H., Luddington, O. S., Culleton, S. R., Francis, R. J., & Boucek, J. A. (2014). A gelatin liver phantom of suspended 90Y resin microspheres to simulate the physiologic microsphere biodistribution of a postradioembolization liver. Journal of nuclear medicine technology, 42 (4), 265-268. DOI: 10.2967/jnmt.114.145292.

[24] Javan, R., & Zeman, M. N. (2018). A prototype educational model for hepatobiliary interventions: unveiling the role of graphic designers in medical 3D printing. Journal of digital imaging,

31(1), 133-143. DOI: 10.1007/s10278-017-0012-4.

[25] Qiu, K., Haghiashtiani, G., & McAlpine, M. C. (2018). 3D printed organ models for surgical applications. Annual Review of Analytical Chemistry, 11, 287-306. DOI: 10.1146/annurev-anchem-061417-125935.

[26] Shevchenko, N., Schwaiger, J., Markert, M., Flatz, W., & Lueth, T. C. (2011, January). Evaluation of a resectable ultrasound liver phantom for testing of surgical navigation systems. In 2011 Annual International Conference of the IEEE Engineering in Medicine and Biology Society (pp. 916-919). IEEE. DOI: 10.1109/IEMBS.2011.6090205.

[27] Chmarra, M. K., Hansen, R., Mårvik, R., & Langø, T. (2013). Multimodal phantom of liver tissue. PloS one, 8(5), e64180. DOI: 10.1371/journal.pone.0064180.

[28] Zein, N. N., Hanouneh, I. A., Bishop, P. D., Samaan, M., Eghtesad, B., Quintini, C., ... & Klatte, R. (2013). Three-dimensional print of a liver for preoperative planning in living donor liver transplantation. Liver transplantation, 19(12), 1304-1310. DOI: 10.1002/lt.23729.

[29] Bazrafshan, B., Hübner, F., Farshid, P., Hammerstingl, R., Paul, J., Vogel, V., ... & Vogl, T. J. (2014). Temperature imaging of laser-induced thermotherapy (LITT) by MRI: Evaluation of different sequences in phantom. Lasers in medical science, 29(1), 173-183. DOI: 10.1007/s10103-013-1306-5.

[30] Li, K., Su, Z., Xu, E., Huang, Q., Zeng, Q., & Zheng, R. (2017). Evaluation of the ablation margin of hepatocellular carcinoma using CEUS-CT/MR image fusion in a phantom model and in patients. BMC cancer, 17(1), 1-10. DOI: 10.1186/s12885-017-3061-7.

[31] Shulman, M., Cho, E., Aasi, B., Cheng, J., Nithiyanantham, S., Waddell, N., & Sussman, D. (2020). Quantitative analysis of fetal magnetic resonance phantoms and recommendations for an anthropomorphic motion phantom. Magnetic Resonance Materials in Physics, Biology and Medicine, 33(2), 257-272. DOI: 10.1007/s10334-019-00775-x.

[32] Kamphuis, M. E., Greuter, M. J., Slart, R. H., & Slump, C. H. (2020). Quantitative imaging: systematic review of perfusion/flow phantoms. European radiology experimental, 4(1), 1-13. DOI: 10.1186/s41747-019-0133-2.

[33] Makhamrah, O., Ahmad, M. S., & Hjouj, M. (2019, November). Evaluation of Liver Phantom for Testing of the Detectability Multimodal for Hepatocellular Carcinoma. In Proceedings of the 2019 2nd International Conference on Digital Medicine and Image Processing (pp. 17-21). DOI: 10.1145/3379299.3379307.

[34] Ahmad, M. S., Makhamrah, O., Suardi, N., Shukri, A., Ab Razak, N. N. A. N., Oglat, A. A., & Mohammad, H. (2021). Hepatocellular Carcinoma Liver Dynamic Phantom For Mri. Radiation Physics and Chemistry, 109632. DOI: 10.1016/j.radphyschem.2021.109632.

[35] EUCLID SEERAM. Computed Tomography: Physical Principles, Clinical Applications, And Quality Control. 4th Edition.Elsevier Health Sciences. 2016. DOI: 978-0-323-31288-2.

[36] Hattori, K., Ikemoto, Y., Takao, W., Ohno, S., Harimoto, T., Kanazawa, S., ... & Kato, H. (2013). Development of MRI phantom equivalent to human tissues for 3.0-T MRI. Medical physics, 40(3), 032303. DOI: 10.1118/1.4790023.

[37] Ahmad, M. S., Suardi, N., Shukri, A., Ab Razak, N. N. A. N., Oglat, A. A., & Mohammad, H. (2020). A recent

short review in non-invasive magnetic resonance imaging on assessment of HCC stages: MRI findings and pathological diagnosis. Journal of Gastroenterology and Hepatology Research, 9(2), 3113-3123.

[38] Madsen, E. L., Hobson, M. A., Shi, H., Varghese, T., & Frank, G. R. (2006). Stability of heterogeneous elastography phantoms made from oil dispersions in aqueous gels. Ultrasound in medicine & biology, 32(2), 261-270. DOI: 10.1016/j.ultrasmedbio.2005.10.009.

[39] Blechinger, J. C., Madsen, E. L., & Frank, G. R. (1988). Tissue-mimicking gelatin–agar gels for use in magnetic resonance imaging phantoms. Medical physics, 15(4), 629-636. DOI: 10.1118/1.596219.

[40] Hopper, T. A., Vasilić, B., Pope, J. M., Jones, C. E., Epstein, C. L., Song, H. K., & Wehrli, F. W. (2006). Experimental and computational analyses of the effects of slice distortion from a metallic sphere in an MRI phantom. Magnetic resonance imaging, 24(8), 1077-1085. DOI: 10.1016/j.mri.2006.04.019.

[41] Niculescu, G., Nosher, J. L., Schneider, M. B., & Foran, D. J. (2009). A deformable model for tracking tumors across consecutive imaging studies. International journal of computer assisted radiology and surgery, 4(4), 337-347. DOI: 10.1007/s11548-009-0298-x.

[42] Mano, I., Goshima, H., Nambu, M., & Iio, M. (1986). New polyvinyl alcohol gel material for MRI phantoms. Magnetic resonance in medicine, 3(6), 921-926. DOI: 10.1002/mrm.1910030612.

[43] Groch, M. W., Urbon, J. A., Erwin, W. D., & Al-Doohan, S. (1991). An MRI tissue equivalent lesion phantom using a novel polysaccharide material. Magnetic resonance imaging, 9(3), 417-421. DOI: 10.1016/0730-725X(91)90430-T.

[44] Mazzara, G. P., Briggs, R. W., Wu, Z., & Steinbach, B. G. (1996). Use of a modified polysaccharide gel in developing a realistic breast phantom for MRI. Magnetic resonance imaging, 14(6), 639-648. DOI: 10.1016/0730-725X(96)00054-9.

[45] De Luca, F., Maraviglia, B., & Mercurio, A. (1987). Biological tissue simulation and standard testing material for MRI. Magnetic resonance in medicine, 4(2), 189-192. DOI:10.1002/mrm.1910040213.

[46] Goldstein, D. C., Kundel, H. L., Daube-Witherspoon, M. E., Thibault, L. E., & Goldstein, E. J. (1987). A silicone gel phantom suitable for multimodality imaging. Investigative radiology, 22(2), 153-157. DOI: 10.1097/00004424-198702000-00013.

[47] Yoshimura, K., Kato, H., Kuroda, M., Yoshida, A., Hanamoto, K., Tanaka, A., ... & Hiraki, Y. (2003). Development of a tissue-equivalent MRI phantom using carrageenan gel. Magnetic Resonance in Medicine: An Official Journal of the International Society for Magnetic Resonance in Medicine, 50(5), 1011-1017. DOI: 10.1002/mrm.10619.

[48] Talari, A. C. S., Martinez, M. A. G., Movasaghi, Z., Rehman, S., & Rehman, I. U. (2017). Advances in Fourier transform infrared (FTIR) spectroscopy of biological tissues. Applied Spectroscopy Reviews, 52(5), 456-506. DOI: 10.1080/05704928.2016.1230863.

[49] Lohumi, S., Lee, S., Lee, H., & Cho, B. K. (2015). A review of vibrational spectroscopic techniques for the detection of food authenticity and adulteration. Trends in Food Science & Technology, 46(1), 85-98. DOI: 10.1016/j.tifs.2015.08.003.

[50] Kozicki, M., Jaszczak, M., Maras, P., Dudek, M., & Cłapa, M. (2017). On the development of a VIPARnd radiotherapy 3D polymer gel dosimeter.

Physics in Medicine & Biology, 62(3), 986. DOI: 10.1088/1361-6560/aa5089.

[51] Brunner, A. J., Blackman, B. R. K., & Davies, P. (2008). A status report on delamination resistance testing of polymer–matrix composites. Engineering Fracture Mechanics, 75(9), 2779-2794. DOI: 10.1016/j.engfracmech.2007.03.012.

[52] Tanikella, N. G., Wittbrodt, B., & Pearce, J. M. (2017). Tensile strength of commercial polymer materials for fused filament fabrication 3D printing. Additive Manufacturing, 15, 40-47. DOI: 10.1016/j.addma.2017.03.005.

[53] Bitar, R., Leung, G., Perng, R., Tadros, S., Moody, A. R., Sarrazin, J., ... & Roberts, T. P. (2006). MR pulse sequences: what every radiologist wants to know but is afraid to ask. Radiographics, 26(2), 513-537. DOI: 10.1148/rg.262055063.

[54] Chen, B. B., Hsu, C. Y., Yu, C. W., Liang, P. C., Hsu, C., Hsu, C. H., ... & Shih, T. T. F. (2016). Dynamic contrast-enhanced MR imaging of advanced hepatocellular carcinoma: comparison with the liver parenchyma and correlation with the survival of patients receiving systemic therapy. Radiology, 281(2), 454-464. DOI: 10.1148/radiol.2016152659.

[55] He, Y., Qin, S., Dyer, B. A., Zhang, H., Zhao, L., Chen, T., ... & Qiu, J. (2019). Characterizing mechanical and medical imaging properties of polyvinyl chloride-based tissue-mimicking materials. Journal of applied clinical medical physics, 20(7), 176-183. DOI: 10.1002/acm2.12661.

[56] Oglat, A. A., Matjafri, M. Z., Suardi, N., Oqlat, M. A., Abdelrahman, M. A., Oqlat, A. A., ... & Abujazar, M. Y. (2018). Chemical items used for preparing tissue-mimicking material of wall-less flow phantom for doppler ultrasound imaging. Journal of medical ultrasound, 26(3), 123. DOI: 10.4103/JMU.JMU_13_17.

[57] Amin, N. B., Abualroos, N. J., & Zainon, R. (2020). Fabrication of anthropomorphic thyroid-neck phantom for dosimetry study in nuclear medicine. Radiation Physics and Chemistry, 166, 108462. DOI: 10.1016/j.radphyschem.2019.108462.

Chapter 4

Hepatocellular Carcinoma: Diagnosis and Surveillance

Aditya Kale

Abstract

Hepatocellular carcinoma arises commonly on the background of liver cirrhosis. Patients presenting with clinical symptoms have advanced stage and often are unsuitable for curative therapies. Diagnosis of hepatocellular carcinoma is commonly performed by multiphase computed tomography (CT) and / or magnetic resonance imaging scans (MRI). Contrast enhanced ultrasound and MRI with hepatobiliary contrast agents are better in characterizing small lesions. Tumor markers play an adjunct role in diagnosis. For HCC in cirrhotic liver biopsy is seldom required and diagnosis is based on typical imaging features of non-rim arterial phase hyperenhancement and washout on delayed phase and pseudocapsule appearance. This is due to differential blood supply of liver parenchyma, regenerative nodules and tumor. Biopsy is only required in noncirrhotic liver, vascular liver diseases, atypical imaging features. Surveillance programs involving high risk groups can help in early detection of lesions which are amenable for curative therapies. Biannual ultrasound with or without alfa fetoprotein are commonly used surveillance tests. Multidisciplinary teams provide platform for care coordination, reassessments of clinical course, and fine changes in treatment plans required for management of this complex group of patients.

Keywords: hepatocellular carcinoma, surveillance, tumor markers, multiphase computed tomography, multiphase magnetic resonance imaging, LI-RADS, multidisciplinary team

1. Introduction

Hepatocellular carcinoma (HCC) is the most common primary malignant tumor of liver. It is sixth most commonly diagnosed cancer and fourth leading cause of cancer related mortality worldwide [1]. Most cases are diagnosed late in course of disease so that curative treatments could not be offered to such patients and hence incidence to mortality ratio for HCC approaches 1 [2]. Incidence of HCC is likely to increase due to increase in population and aging, as well as changing distribution of risk factors like obesity, hepatitis B and C virus infection and alcohol consumption [3]. Diagnosis at early stages and implementing surveillance programs in high risk population may reduce mortality [3]. This chapter focuses on diagnosis and surveillance for HCC.

2. Diagnosis of hepatocellular carcinoma

Diagnosis of hepatocellular carcinoma is primarily based on imaging with multiphase computed tomography (CT) scan and/or multiphase magnetic resonance

IntechOpen

imaging (MRI) scan. Like in other cancers, biopsy is required in selective cases where there is diagnostic dilemma. HCC usually becomes symptomatic only in advanced stages of the disease hence clinical features are seldom useful for the diagnosis of disease. Tumor markers are useful blood test in supporting diagnosis and prognostication of most of HCC however, they have their own limitations in early diagnosis of HCC. This section throws light on clinical features, imaging investigations and tumor markers and there role in diagnosis of hepatocellular carcinoma.

2.1 Clinical features of HCC

Early HCC are asymptomatic and are usually picked up during surveillance imaging. Classic clinical triad of right upper quadrant abdominal pain, palpable lump and weight loss is noted in 90% of the symptomatic patients [4]. New onset of abdominal pain and abdominal distension due to ascites are common in patients with underlying liver cirrhosis [5, 6]. Rapid worsening of portal hypertension indicates invasion of portal vein by tumor leading to tumor thrombosis [6]. Generalized weakness, anorexia and weight loss are common symptoms noted in 90%, 74% and 55% patients respectively [7]. Catastrophic presentation in the form of tumor rupture, hemoperitoneum and shock occurs in 3–15% of cases [8]. Hepatomegaly with irregular or nodular surface is common finding in nearly 84% cases [7]. Arterial bruit is present in minority of cases (2.6%) [9]. Ascites in HCC is most commonly due to underlying decompensated cirrhosis or due to tumor invasion of hepatic veins, portal vein or peritoneum and is often hemorrhagic [9]. Paraneoplastic manifestations of HCC include type B hypoglycemia due to increased production of insulin like growth factors by tumor, hypercalcemia, hypertension, carcinoid syndrome, clubbing, polycythemia, porphyria, thyrotoxicosis, migratory thrombophlebitis, watery diarrhea, sexual changes like feminization, gynecomastia [9].

2.2 Imaging diagnosis of hepatocellular carcinoma

Almost 90% of HCC develop on the background cirrhotic liver [10]. Regenerative nodules form in cirrhotic livers obtain majority of blood supply from portal vein, like the normal liver parenchyma. As the nodule progresses from regenerative to dysplastic and then into HCC, there is shift in blood supply from portal vein to hepatic artery [10]. Hence HCC obtains majority of the blood supply from hepatic artery. This forms the basis of diagnosis of HCC by non-invasive methods using multiphase computed tomography scan (CT) and magnetic resonance imaging (MRI). Radiology forms the cornerstone in diagnosis of HCC in cirrhotic liver. Non-invasive methods are applied to nodule ≥1 cm in cirrhotic liver due to high pretest probability [10].

Technical details related to machine, required images and additional images to be taken while evaluating liver nodule are mentioned in **Table 1**.

2.2.1 Typical appearance of hepatocellular carcinoma in cirrhotic liver on multiphase CT or MRI scans include

1. Non-rim arterial phase hyperenhancement AND

2. Non-rim washout in portal venous phase

3. Enhancing capsule appearance in portal venous phase or delayed venous phase

Technical details	Multiphase CT scan	MRI scan
Machine specifications	• Multidetector CT with more than 8 detector rows • Slice thickness 3 mm • Injection rate 4 milliliter/second	• 1.5 T or 3 T • Torso phased array coil
Required images	• Non-contrast • Arterial phase at 30 seconds with bolus tracking • Venous phase at 65 seconds • Delayed phase at 240 seconds	• Unenhanced T1 weighted in phased and opposed phase imaging • T2 weighted imaging (fat suppression per institutional preference) • All contrast agents in T1 weighted imaging. • Precontrast imaging • Arterial phase • Portal venous phase • Delayed venous phase
Additional images	• Multiplanar reformations • Precontrast in patients with locoregional treatment	• Diffusion weighted images • Subtraction imaging • Multiplanar acquisition

Table 1.
Technical details, required images and additional images to be obtained while evaluating liver space occupying lesion [11].

4. Increase in size of mass > 50% in <6 months measured in same phase sequence and plane (if possible). To measure the size of lesion largest outer edge to outer edge dimensions should be taken.

5. Ancillary features for diagnosis of HCC include hyperintensity on T2-weighted MRI, hyperintensity on diffusion-weighted MRI, intra-lesional fat, lesional iron sparing, corona enhancement, presence of capsule, mosaic architecture, nodule-in-nodule architecture, intralesional hemorrhage however, these features do not have specificity of 100% and do not allow conclusive diagnosis of HCC.

2.2.2 Comparison of multiphase CT and MRI with extracellular contrast agents performance in detecting HCC

Table 2 shows comparative performance of multiphase CT and MRI in HCC with various sizes [12].

For all sizes and tumors with <1 cm MRI with extracellular contrast agents appears to be more sensitive than CT scan with comparable specificity and diagnostic odds. Hence for small lesions MRI with extracellular contrast agents may be preferred modality over CT scan. Having said this availability, cost, longer scan times, more technical complexities, expertise, several patient factors like ascites, difficulty in breath holding, claustrophobia may limit its use as the first investigation for evaluation of liver lesion in cirrhotic patients. CT scan on the other had is technically relatively simple, less number and short duration of sequences, widely available and less costly than MRI. However, radiation exposure is the disadvantage of the CT scan. Hence multiple factors like availability, cost, patient related factors, tumor size, radiation are necessary to be considered to choose between CT scan and MRI as first investigation for evaluation of liver lesion [12].

Tumor size	Sensitivity (CT vs. MRI)	Specificity (CT vs. MRI)	Diagnostic odds CT vs. MRI
All sizes	0.69 vs. 0.84 (p = 0.0003)	0.92 vs. 0.94 (p = 0.83)	22 vs. 43 (p = 0.24)
< 1 cm	0.48 vs. 0.69 (p = 0.049)	0.46 vs. 0.69 (p = 0.08)	2.05 vs. 2.3 (p = 0.8)
1–2 cm	0.64 vs. 0.7 (p = 0.15)	0.87 vs. 0.88 (p = 0.78)	13 vs. 17 (p = 0.78)
2 cm	0.79 vs. 0.88 (p = 0.09)	0.9 vs. 0.87 (p = 0.71)	25.79 vs. 64.66 (p = 0.47)

Table 2.
Comparative performance of multiphase CT and MRI in HCC with various sizes.

2.2.3 Role of MRI with hepatocyte specific contrast agents in diagnosis of HCC

This technique uses Gadoxetic acid as a contrast agent. Approximately 50% of the administered dose is taken up by hepatocyte and excreted into the bile ducts and remaining half was excreted by kidneys [13]. Images are taken in two phases: Transitional phase taken at 2–5 minutes after contrast agent and hepatobiliary phase taken after 20 minutes of contrast injection [13]. Lesions with functional hepatocytes take up the contrast in hepatobiliary phase and appear hyperintense. Those without functional hepatocytes like high grade dysplastic nodules or HCC do not take the contrast in hepatobiliary phase and appear hypointense compared to background liver parenchyma [13]. These early HCC or high grade dysplastic nodules may not show typical arterial hyperenhancement resulting in missing some of the early HCC lesions. Addition of hepatobiliary phase to conventional dynamic MRI sequences increases likelihood of identifying malignant nodules and reduces the risk of overlooking malignant lesions [13–15]. Signal intensity of lesion on hepatobiliary phase is also a prognostic factor with hypointense lesions on hepatobiliary phase which are non-hypervascular, non-HCC have a higher risk of progression to typical HCC as compared to those lesions which are iso- or hyper-intense [16, 17].

2.2.4 Role of contrast enhanced ultrasound in diagnosis of HCC

It is performed with intravenous injection of a microbubble contrast agent. Real-time imaging is performed continuously for the 1st minute to capture the arterial phase. This is followed by intermittent scanning every 30–60 seconds for up to about 5 minutes to evaluate washout [11]. Typical appearance of HCC on Contrast enhanced ultrasound (CEUS) shows non rim arterial phase hyperenhancement and washout in delayed phase >60 seconds to differentiate it from mass forming cholangiocarcinoma which show early washout. It requires expertise and cannot scan entire liver at a time like CT or MRI [11]. CEUS has low sensitivity for detection of lesion as compared to CT and MRI but has higher specificity as compared to CT and MRI especially for small nodules (< 20 mm) 92.9% vs. 76.8% vs. 83.2% [18]. CEUS as second imaging modality has highest specificity 76.8% (after MRI) and 70.7% (after CT) for diagnosis of HCC [19].

2.2.5 Liver imaging reporting and data system (Li-RADS)

Liver imaging reporting and data system (Li-RADS) provides standardization for hepatocellular carcinoma (HCC) imaging. Li-RADS defines eight unique diagnostic categories LR 1 to 5, LR-M for malignant but not specific for HCC, LR-TIV for tumor in vein, LR-TR for treated lesion, based on imaging appearance that reflect the probability of HCC or malignancy with or without tumor in vein. Term LR-NC (non-categorizable observation) is used when observation that cannot be meaningfully categorized due to lack of one or more major criteria. LI-RADS criteria are to be applied for liver nodules in cirrhotic livers and lesion >1 cm. **Table 3** describes the each Li-RADS category and risk of HCC and non-HCC malignancy [11].

LI-RADS is not applicable for liver lesions in noncirrhotic liver, vascular liver diseases, sinusoidal obstruction syndrome, chronic inflow obstruction and hereditary hemorrhagic telangiectasia.

2.2.6 Role of Fluorodeoxyglucose positron emission tomography (FDG-PET) in diagnosis of HCC

FDG uptake is seen only in 40% of patients with HCC, so FDG-PET scan is not useful for diagnosis of HCC [20]. Uptake on 18F-FDG-PET has some potential prognostic significance and is associated with poor prognosis, increased serum alpha-fetoprotein and vascular invasion. Therefore, it may facilitate the selection of patients for surgical resection or liver transplantation [21].

2.2.7 Diagnosis of portal vein thrombosis- tumoral vs. non-tumoral (bland thrombus)

Cirrhosis without HCC is associated with portal vein thrombosis with prevalence ranging from 1% in compensated cirrhosis to as high as 25% in patients with advanced liver disease requiring liver transplantation [22]. Macrovascular invasion of the portal vein is a major prognostic factor frequently seen in HCC. Portal vein thrombosis may create diagnostic dilemma in patients with cirrhosis and HCC. Presence of arterial phase hyperenhancement, diffusion weighted MRI with high b values, venous expansion with diameter > 23 mm, thrombus in continuity with parenchymal HCC are the findings which point towards the diagnosis of tumoral portal vein thrombosis [23, 24].

2.3 Pathological diagnosis of hepatocellular carcinoma

HCC diagnosis in cirrhotic liver is based on imaging criteria mentioned above. However biopsy is required in patients with vascular liver diseases, non-cirrhotic livers, inconclusive radiological investigations, elevation of CA 19.9 or carcinoembryonic antigen (CEA) and liver lesion without HCC risk factors [24]. Samples for histological diagnosis of HCC can be obtained by image guided (ultrasound / CT scan) biopsy sometimes by diagnostic laparoscopy. Resected specimens and explants after liver transplants need evaluation for resection margin and histological assessment [24].

2.3.1 Gross appearance

HCC takes three forms nodular, massive or diffusely infiltrating type. Nodular form is often associated with liver cirrhosis. Massive form is associated with satellite nodules and has potential to rupture. Diffuse infiltrating type causes involvement of large part of liver and its vascular structures mainly portal vein, and is associated with poor prognosis [25].

Li-RADS category	Description	Interpretation	Risk of overall malignancy	Risk of HCC
LR-NC	Observation that cannot be categorized into specific category due to inability to assess one or more major criteria.	Noncategoriz-able observation	—	—
LR-1	Benign observation with 100% certainty	Benign	0%	0%
LR-2	High probability of being benign observation. No major features, LR-M features, ancillary features favoring malignancy	Probably benign	13%	14%
LR-3	Nonmalignant and malignant entities each have moderate probability. Nonrim APHE without any other major features OR Arterial phase iso/ hypoenhancement with size <20 mm and ≤ 1 additional major feature or > 20 mm and no major feature.	Moderate probability of being malignant or nonmalignant	38%	40%
LR-4	High probability of HCC but not 100% certainty. Non rim APHE and < 10 mm and ≥ 1 additional major feature 10–19 mm with capsule >20 mm with ≥1 additional major feature OR <20 mm with 2 additional major features	Probably HCC	74%	80%
LR-5	100% certainty of being HCC Nonrim APHE and 10–19 mm with non-peripheral washout OR 10–19 mm with ≥50% size increase in <6 months >20 mm with ≥1 additional feature	Definitely HCC	94%	97%
LR-TIV	Presence of soft tissue in vein regardless of mass in parenchyma	Malignancy with tumor in vein	—	—
LR-M	Targetoid mass with: Rim APHE Peripheral washout Delayed central enhancement Targetoid diffusion restriction Nontargetoid mass not meeting LR-5 criteria and without TIV with >1 of following Infiltrative appearance Marked diffusion restriction Necrosis or ischemia	Probably or definitely malignant but not specific for HCC	36%	93%

Table 3.
LI-RADS criteria with description of terminologies, risk of overall malignancy and risk of HCC. [APHE – Arterial phase hyperenhancement, TIV- tumor in vein].

2.3.2 Microscopic appearance

Microscopically HCC can be well differentiated, moderately differentiated, undifferentiated and progenitor cell. Most common variety is well differentiated type. It can be of trabecular type or acinar type (pseudoglandular type). Malignant hepatocytes are polygonal with large hyperchromatic nuclei. Bile production is present. Moderately differentiated HCC can be of solid, scirrhous, sarcomatoid and clear cell varieties. Solid type tumor shows small hepatocytes with areas of necrosis, inconspicuous fibrous tissue and absent bile production. In scirrhous variety abundant connective tissue stroma is noted separating hepatocytes. Clear cell variety has cells having high glycogen content. Undifferentiated HCC has pleomorphic cells with variable sized nuclei. Progenitor cell HCC have their origin from stem cells of liver. These tumors may appear similar to HCC or mixed cholangiohepatocellular carcinoma [25]. On biopsy specimens differentiation of small HCC from high grade dysplastic nodules is challenging. Diagnosis of HCC needs to be supplemented with three marker panel as recommended by International Consensus Group of Hepatocellular Neoplasia and the World Health Organization. This is because features of interstitial and vascular invasion can be missed on biopsy specimens. Combination of HSP70 (HSPA7), glypican 3 (GPC3), and glutamine synthetase (GS) has sensitivity and specificity of 72% and 100%, respectively in surgically resected specimens and its specificity is validated in biopsy specimens [26, 27]. Several immunohistochemical markers useful in diagnosis of hepatocellular carcinoma include Arginase-1 which is most sensitive and specific marker for hepatocellular differentiation. Hepatocyte paraffin-1 (Hep Par-1) has both sensitivity and specificity greater than 80% for HCC. Polyclonal carcinoembryonic antigen (pCEA) shows typical canalicular pattern and has sensitivity of 92% and 88% for well differentiated and moderately differentiated HCC [28].

HCC is heterogenous tumor in pathogenesis, behavior, phenotype and has different genetic signatures as described by recent studies. As mentioned above several different subtypes are described. 5th edition of world health organization classification of digestive system tumors integrates histopathologic features and molecular signatures of these tumors. **Table 4** shows morphological features, molecular signatures of different HCC subtypes as per 5th Edition of WHO Classification of Digestive system tumors [29, 30].

2.3.3 Risks associated with biopsy of the lesion

Biopsy is associated with risk of bleeding in 3–4% cases and severe bleeding requiring transfusion in 0.5% cases [31]. Risk of needle track seeding of tumor cells is about 2.7% [32]. Sampling errors can occur for small lesions <2 cm [33].

2.4 Role of tumor markers in diagnosis of HCC

Tumor markers are the substances which can be measured in cells, tissues, body fluids, indicate presence of cancer and help in prognostication. Ideal tumor marker should be highly sensitive and specific so as to diagnose lesions early HCC. Alfa fetoprotein (AFP) is used since long time for surveillance and diagnosis of hepatocellular carcinoma [34]. Now with identification of new molecular signatures, our understanding of pathological processes involved in HCC is improved leading development of newer biomarkers. This section will through light on old and new tumor markers and their utility in diagnosis of HCC [34].

2.4.1 Alfa fetoprotein (AFP)

AFP is a glycoprotein produced by fetal liver. After birth levels of AFP fall and its synthesis is repressed in adult life. It is expressed under some pathological conditions like chronic liver disease, cirrhosis, HCC, germ cell tumors and cholangiocarcinoma [35]. It is the most extensively studied biomarker for surveillance and diagnosis of

Variant	Histopathology	Molecular signature	Comments
Steatohepatic	Features of steatohepatitis in tumor.	IL-6/JAK/STAT activation	Less often vascular invasion or satellite nodules. Prognosis similar to conventional HCC
Clear cell	>80% cells demonstrates clear cytoplasm due to glycogen.	Not known	Slightly better prognosis compared to conventional HCC. Needs differentiation from clear cell type of renal cell carcinoma.
Macrotrabecular	Prominent thick trabeculae.	TP53 mutation FGF9 amplification.	Associated with HBV infection, vascular invasion, poor differentiation, high alfa-fetoprotein.
Scirrhous	Tumor cells mixed with dense fibrous stroma.	TSC1/TSC2 mutations, transforming growth factor beta activation.	Large tumors, vascular invasion, infiltrative growth.
Chromophobe	Cells have clear cytoplasm, focal areas of nuclear atypia.	Alternate lengthening of telomere phenotype.	Prognosis similar to conventional HCC.
Neutrophil rich	Diffuse tumoral infiltration by neutrophils.	Granulocyte monocyte colony stimulating factor production.	Elevated leucocyte count, interleukin-6. Poor prognosis.
Lymphocyte rich	Lymphocytic infiltration of tumor.	Not known.	Favorable outcome to conventional HCC.

Table 4.
Shows morphological features, molecular signatures of different HCC subtypes as per 5th edition of WHO classification of digestive system tumors.

HCC. AFP is elevated in nearly 70% patients with HCC. When cut-off value of 20 ng/ml is used AFP has sensitivity of 59.9% and specificity of 93% while at the cut-off value of 200 ng/ml sensitivity drops to 22% and specificity of 100% [35, 36]. AFP can be falsely elevated in patients with viral infections like hepatitis B and C. Positive predictive value of AFP in diagnosing HCC in patients with viral etiologies and non-viral etiologies was 70% vs. 94% in one study using cut-off of 20 ng/ml [34]. AFP also has prognostic significance with values ≥400 ng/ml have higher tumor burden, bilobar involvement, tumoral portal vein thrombosis and diffuse and massive variety of tumors [35]. Limitations of AFP measurement include false negative in small HCC and 30% of large tumors do not have elevated levels [35]. False positive in chronic liver disease, cirrhosis, HCC, germ cell tumors and cholangiocarcinoma [34, 35]. AFP-L3 glycoform of AFP is detected in approximately 35% of <3 m size HCC. Cut-off level of 15% has sensitivities ranging from 75%–96.9% and specificities of 90–92% [35]. Higher levels of AFP-L3 are associated with worse liver function, poor histology and large tumor mass and portal vein invasion [35].

2.4.2 Glypican-3

It is proteoglycan in plasma membrane. It produced by tumor cells but not elevated in non-HCC liver diseases. It can be detected in 40–53% of HCC patients and 33% of HCC patients with negative for both AFP and PIVKA-II. Addition of Glypican-3 measurements to AFP improves sensitivity from 50–72% [34, 35].

2.4.3 Des-gamma-carboxyprothrombin or protein induced by vitamin K absence or antagonist II (PIVKA-II)

It is abnormal product from liver carboxylation disturbance during the formation of thrombogen [34, 35]. It is overproduced in HCC patients. Sensitivity and specificity of PIVKA-II at the cut-off level 40 mAU/ml is 51.7% and 86.7% while at the cut-off value of 125 mAU/mL in discriminating HCC from nonmalignant hepatopathy sensitivities and specificities were 89% and 86.7% [37, 38]. In combination AFP-L3, AFP and DCP achieved 60.6% sensitivity and 100% specificity while DCP combined with AFP alone increased sensitivity from 65–87%, but specificity dropped from 84–69% [39, 40]. Japanese clinical guidelines recommend the combined use of PIVKA-II and AFP for the diagnosis of HCC, management of high-risk population, and prognosis of anticancer treatment [41].

2.4.4 Long noncoding RNAs (Inc RNAs)

Recent evidences have shown that long noncoding RNAs (lncRNAs) are involved in cancer diagnosis and prognosis. Pooled sensitivity, specificity, positive likelihood ratio (PLR), negative likelihood ratio (NLR), diagnostic odds ratio (DOR), and AUC for lncRNAs in the diagnosis of HCC were 0.83, 0.80, 4.2, 0.21, 20, and 0.88, respectively [42].

Table 5 summarizes newer biomarkers under evaluation for diagnosis of HCC.

2.5 Fibrolamellar hepatocellular carcinoma (FL-HCC)

Rare variant of HCC accounting for only 1% cases. In contrast to conventional HCC, FL-HCC is common in young patients aged <40 years, occurs in normal liver and has normal AFP levels [53]. FL-HCC is chromosomally stable tumor and displays genomic homogeneity in contrast to conventional HCC. Mutations in AFP, TP53 beta-catenin and surviving are not seen in FL-HCC, however increased expression of anterior gradient-2, CD133, CD44 and nuclear factor-kB pathway are seen in FL-HCC. Chromosomal imbalances involving chromosomes 1, 7 and 8 are noted in aggressive FL-HCC [54–56]. FL-HCC is typically large tan colored well-circumscribed firm mass without underlying chronic liver disease or cirrhosis. Central stellate scar is seen in 75% cases. Microscopically it is composed of cluster or sheets of large polygonal or spindle shaped cells with eosinophilic cytoplasm and prominent nuclei. Fibrous stroma is seen around the tumor cells. It has capsule and central scar [57, 58]. On immunohistochemistry it shows hepatocyte paraffin 1, CK7, CD133, CD44, α-1-antitrypsin, fibrinogen, C-reactive protein, carcinoembryonic antigen and copper [55, 59]. Patient presents with abdominal pain, malaise, weight loss and abdominal lump [57]. On ultrasound FL-HCC has no specific features [60]. On computed tomography scan tumors are well defined with lobulated outline. It has hypodense large >2 cm central scar and radiating fibrotic bands are more common. Central scar may show calcification. On contrast enhancement in arterial phase it shows heterogenous hyperattenuation. On the portal venous phase and delayed phase, approximately 50% of fibrolamellar HCCs become isoattenuating to liver. However, they may also be hyperattenuating (36%) or hypoattenuating (16%). Central scar may show delayed enhancement in 25–65% cases. Venous and biliary obstruction is rare [60]. On MRI, FL-HCC is hypointense on T1 imaging and hyperintense on T2 images. Central scar is hypointense on T1 and T2 weighted images. On contrast injection, it shows heterogenous enhancement which becomes iso or hypointense in delayed phase [60]. Nodal metastasis occur in 50–65% of FL-HCC and commonly occur in hepatoduodenal ligament and hepatic hilum. Cornerstone for treatment is surgical resection with

Serial Number	Tumor marker	Comments
1	Serum Gamma-glutamyl transferase II isoenzyme [43]	74% for all HCC and 34% for small HCC. In combination with AFP, PIVKA-II sensitivity may be improved.
2	Alpha-I-fucosidase [44]	Activity increases in HCC patients. Sensitivity and specificity at 870 nmol/ml per hour is 81.7% and 70.7% respectively
3	Alfa-fetoprotein mRNA [45, 46]	Serum AFP mRNA detected by reverse-transcription polymerase chain reaction (RTPCR) is correlated with portal vein thrombosis, number of nodules of tumor, tumor diameter, stage and post-operative recurrence.
4	Human telomerase reverse transcriptase mRNA (hTERT) [47, 48]	It has sensitivity and specificity of 88.2% and 70% and levels correlate with AFP concentration, tumor size, tumor differentiation.
5	Vascular endothelial growth factor(VEGF) [49]	Serum VEGF levels per platelet count are increased >1.4 picogram/10^6 in patients with HCC and correlate with stage, portal vein thrombosis, response to therapy and survival.
6	Interleukin-8 [50]	It is chemokine having direct effect on tumor cells, angiogenesis, tumor migration. Serum levels are significantly elevated in HCC patients compared to healthy adults and correlate with tumor size, venous invasion, advanced stage, absence of capsule and poor prognosis
7	Transforming growth factor-beta 1 [51]	Serum levels elevated in HCC. At cut-off 800 pg./ml sensitivity and specificity is 68% and 95%.
8	Tumor-specific growth factor (TSGF) [52]	Serum TSGF reflects the existence of tumor. It has been indicated that TSGF can be used as a diagnostic marker in detecting HCC, and its sensitivity can reach 82% at the cut-off value of 62 U/mL. With other markers like AFP, ferritin sensitivity and specificity can reach up to >90%

Table 5.
Summary of new tumor markers in HCC.

adequate lymph node dissection. The 5 year overall survival rate after partial hepatectomy was 70%. Radioembolization using ^{90}Y is helpful in unresectable FL-HCC. Liver transplantation is therapeutic option in selected patients [60, 61].

2.6 Diagnosis of HCC in noncirrhotic liver

About 10% HCC can occur in noncirrhotic liver. Risk factors include alcohol (21%), chronic hepatitis B(30.60%), chronic hepatitis C infection (14.36%), diabetes (40%), family history (13.85%) and cryptogenic (39%). Other risk factors include aflatoxin B, metabolic liver diseases, chemical and industrial carcinogens like vinyl chloride. HCC in noncirrhotic liver present as advanced disease, larger in size [62]. Male to female ratio is 2:1. Hepatomegaly, abdominal pain, malaise, weight loss and anorexia are common presenting features [62, 63]. On ultrasound, lesion can be hypoechoic, hyperechoic due to intralesional fat or mixed echogenicity due to necrosis. On unenhanced CT, lesions appear as hypodense circumscribed masses. Few of them show calcifications, hemorrhagic areas and necrosis. On contrast injection, it does show arterial phase hyperenhancement and washout in delayed phase but specificity is lower as other lesions like hepatocellular adenoma and hypervascular metastasis. On MRI these tumors have variable T1 and T2 weighted images depending on degree of fat, necrosis and fibrosis. On contrast injection, features are similar to CT scan. Liver biopsy is often required for diagnosis [62, 63].

3. Surveillance for hepatocellular carcinoma

Surveillance is defined as periodic application of diagnostic test to individuals who have specific risk factors for disease. Surveillance depends on the incidence of the surveyed disease in the target population, the availability of efficient diagnostic test(s) at bearable costs and acceptability for the target population, and the availability of treatments and their effectiveness if disease is diagnosed early in course of disease. Primary objective of surveillance program is early diagnosis of disease so that curative treatments can be offered to the patients [64].

3.1 Target population for surveillance

While deciding the appropriate population it is necessary to consider incidence of HCC in the population, probability that curative therapies can be offered to the patients who are diagnosed as having the disease and cost effectiveness of surveillance. In case of HCC, application of curative therapies not only depend on extent of tumor but also on underlying liver function. Hence appropriate patients should be enrolled in the surveillance program [3, 24].

3.1.1 Cirrhotic patients

Nearly 90% HCC develop on the background of cirrhosis of liver. The annual incidence of HCC is 2.0–6.6% in patients with cirrhosis [24]. Cost-effectiveness studies in western patients have shown that surveillance for HCC would be beneficial if the incidence is 1.5%/year or greater, irrespective of etiology of cirrhosis [65]. However, advanced cirrhosis with Child score C or Child score B with gross ascites, hepatorenal syndrome, clinical jaundice do not qualify for curative therapies for HCC and do not warrant surveillance unless they are considered for liver transplantation. Child A cirrhotic patients or those decompensated cirrhotic patients who are listed for liver transplant warrant surveillance as diagnosis of HCC modifies the priority and decision to transplant [66–68].

3.1.2 Noncirrhotic patients

HCC can develop in noncirrhotic liver in patients infected with hepatitis B virus. The risk varies with geographical distribution and is higher in Asia and Africa than Western countries. Higher levels of HBV replication, age and gender (males higher than females) are the risk factors for development of HCC which is lower than cirrhotic but definitely higher than general population [69, 70]. In a cohort study of males belonging to multiple race and age-groups, risk of HCC was highest among Asian Pacific Islanders, followed by whites and African Americans. Also, regardless of race, annual incidence of HCC was more than 0.2% for all patients older than 40 years with high levels of alanine aminotransferase [71]. A similar HCC incidence rate of 0.2 per 100 person-years has been observed in inactive carriers with chronic HBV infection from East Asian countries. Asian females >50 years of age and patients with family history of HCC are also at increased risk of HCC. Hence, surveillance should be offered in the above subset of patients as these patients are noncirrhotic with preserved liver function and fit for curative resection for HCC [66, 67]. Patients with chronic hepatitis B on therapy with advanced fibrosis or cirrhosis at baseline should also be enrolled under surveillance program [72, 73]. Various scoring systems are available which can help in stratifying the patients based on risk of HCC and those with significant risk should be offered surveillance [74]. Examples of such scoring systems include GAG-HCC score, LSM-HCC score, PAGE-B score, REACH-B score. REVEAL risk model [74].

Patients with chronic hepatitis C infection with bridging fibrosis are at increased risk of development of HCC. Transition from advanced fibrosis to cirrhosis cannot be accurately determined [75]. Several studies show that liver stiffness assessment performed by transient elastography correlates with risk of development of HCC [76, 77]. Hence these patients warrant surveillance for HCC. Patients with chronic HCV infection previously treated, who have achieved sustained virological response but had advanced fibrosis or cirrhosis need HCC surveillance [74].

Prevalence of nonalcoholic fatty liver disease (NAFLD) is increasing in all part of the world. Nonalcoholic steatohepatitis (NASH) is associated with morbidity and mortality due to cirrhosis and its complications and development of HCC [3]. Similar to cirrhotic patients with other etiologies, patients with NASH cirrhosis should be included in surveillance program. A systematic review and metanalysis of studies on HCC in noncirrhotic NASH subjects showed that these subjects were at greater odds of developing HCC than non-cirrhotic subjects of other etiologies (OR 2.61, 95% CI 1.27–5.35, P = 0.009) [78]. The incidence of HCC in patients with non-advanced fibrosis is expected to be insufficiently high to deserve universal surveillance, given the large prevalence of NAFLD in the general population [79]. American society of gastroenterology clinical practice update on screening and surveillance of HCC in NAFLD suggest to use two noninvasive tests to assess level of fibrosis [79]. Those patients with significant fibrosis on both tests to be enrolled in the screening program. Genetic studies have shown the presence of the PNPLA3 risk allele is increased in those NAFLD with HCC. However limited availability of the test restricts its use in clinical practice [79].

Patients with Wilson's disease, autoimmune liver disease and alpha 1- antitrypsin deficiency have lower risk of developing HCC unless cirrhosis is developed. Hence routine surveillance is not recommended [24].

3.2 Surveillance tests

Surveillance tests should be sensitive, easily available to large population, less costly, safe, acceptable to the people and permits early diagnosis of disease. Surveillance tests used for HCC surveillance can be classified as radiological, serological or combination of both. Section 2.2 and 2.4 describe imaging and tumor markers, their sensitivity, specificity and accuracy.

3.2.1 Radiologic surveillance tests

Ultrasonography (USG) of liver is the most commonly used method for surveillance. It is non-invasive, relatively inexpensive, easily available and without any associated risk of radiation. It has the sensitivity of 84% for any stage HCC and 63% for early-stage HCC [80]. In patients with cirrhosis, USG may have a suboptimal performance due to the presence of fibrous septa and regenerative nodules, which appear as a coarse pattern on ultrasound and may mask the presence of a small tumor. In a meta-analysis, the sensitivity and specificity of USG for detection of HCC at any stage were 84% (95% CI, 76–92%) and 91% (95% CI, 86–94%), respectively, but, the pooled sensitivity of ultrasound was only 47% (95% CI, 33–61%) for detection of early-stage HCC [81]. Hence, it is recommended that USG of liver for HCC surveillance should be done by an expert radiologist. Compared to ultrasonography, computed tomography and MRI had better sensitivity and specificity for diagnosis of early HCC (Refer to Section 2.2 for details). However use of radiation, complex imaging techniques, availability, cost of imaging are the important limiting factors. While comparing 6-monthly USG and yearly triphasic CT for HCC surveillance, it was found that biannual ultrasound was more sensitive (71.4%) when compared to CT (66.7%) with lower overall cost [82].

3.2.2 Serological tests

Serological test for early diagnosis of HCC include AFP, PIVKA II, AFP-L3, alpha fucosidase and glypican. (Refer to Section 2.4). Out of all AFP is most widely studied. In a study evaluating the biomarkers AFP had the best area under the receiver operating characteristic curve (0.80, 95% confidence interval [CI]: 0.77–0.84), followed by des-gamma carboxy-prothrombin (DCP) (0.72, 95% CI: 0.68–0.77) and lectin-bound AFP (AFP-L3%) (0.66, 95% CI: 0.62–0.70) for early-stage HCC and the sensitivity of AFP was 66% [83]. As a serological test alone for surveillance AFP has suboptimal performance however, it may used if ultrasound is not easily available [84, 85]. One problem with use of AFP as surveillance test is that only in 10–20% of early HCC have elevated AFP and on the other hand AFP can be falsely elevated in chronic hepatitis B and C infections [24]. Instead of single biomarker for surveillance combination of multiple biomarkers are being increasingly studied. GALAD, which includes gender, age, lectin-bound AFP % (AFPL3%), AFP, and des-gamma carboxy prothrombin (DCP) studied in a multinational phase II study involving 6,834 patients (2,430 HCC and 4,404 chronic liver disease), achieved sensitivities ranging from 60–80% for early HCC detection. Another panel including AFP, fucosylated kininogen, age, gender, alkaline phosphatase, and alanine aminotransferase demonstrated a c-statistic of 0.97 (95% CI 0.95–0.99) for early HCC detection. A methylated DNA marker panel had a c-statistic of 0.96 (95% CI 0.93–0.99), with a sensitivity exceeding 90%, for early HCC detection in a phase II study. Although these studies appear promising further research is needed in this field [3].

3.2.3 Combination of both

Meta-analysis had shown that combination of AFP and USG to be superior to only USG or AFP alone. Ultrasound with vs. without AFP detected early-stage HCC with 63% sensitivity (95% CI, 48–75%) and 45% sensitivity (95% CI, 30–62%), respectively (P = .002) [86]. The benefit of AFP in addition to ultrasound was consistent across subgroups, including prospective studies, studies conducted in the United States, and studies conducted after the year 2000 [86]. Counter argument to this approach is that, although addition of AFP to USG helps in detection of 6–8% additional tumors does not balance the increase in false positive results resulting due to active inflammation causing raise in AFP levels in absence of HCC, adding to cost of screening without significant benefit [24].

3.3 Surveillance interval

It depends on rate of tumor growth and incidence of cancer in the population [24]. Median doubling time of an HCC lesion is 6.5 months +/− 5.7 months [87]. Analysis of prospectively maintained multi-center Italian database showed a better overall median survival of 40.3 months in the 6-monthly surveillance group, compared to 30 months in the 12-monthly surveillance group (P = 0.03) [88]. Subsequently a French study evaluated impact of shortening of surveillance to 3 months. It showed that 3-months surveillance group had higher incidence of non-malignant lesions, similar number of patients in both 3-months and 6-months group were detected with HCC at an early stage (79% vs. 71%; P = 0.40) and similar proportions received curative therapies (62% vs. 58%; P = 0.88) [89]. Hence it appears that 6 months interval is optimal.

3.4 Benefits of surveillance

Cancer surveillance programs are aimed to detect tumors early so that curative treatments can be provided to patients. Evidence in favor of surveillance programs

	EASL	AASLD	APASL	JSH	INASL
Target population	• Cirrhotic Child A and B • Child C listed for transplant • Noncirrhotic • HBV high risk for HCC • Noncirrhotic F3 fibrosis as per risk	• All cirrhotic patients • HCV cirrhotic post antivirals SVR achieved.	• Cirrhosis any etiology. • Chronic HBV and HCV infection with high risk.	• **Extremely high risk**: Cirrhosis related HBV and HCV • **High risk:** Cirrhosis nonviral, Chronic hepatitis B and C	• Child A and B cirrhotics • Child C cirrhotics on transplant list • High risk noncirrhotic chronic HBV and HCV
Ultrasound	✓	✓	✓	✓	✓
CT/MRI	X	X	X	✓ **In extremely high risk group 6–12 monthly.**	X
AFP	X	✓+/–	✓ Cut-off 200 ng/ml	✓	✓
Other markers	X	X	X	**PVIKA II AFP-L3**	X
Surveillance Interval	6 months	6 months	6 months	**Extremely high risk-** 3–4 monthly. **High risk** – 6 months	6 months

Table 6.
Recommendations, screening tests, screening interval by various societies across the world. (SVR-sustained virological response).

in HCC has remained controversial. One randomized controlled trial supporting HCC surveillance with 6-monthly abdominal ultrasound was performed in more than 18,000 Chinese patients and showed a 37% reduction in mortality risk in screened patients [90]. Other studies are retrospective, observational and has suffered some biases. Lead time which means the given proportion of survival benefit is due to early diagnosis due to surveillance and length time bias arises due to detection of slow growing tumors during surveillance programs where as fast growing tumors become symptomatic early in their course [3]. Surveillance programs can create a state of anxiety in mind of patients. Additional tests and financial burden if screening tests are indeterminate. There is also possibility of overtreatment of tumor which might never become symptomatic [3]. Considering dismal prognosis of HCC, all societies recommend screening of at risk patients for HCC [24, 33, 91–93].

3.5 Summary of recommendations by various societies

Table 6 summarizes recommendations, screening tests, screening interval by various societies across the world [24, 33, 91–93].

4. Role of multidisciplinary team in surveillance and diagnosis of HCC

Optimal care of patients with HCC involves specialists from multiple disciplines like gastroenterology/hepatology, surgical oncologist, liver transplant team, medical oncologist, radiologist, interventional radiologist, primary care physician, radiation oncologist, pathologists, palliative care specialist, nursing staff and dieticians. Multidisciplinary teams (MDTs) have evolved to facilitate care coordination, reassessments of clinical course, and fine changes in treatment plans required for these complex group of patients. MDTs provide platform to facilitate prompt diagnosis of HCC by reviewing patients imaging, tumor markers and also assessing the need for biopsy which is associated with complications like bleeding and needle track seeding. As mentioned in previous sections, diagnosis of HCC is primarily based on imaging and there are restricted indications for biopsy of lesion. Experts in MDTs can also play a role in suggesting next investigation if one of the diagnostic investigation is inconclusive [94].

5. Conclusion

To conclude, small HCC rarely become symptomatic. HCC can be a cause for new onset decompensation. Diagnosis of HCC requires multiphase computed tomography or MRI scan. In cirrhotic liver, diagnosis of HCC is based on typical imaging features and rarely needs biopsy. In noncirrhotic liver and vascular liver diseases biopsy may be required to confirm diagnosis. Contrast enhanced ultrasound and MRI with hepatobiliary contrast agents are promising modalities for evaluation of small and indeterminate nodules. Tumor markers play adjunct role in diagnosis but has prognostic significance. Pathologically HCC is heterogenous tumor with multiple subtypes with distinct molecular signatures. HCC surveillance in high risk groups with biannual ultrasound with or without alfa-fetoprotein helps in early detection of lesions which are amenable to curative treatment. Multidisciplinary teams provide platform for care coordination, reassessments of clinical course, and fine changes in treatment plans required for this complex group of patients.

Conflict of interest

The author declare no conflict of interest.

Author details

Aditya Kale
Department of Gastroenterology, Seth G. S. Medical College and KEM Hospital, Mumbai, India

*Address all correspondence to: adityapkale@yahoo.com

References

[1] Wang H, Naghavi M, Allen C, Barber RM, Bhutta ZA, et al. Mortality and Causes of Death Collaborators. Global, regional, and national life expectancy, allcause mortality, and cause-specific mortality for 249 causes of death, 1980-2015: a systematic analysis for the Global Burden of Disease Study 2015. Lancet 2016; 388:1459-1544.

[2] Akinyemiju T, Abera S, Ahmed M, Alam N, Alemayohu MA, et al. The burden of primary liver cancer and underlying etiologies from 1990 to 2015 at the global, regional, and national level: results from the global burden of disease study 2015. JAMA Oncol 2017;3:1683-1691

[3] Singal A, Lampertico P, Nahon P. Epidemiology and surveillance for hepatocellular carcinoma:New trends. Journal of Hepatology 2020 vol. 72 j 250-261.

[4] Bartlett D, Carr B, Marsh J. Cancer of the liver. In: DeVita J, Vincent T, Hellman S, Rosenberg S, editors. Cancer: Principles & practice of oncology. 7th ed. Philadelphia: Lippincott Williams & Wilkins; 2005. p. 986-1008.

[5] Aljumah AA, Kuriry H, Alzunaitan M, Al Ghobain M, Al Muaikeel M, Al Olayan A, et al. Clinical Presentation, Risk Factors, and Treatment Modalities of Hepatocellular Carcinoma: A Single Tertiary Care Center Experience. Gastroenterol Res Pract. 2016;2016.

[6] Charach L, Zusmanovitch L, Gideon C. Hepatocellular Carcinoma. Part 2: Clinical Presentation and Diagnosis. Eur Med J. 2017;5(1):81-88.

[7] Kumar R, Saraswat MK, Sharma BC, Sakhuja P, Sarin SK. Characteristics of hepatocellular carcinoma in India: a retrospective analysis of 191 cases. QJM: An International Journal of Medicine, Volume 101, Issue 6, June 2008, Pages 479-485.

[8] Eric C. H. Lai, W. Y. Lau. Spontaneous Rupture of Hepatocellular Carcinoma A Systematic Review. Arch Surg. 2006;141(2):191-198

[9] Bisceglie AMD, Befeler AS. Chapter 96. Hepatic Tumors and Cysts. Section IX Liver, Slesinger and Fordtran Text book of Gastroenterology. Elsevier 2016, Page no 1604-1627.

[10] Jeong YY, Yim NY, Kang HK. Hepatocellular Carcinoma in the Cirrhotic Liver with Helical CT and MRI: Imaging Spectrum and Pitfalls of Cirrhosis-Related Nodules. AJR 2005;185:1024-1032.

[11] Chernyak V, Fowler KJ, Kamaya A, Kielar AZ, Elsayes KM, Mustafa R. Bashir MR, et al. Liver Imaging Reporting and Data System (LI-RADS) Version 2018: Imaging of Hepatocellular Carcinoma in At-Risk Patients. Radiology 2018; 289:816-830.

[12] Roberts L, Sirlin CB, Zaiem F, Almasri J, Prokop LJ, Heimbach JK et al. Imaging for the Diagnosis of Hepatocellular Carcinoma: A Systematic Review and Meta-analysis. HEPATOLOGY, VOL. 67, NO. 1, 2018.

[13] Chanyaputhipong J, Su-Chong Albert Low, Chow PKH. Gadoxetate Acid-Enhanced MR Imaging for HCC: A Review for Clinicians. International Journal of Hepatology. Volume 2011, Article ID 489342, 13 pages. doi:10.4061/2011/489342.

[14] Di Martino M, De Filippis G, De Santis A, Geiger D, Del Monte M, Lombardo CV, et al. Hepatocellular carcinoma in cirrhotic patients: prospective comparison of US, CT and

MR imaging. Eur Radiol 2013;23:887-896.

[15] Phongkitkarun S, Limsamutpetch K, Tannaphai P, Jatchavala J. Added value of hepatobiliary phase gadoxetic acid-enhanced MRI for diagnosing hepatocellular carcinoma in high-risk patients. World J Gastroenterol 2013;19:8357.

[16] Kim H-D, Lim Y-S, Han S, An J, Kim G-A, Kim SY, et al. Evaluation of early-stage hepatocellular carcinoma by magnetic resonance imaging with gadoxetic acid detects additional lesions and increases overall survival. Gastroenterology 2015;148:1371-1382.

[17] Joo I, Lee JM. Recent advances in the imaging diagnosis of hepatocellular carcinoma: value of gadoxetic acid-enhanced MRI. Liver Cancer 2016;5:67-87.

[18] Forner A, Vilana R, Ayuso C, Bianchi L, Solé M, Ayuso JR, et al. Diagnosis of hepatic nodules 20 mm or smaller in cirrhosis: Prospective validation of the noninvasive diagnostic criteria for hepatocellular carcinoma. Hepatology 2008;47:97-104.

[19] Aubé C, Oberti F, Lonjon J, Pageaux G, Seror O, N'Kontchou G, et al. EASL and AASLD recommendations for the diagnosis of HCC to the test of daily practice. Liver Int 2017;37: 1515-1525.

[20] Chotipanich C, Kunawudhi A, Promteangtrong C, Tungsuppawattanakit P, Sricharunrat T, Wongsa P. Diagnosis of hepatocellular carcinoma using C11 CHOLINE PET/CT: comparison with F18 FDG, contrast enhanced MRI and MDCT. Asian Pac J Cancer Prev 2016;17:3569-3573.

[21] Lin C, Liao C, Chu L, Yen K, Jeng L, Hsu C, et al. Predictive value of 18FFDG PET/CT for vascular invasion in patients with hepatocellular carcinoma before liver transplantation. Clin Nucl Med 2017;42:e183–e187.

[22] Faccia M, Ainora ME, Ponziani FR, Riccardi L, Garcovich M, Gasbarrini M et al. Portal vein thrombosis in cirrhosis: Why a well-known complication is still matter of debate. World J Gastroenterol. Aug 21, 2019; 25(31): 4437-4451.

[23] Tublin ME, Dodd GD, Baron RL. Benign and Malignant Portal Vein Thrombosis: Differentiation by CT Characteristics. AJR:168, March 1997.

[24] Galle PR, Forner A, Llovet JM, Mazzaferro V, Piscaglia F, Raoul JL et al. EASL Clinical Practice Guidelines: Management of hepatocellular carcinoma. Journal of Hepatology 2018 vol. xxx j xxx–xxx.

[25] Bisceglie AMD, Befeler AS. Chapter 96. Hepatic Tumors and Cysts. Slesinger and Fordtran Text book of Gastroenterology Chapter 96, Hepatic tumours and cysts. Section IX Liver Page no 1604-1627.

[26] Di Tommaso L, Franchi G, Park YN, Fiamengo B, Destro A, Morenghi E et al. Diagnostic value of HSP70, Glypican 3, and Glutamine Synthetase in hepatocellular nodules in cirrhosis. Hepatology 2007;45:725-734.

[27] Tremosini S, Forner A, Boix L, Vilana R, Bianchi L, Reig M, et al. Prospective validation of an immunohistochemical panel (glypican 3, heat shock protein 70 and glutamine synthetase) in liver biopsies for diagnosis of very early hepatocellular carcinoma. Gut 2012;61:1481-1487.

[28] Choi WT, Kakar S. Immunohistochemistry in the Diagnosis of Hepatocellular Carcinoma. Gastroenterol Clin N Am 46 (2017) 311-325.

[29] Torbenson MS, Ng IOL, Park YN, Roncalli M, Sakamoto M. Hepatocellular

carcinoma. In: WHO Classification of Tumours Editorial Board, editor. Digestive system tumours. WHO classification of tumours series. 5th ed. Lyon: International Agency for Research on Cancer; 2019; 229-239.

[30] Kim H, Jang M, Park YN. Histopathological Variants of Hepatocellular Carcinomas: an Update According to the 5th Edition of the WHO Classification of Digestive System Tumors. J Liver Cancer 2020; 20(1):17-24.

[31] Rockey DC, Caldwell SH, Goodman ZD, Nelson RC, Smith AD. American Association for the Study of Liver Diseases. Liver biopsy. Hepatology 2009;49:1017-1044.

[32] Silva MA, Hegab B, Hyde C, Guo B, Buckels JAC, Mirza DF. Needle track seeding following biopsy of liver lesions in the diagnosis of hepatocellular cancer: a systematic review and meta-analysis. Gut 2008;57:1592-1596.

[33] Kumar A, Acharya SK, Singh SP, Arora A, Dhiman RK, Aggarwal R et al. 2019 Update of Indian National Association for Study of the Liver Consensus on Prevention, Diagnosis, and Management of Hepatocellular Carcinoma in India: The Puri II Recommendations. Journal of Clinical and Experimental Hepatology January–February 2020, Vol. 10, No. 1,43-80.

[34] Zacharakis G, Aleid A, Aldossari KA. New and old biomarkers of hepatocellular carcinoma. Hepatoma Res 2018;4:65.

[35] Zhou L, Liu J, Luo F. Serum tumor markers for detection of hepatocellular carcinoma. World J Gastroenterol 2006 February 28; 12(8):1175-1181.

[36] Chang TS, Wu YC, Tung SY, Wei KL, Hsieh YY, Huang HC et al. Alpha-Fetoprotein Measurement Benefits Hepatocellular Carcinoma Surveillance in Patients with Cirrhosis. Am J Gastroentero April 2015.

[37] Cui R, Wang B, Ding H, Shen H, Li Y, Chen X. Usefulness of determining a protein induced by vitamin K absence in detection of hepatocellular carcinoma. Chin Med J (Engl) 2002; 115:42-45.

[38] Marrero JA, Su GL, Wei W, Emick D, Conjeevaram HS, Fontana RJ, Lok AS. Des-gamma carboxyprothrombin can differentiate hepatocellular carcinoma from nonmalignant chronic liver disease in american patients. Hepatology 2003; 37:1114-1121.

[39] Marrero JA, Feng Z, Wang Y, Nguyen MH, Befeler AS, Roberts LR, Reddy KR, Harnois D, Llovet JM, Normolle D, Dalhgren J, Chia D, Lok AS, Wagner PD, Srivastava S, Schwartz M. Alpha-fetoprotein, des-gamma carboxyprothrombin, and lectin-bound alpha-fetoprotein in early hepatocellular carcinoma. Gastroenterology 2009;137:110-118.

[40] Lok AS, Sterling RK, Everhart JE, Wright EC, Hoefs JC, et al. Des-gamma-carboxy prothrombin and alpha-fetoprotein as biomarkers for the early detection of hepatocellular carcinoma. Gastroenterology 2010;138:493-502.

[41] Kudo M, Izumi N, Kokudo N, et al. Management of hepatocellular carcinoma in Japan: Consensus-Based Clinical Practice Guidelines proposed by the Japan Society of Hepatology (JSH) 2010 updated version. Dig Dis Basel Switz. 2011;29(3):339-364. doi:10.1159/000327577.

[42] Hao Q-Q, Chen G-Y, Zhang J-H, Sheng J-H, Gao Y. Diagnostic value of long noncoding RNAs for hepatocellular carcinoma: A PRISMA-compliant metaanalysis. Medicine (Baltimore). 2017;96(28):e7496. doi:10.1097/MD.0000000000007496.

[43] Cui R, He J, Zhang F, Wang B, Ding H, Shen H, Li Y, Chen X. Diagnostic value of protein induced by vitamin K absence (PIVKAII) and hepatoma-specific band of serum gammaglutamyl transferase (GGTII) as hepatocellular carcinoma markers complementary to alpha-fetoprotein. Br J Cancer 2003; 88: 1878-1882.

[44] Ishizuka H, Nakayama T, Matsuoka S, Gotoh I, Ogawa M, Suzuki K, et al. Prediction of the development of hepato-cellular-carcinoma in patients with liver cirrhosis by the serial determinations of serum alpha-L-fucosidase activity. Intern Med 1999; 38: 927-931.

[45] Minata M, Nishida N, Komeda T, Azechi H, Katsuma H, Nishimura T, et al. Postoperative detection of alpha-fetoprotein mRNA in blood as a predictor for metastatic recurrence of hepatocellular carcinoma. J Gastroenterol Hepatol 2001; 16:445-451.

[46] Yang SZ, Dong JH, Li K, Zhang Y, Zhu J. Detection of AFPm-RNA and melanoma antigen gene-1mRNA as markers of disseminated hepatocellular carcinoma cells in blood. Hepatobiliary Pancreat Dis Int 2005; 4: 227-233.

[47] Miura N, Maeda Y, Kanbe T, Yazama H, Takeda Y, Sato R et al. Serum human telomerase reverse transcriptase messenger RNA as a novel tumor marker for hepatocellular carcinoma. Clin Cancer Res 2005; 11: 3205-3209.

[48] Miura N, Shiota G, Nakagawa T, Maeda Y, Sano A, Marumoto A, et al Sensitive detection of human telomerase reverse transcriptase mRNA in the serum of patients with hepatocellular carcinoma. Oncology 2003; 64: 430-434.

[49] Kim SJ, Choi IK, Park KH, Yoon SY, Oh SC, Seo JH, et al. Serum vascular endothelial growth factor per platelet count in hepatocellular carcinoma: correlations with clinical parameters and survival. Jpn J Clin Oncol 2004; 34: 184-190.

[50] Ren Y, Poon RT, Tsui HT, Chen WH, Li Z, Lau C, et al. Interleukin-8 serum levels in patients with hepatocellular carcinoma: correlations with clinicopathological features and prognosis. Clin Cancer Res 2003; 9: 5996-6001.

[51] Song BC, Chung YH, Kim JA, Choi WB, Suh DD, Pyo SI, et al. Transforming growth factorbeta1 as a useful serologic marker of small hepatocellular carcinoma. Cancer 2002; 94: 175-180.

[52] Pan L, Lei JI, Pan BI, Kong FL, Lin M, Liu SQ, et al. Significance of detection of 3 serum tumor markers in the diagnosis of primary hepatocellular carcinoma. Zhongguo Zhongliu Linchuang Yu Kangfu 2004; 11: 401-402.

[53] El-Serag HB, Davila JA. Is fibrolamellar carcinoma different from hepatocellular carcinoma? A U.S. population-based study. Hepatology 2004; 39:798-803.

[54] Vivekanandan P, Micchelli ST, Torbenson M. Anterior gradient-2 is overexpressed by fibrolamellar carcinomas. Hum Pathol 2009; 40:293-299

[55] Zenali MJ, Tan D, Li W, Dhingra S, Brown RE. Stemness characteristics of fibrolamellar hepatocellular carcinoma: immunohistochemical analysis with comparisons to conventional hepatocellular carcinoma. Ann Clin Lab Sci 2010; 40:126-134

[56] Kakar S, Chen X, Ho C, et al. Chromosomal changes in fibrolamellar hepatocellular carcinoma detected by array comparative genomic hybridization. Mod Pathol 2009; 22:134-141

[57] Berman MA, Burnham JA, Sheahan DG. Fibrolamellar carcinoma of the liver: an immunohistochemical study of nineteen cases and a review of the literature. Hum Pathol 1988; 19:784-794.

[58] Ichikawa T, Federle MP, Grazioli L, Madariaga J, Nalesnik M, Marsh W. Fibrolamellar hepatocellular carcinoma: imaging and pathologic findings in 31 recent cases. Radiology 1999; 213: 352-361.

[59] Ward SC, Waxman S. Fibrolamellar carcinoma: a review with focus on genetics and comparison to other malignant primary liver tumors. Semin Liver Dis 2011; 31:61-70.

[60] Ganeshan D, Szklaruk J, Kundra V, Kaseb A, Rashid A, et al. Imaging Features of Fibrolamellar Hepatocellular Carcinoma. AJR 2014; 202:544-552.

[61] Mavros MN, Mayo SC, Hyder O, Pawlik TM. A systematic review: treatment and prognosis of patients with fibrolamellar hepatocellular carcinoma. J Am Coll Surg 2012; 215:820-830.

[62] Desai A, Sandhu S, Jin-Ping Lai, Sandhu DS. Hepatocellular carcinoma in non-cirrhotic liver: A comprehensive review. World J Hepatol 2019 January 27; 11(1): 1-18.

[63] Gaddikeri S, McNeeley MF, Wang CL, Bhargava P, Dighe MK, Yeh MMC, et al Hepatocellular Carcinoma in the Noncirrhotic Liver. AJR 2014; 203:W34–W47.

[64] Prorok PC. Epidemiologic approach for cancer screening. Problems in design and analysis of trials. Am J Pediatr Hematol Oncol 1992;14:117-128.

[65] Sarasin FP, Giostra E, Hadengue A. Cost-effectiveness of screening for detection of small hepatocellular carcinoma in western patients with Child-Pugh class A cirrhosis. Am J Med 1996;101:422-434.

[66] Sherman M, Furlan A, Marin D, Agnello F, Martino Di M, Marco Di V, et al. Surveillance for hepatocellular carcinoma. Best Pract Res Clin Gastroenterol 2014;28:783-793.

[67] Díaz-González Á, Forner A. Surveillance for hepatocellular carcinoma. Best Pract Res Clin Gastroenterol 2016;30:1001-1010.

[68] Trevisani F, Santi V, Gramenzi A, Di Nolfo MA, Del Poggio P, Benvegnù L, et al. Surveillance for early diagnosis of hepatocellular carcinoma: is it effective in intermediate/advanced cirrhosis? Am J Gastroenterol 2007;102:2448-2457.

[69] Chen CJ, Yang HI, Iloeje UH. Hepatitis B virus DNA levels and outcomes in chronic hepatitis B. Hepatology 2009;49:S72–S84.

[70] Yang HI, Yuen MF, Chan HL, Han KH, Chen PJ, Kim DY, et al. Risk estimation for hepatocellular carcinoma in chronic hepatitis B (REACH B): development and validation of a predictive score. Lancet Oncol 2011;12:568-574.

[71] Mittal S, Kramer JR, Omino R, Chayanupatkul M, Richardson PA, El-Serag HB, Kanwal F. Role of Age and Race in the Risk of Hepatocellular Carcinoma in Veterans With Hepatitis B Virus Infection. Clin Gastroenterol Hepatol. 2018 Feb;16(2):252-259.

[72] Wong GL-H, Chan HL-Y, Chan H-Y, Tse PC-H, Tse Y-K, Mak CW-H, et al. Accuracy of risk scores for patients with chronic hepatitis B receiving entecavir treatment. Gastroenterology 2013;144:933-944.

[73] Sung JJY, Tsoi KKF, Wong VWS, Li KCT, Chan HLY. Meta-analysis: treatment of hepatitis B infection reduces risk of hepatocellular

carcinoma. Aliment Pharmacol Ther 2008;28:1067-1077.

[74] Wong V, Janssen HLA. Can we use HCC risk scores to individualize surveillance in chronic hepatitis B infection? Journal of Hepatology 2015 vol. 63 j 722-732.

[75] Lok AS, Seeff LB, Morgan TR, di Bisceglie AM, Sterling RK, Curto TM, et al. Incidence of hepatocellular carcinoma and associated risk factors in hepatitis C-related advanced liver disease. Gastroenterology 2009;136:138-148.

[76] Masuzaki R, Tateishi R, Yoshida H, Goto E, Sato T, Ohki T, et al. Prospective risk assessment for hepatocellular carcinoma development in patients with chronic hepatitis C by transient elastography. Hepatology 2009;49:1954-1961.

[77] Singh S, Fujii LL, Murad MH, Wang Z, Asrani SK, Ehman RL, et al. Liver stiffness is associated with risk of decompensation, liver cancer, and death in patients with chronic liver diseases: a systematic review and meta-analysis. Clin Gastroenterol Hepatol 2013;11:1573-84-2-9.

[78] Stine JG, Wentworth BJ, Zimmet A, Rinella ME, Loomba R, Caldwell SH, Argo CK. Systematic review with meta-analysis: risk of hepatocellular carcinoma in non-alcoholic steatohepatitis without cirrhosis compared to other liver diseases. Aliment Pharmacol Ther. 2018 Oct;48(7):696-703.

[79] Loomba R, Lim JK, Patton H, El-Serag HB. AGA Clinical Practice Update on Screening and Surveillance for Hepatocellular Carcinoma in Patients With Nonalcoholic Fatty Liver Disease: Expert Review. Gastroenterology 2020;158:1822-1183.

[80] Zhang B, Yang B. Combined alpha fetoprotein testing and ultrasonography as a screening test for primary liver cancer. J Med Screen. 1999;6(2):108-110.

[81] Tzartzeva K, Obi J, Rich NE, Parikh ND, Marrero JA, Yopp A, Waljee AK, Singal AG. Surveillance Imaging and Alpha Fetoprotein for Early Detection of Hepatocellular Carcinoma in Patients With Cirrhosis: A Meta-analysis. Gastroenterology. 2018 May;154(6):1706-1718.e1.

[82] Pocha C, Dieperink E, McMaken KA, Knott A, Thuras P, Ho SB. Surveillance for hepatocellular cancer with ultrasonography vs. computed tomography -- a randomised study. Aliment Pharmacol Ther. 2013 Aug;38(3):303-312.

[83] Marrero JA, Feng Z, Wang Y, Nguyen MH, Befeler AS, Roberts LR, et al. Alpha-fetoprotein, des-gamma carboxyprothrombin, and lectin-bound alpha-fetoprotein in early hepatocellular carcinoma. Gastroenterology. 2009 Jul;137(1):110-8.46

[84] Chen JG, Parkin DM, Chen QG, Lu JH, Shen QJ, Zhang BC, et al. Screening for liver cancer: results of a randomised controlled trial in Qidong, China. J Med Screen 2003;10:204-209.

[85] McMahon BJ, Holck P, Bulkow L, Snowball M. Serologic and clinical outcomes of 1536 Alaska Natives chronically infected with hepatitis B virus. Ann Intern Med 2001;135:759-768.

[86] Tzartzeva K, Obi J, Rich NE, Parikh ND, Marrero JA, Yopp A, et al. Surveillance Imaging and Alpha Fetoprotein for Early Detection of Hepatocellular Carcinoma in Patients With Cirrhosis: A Meta-analysis. Gastroenterology. 2018 May; 154(6): 1706-1718.e1.

[87] Ebara M, Hatano R, Fukuda H, Yoshikawa M, Sugiura N, Saisho H. Natural course of small hepatocellular

carcinoma with underlying cirrhosis. A study of 30 patients. Hepatogastroenterology. 1998 Aug;45 Suppl 3:1214-20.

[88] Santi V, Trevisani F, Gramenzi A, Grignaschi A, Mirici-Cappa F, Del Poggio P, et al; Italian Liver Cancer (ITA.LI.CA) Group. Semiannual surveillance is superior to annual surveillance for the detection of early hepatocellular carcinoma and patient survival. J Hepatol. 2010 Aug;53(2):291-297.

[89] Santi V, Trevisani F, Gramenzi A, Grignaschi A, Mirici-Cappa F, Del Poggio P, et al; Italian Liver Cancer (ITA. LI.CA) Group. Semiannual surveillance is superior to annual surveillance for the detection of early hepatocellular carcinoma and patient survival. J Hepatol. 2010 Aug;53(2):291-297.

[90] Zhang BH, Yang BH, Tang ZY. Randomized controlled trial of screening for hepatocellular carcinoma. J Cancer Res Clin Oncol 2004;130:417-422.

[91] Heimbach JK, Kulik LM, Finn RS, Sirlin CB, Abecassis MM, Roberts LR, et al. AASLD Guidelines for the Treatment of Hepatocellular Carcinoma. Hepatology, VOL. 67, NO. 1, 2018.

[92] Omata M, Cheng AL, Kokudo N, Kudo M, Lee JM, Jia J, Tateishi R et al.Asia–Pacific clinical practice guidelines on the management of hepatocellular carcinoma: a 2017 update. Hepatol Int (2017) 11:317-370.

[93] Kokudo N, Takemura N, Hasegawa K, Takayama T, Kubo S, Shimada M et al. Clinical practice guidelines for hepatocellular carcinoma: The Japan Society of Hepatology 2017 (4th JSH-HCC guidelines) 2019 update. Hepatology Research 2019.

[94] Siddique O, Yoo ER, Perumpail RP, Perumpail BJ, Liu A, Cholankeril G. et al. The importance of a multidisciplinary approach to hepatocellular carcinoma. J Multidiscip Healthc. 2017; 10: 95-100.

Chapter 5

Circulating Biomarkers for Early Diagnosis of Hepatocellular Carcinoma

Hoang Van Tong, Pham Van Dung,
Nguyen Thi Mong Diep and Nguyen Linh Toan

Abstract

Hepatocellular carcinoma (HCC) is one of the most common malignant tumors, which is also often fatal. An early and accurate diagnosis is a decisive step towards the survival of the patients. Molecular biology improved significantly the prognosis of liver cancers through learned use of tumor markers like proteantigens, cytokines, enzymes, isoenzymes, circulating RNAs, gene mutations and methylations. Nevertheless, much improvement is still achievable and needed in this area, which is crucial in order to make an early diagnosis and monitor the progression of the disease. We present in this review what we believe to be the most relevant data regarding tissue and serum biomarkers related to HCC.

Keywords: Biomarkers, Hepatocellular Carcinoma, Diagnosis, Liver Cancer

1. Introduction

Hepatocellular carcinoma (HCC) is the fifth most common cancer in males, the seventh in females, and the third leading cause of cancer-related deaths. Each year there are approximately 800,000 fatalities [1–3]. In developing countries, morbidity and mortality rates are 84% and 83%, respectively [4]. HCC typically occurs in the context of chronic hepatitis B virus (HBV) or hepatitis C virus (HCV) infection, accounting for 85% of all HCC cases globally [3]. Lower risk factors include non-alcoholic fatty liver disease (NAFLD) and chronic alcohol consumption [4].

Tumor evolution is a complex process implying many stages and involving many factors, such as genetic and chromosomal changes. During tumor development, the number, type, extent, and distribution of markers and variants are closely related to the occurrence, progression, invasion, and metastasis of HCC. Therefore, diagnosis and early detection are highly important in management and treatment because it is only possible to cure the disease when the tumor when it is detected at a small size.

Advances in the understanding of tumor biology, combined with the development of molecular methods in looking for new biomarkers in the early detection of the disease, their invasiveness, likelihood of metastasis and recurrence, has led to the discovery and use of several new markers in this disease. In this review, we discuss the results of the studies that we consider the most relevant, and in particular their diagnostic performance for the detection of HCC at an early stage.

IntechOpen

2. Embryonic antigen

2.1 Alpha-fetoprotein (AFP)

Alpha-fetoprotein (AFP) is a large serum glycoprotein that is synthesized in the liver that occurs during fetal life is repressed during adulthood [5]. Therefore, AFP levels often diminish rapidly after birth and remain low throughout adulthood. Since AFP was discovered in the serum of HCC patients in 1964 [6], it has been regarded as the most useful serum protein for patients at risk for HCC [7–9]. However, the sensitivity and specificity of using AFP for early HCC detection are widely variable as elevated AFP levels are also observed in many other cancers [10]. In addition, AFP levels are below the detection limit in small liver tumors, while it can be above the detection limit when the tumor is large, producing an AFP-negative HCC. AFP is considered to have a screening role in HCC but its role is limited since it does not allow to distinguish between cancerous lesions and some other benign liver damage pathologies, hence causing a high proportion of false positives and false negatives. Patients with hepatitis still have high AFP level even without liver tumors. The positive predictive value of AFP for detecting HCC is 70% for people with hepatitis viruses and 94% for those without. Therefore, AFP is more effective in detecting HCC in cases without hepatitis viruses.

According to the 2010 recommendations of the American Association for the Study of Liver Diseases (AASLD) for the diagnosis and treatment of HCC, the effectiveness of AFP as a test to diagnose HCC was lower than expected. AFP is also increased in biliary carcinoma in the liver or metastases from colon cancer. Biliary cancer in the liver is also quite common in cirrhotic patients, although the incidence of this disease is lower than that of HCC. The fact that these two liver cancers are common in cirrhosis makes it necessary to identify accurately the disease. Because AFP may increase in many cases other than HCC, it is no longer recommended to be used in Europe and the Americas for its diagnosis. The current diagnosis of HCC is based on imaging and histopathology [11]. The Asia Pacific Association for the Study of the Liver (APASL) also stated that AFP alone is not recommended to diagnose HCC. When combined with other methods, the diagnosis threshold of AFP was 200 ng/ml (**Table 1**) [12].

2.2 AFP heterogeneity

AFP exists as three glycoforms, each of them having a different binding capability to lectin *Lens culinaris* agglutinin (LCA): AFP-L1 (non-binding fraction), AFP-L2 (weak binding fraction), and AFP-L3 (binding fraction). AFP-L1 is increased in early stages of liver disease progression, AFP-L2 has an intermediate affinity for lectin and is a major component during pregnancy because it is derived from the yolk sacs. AFP-L3 is only elevated in patients with HCC because it is solely produced by cancer cells, making it a specific biomarker for HCC [13, 14]. However, the drawback of AFP-L3 is that it can only be detected if AFP levels are >20 ng/ml.

AFP-L3 immunoassay sensitivity has been further improved by higher sensitivity analytical methods and advanced microfluidics-based separation science [15]. "Highly sensitive AFP-L3" (hs-AFP-L3) obtained significantly better results than conventional AFP-L3, even when patients had a single and/or small HCC tumor. The sensitivity and specificity of hs-AFP-L3 were 57% and 63.5%, and 40.4% and 81.1% for conventional AFP-L3 [16]. These results make hs-AFP-L3 a valuable biomarker for detecting early-stage HCC (**Table 1**).

Marker	Cut-off value	Sensitivity (%)	Specificity (%)	Reference
AFP	>200 ng/ml	39–45	76–94	ADSSL
AFP-L3	AFP-L3/AFP > 15	55.3	93.9	Taketa [1]
GP73	85,5 mg/l	80	82	Schewegle [2]
GPC3	n.a.	55.2	84.2	Jia [3]
OPN	n.a.	86	86	Wan [4]
SCCA	n.a.	84.2	48.9	Gianneli [5]
DCP	+ AFP	72.7 74.2	90 87.2	Carr et al. [6] Bertino [7]
GGT	5,5 IU/ml	86	n.a.	Yao et al. [8]
hsGGT	n.a.	74	n.a.	Cui et al. [9]
AFU	n.a.	81.5	85.4	Wang et al. [10]
TGF-β1	800 pg./ml	95	n.a.	Song et al. [11]
TGF-β1 mRNA	> 1,2 μg/l	89.5	94	Dong et al. [12]
TSGF	62 IU/ml	82	n.a.	Yin et al. [13]
IGF-II	4,1 mg/l	63	90	Tsai et al. [14]
HGF	>1 ng/ml	100	n.a.	Vejchapipat et al. [15]

Abbreviation: *n.a.: not applicable; AFP, alpha-fetoprotein; GP73, Golgi protein 73; GPC3, Glypican-3; OPN, Osteopontin; SCCA, squamous cell carcinoma antigen; DCP, Des-γ-carboxyprothrombin; GGT, Gamma-glutamyltransferase; AFU, Alpha L fucosidase; TGF-β1, Transforming growth factor-β; IGF-II, insulin-like growth factor-II; HGF, Hepatocyte growth factor.*

Table 1.
Diagnostic performance of biomarkers for HCC.

3. Proteantigen

3.1 Glypican-3 (GPC3)

Glypican-3 (GPC3) is a member of the glycican family of heparan sulfate proteoglycans linked to cell membranes by glycosyl-phosphatidylinositol [17]. It is a fetal glycoprotein that exists on the cell surface to help regulate cell growth during pregnancy. GPC3 is associated with the malignant proliferation of cells but there are currently no studies to prove its association with healthy people and benign conditions. Quite a number of studies have proven the overexpression of GPC3 in malignant diseases such as breast cancer, ovarian cancer, or lung adenocarcinoma [18, 19]. With HCC, its expression is increased through the autocrine/paracrine regulator in conjunction with the Wnt signaling pathway [20]. Some studies have concluded that the sensitivity of GPC3 in HCC diagnosis ranges from 40 to 53%, which is interesting considering that in about 33% of cases, both AFP and DCP serum were within normal limits [21, 22]. GPC3 has been detected in HCC tumor but not in benign liver tissues, so it is likely a marker for early detection of HCC [23]. GPC3 expression does not depend on some clinical features such as tumor size, GPC3 sensitivity in early HCC diagnosis (size <3 cm) was 56% [23]. In a meta-analysis, the sensitivity and specificity of serum GPC3 to diagnose HCC were 55.2% and 84.2%, respectively [24]. A smaller analysis of the early-stage HCC group (BCLC 0 and A or TNM phase I) showed a sensitivity and specificity of GPC3 of 55.1% and 97%, respectively, which are higher than the those obtained with the AFP serum in the same study, that were 34.7% and 87.6%. Combining GPC3 and AFP increased the sensitivity to 76% for early-stage tumors [24]. In short, GPC3 might be a marker for HCC, especially in the early stages, but GPC3 expression also increases in some other malignancies, so the specificity for HCC diagnosis is not high. It can still increase diagnostic sensitivity when combined with other valuable serum markers (**Table 1**).

3.2 Heat shock protein 70 (HSP70)

Heat shock protein (HSP) is an antiapoptotic protein whose overexpression allows cell survival. It protects cells and stimulates the reparation of tissue damage. A study indicated the positive rate of HSP70 and HSP27 in HCC tissues at 56.3% and 61.9%, respectively [25]. There was a correlation between the stained intensity of HSP70 and tumor size, portal vein invasion, and tumor stage, while HSP27 was only associated with hepatitis B virus (HBV) related HCC. In addition, the overexpression of HSP70 and HSP27 in HCC tumors may lead to increased tumor growth and metastasis (**Table 1**) [26].

Data suggest that HSP70 can be used as a prognosis indicator for HCC. Its expression was detected in 282 of 392 HCC cases (71.9%), compared to 14 of 115 non-neoplastic liver tissues [27]. The sensitivity and specificity in the detection of HCC have been measured at 57.5% and 85%, respectively [28]. The expression of HSP70 is also correlated with the differentiation and apoptosis of tumor cells. HSP70 promotes cancer cell growth by stabilizing cyclin D1 and suppressing apoptosis in cancer cells by inhibiting the p53 pathway [29, 30]. This information makes HSP70 and HSP27 potential markers of HCC that should be further investigated.

3.3 Golgi protein 73 (GP73)

Golgi protein 73 (GP73) is a type II Golgi-specific membrane protein, which is normally expressed in epithelial cells of many human tissue types, but not hepatocytes [31]. A study showed that serum GP73 levels of patients with HBV-related HCC were significantly increased compared to patients with HBV and healthy adults [32, 33]. The sensitivity of diagnosis of HCC (76.9%) was significantly higher than that of AFP (48.6%), suggesting that GP73 can be an effective serum biomarker for the diagnosis of HCC [34]. The combination of GP73 and AFP further increased the sensitivity and specificity to 89.2% and 85.2%, respectively, with an AUC of 0.96 (**Table 1**).

FC-GP73 further improves the HCC diagnostic performance made with GP73 from 65 to 90 to 90–100%, respectively. Even when GP73 is at a very low level or absent, FC-GP73 is still detectable [35]. These are encouraging data but there is still a lot of work to be done regarding the correlation between GP73 and tumor size, stage, recurrence, and prognosis before this marker can be used.

3.4 Squamous cell carcinoma antigen (SCCA)

Squamous cell carcinoma antigen (SCCA) belongs to the high molecular weight protease inhibitor family found in the squamous and granular layers of the normal squamous epithelium. It consists of two different isomers, encoded by two highly homologous genes: SCCA1 being neutral, and SCCA2 acid [36]. SCCA2 has been detected in many malignancies such as cervical, lung, head and neck carcinoma, and it has been used as a valuable diagnostic biomarker in clinical practice [37].

Giannelli et al. showed that SCCA expression was higher in the HCC group than in the cirrhotic group. The sensitivity of SCCA is 84.2%, but the specificity is low at

48.9%. In the small tumor group (≤ 3 cm) the sensitivity and specificity of SCCA were 56.1% and 74.9% with a cut-off of 3.2 ng/ml. In their study of SCCA expression in cells, using immunohistochemistry, Guido et al. demonstrated that SCCA expression in cancerous tissues and dysplasia nodules was much higher than that of newly formed nodules in early HCC diagnosis [38]. SCCA was highly sensitive, but its specificity was quite low. Its expression in early HCC tissue and in dysplasia nodules makes SCCA a valuable complementary marker for HCC diagnosis. An alternative biomarker is an immune complex between SCCA and IgM, SCCA-IgM, whose expression increases in early HCC. The immune complex SCCA-IgM has a higher diagnostic performance than the free SCCA and is also more relevant since it is not found in the serum of healthy people. However, the detection rate of SCCA-IgM immune complex is 18% for chronic hepatitis, 26% for cirrhosis and 70% for HCC [39]. Its sensitivity and specificity for HCC diagnosis are 89% and 50% [40]. The concentration of SCCA-IgM immune complex is constantly increasing in patients with cirrhosis who tend to progress to HCC. Sensitivity and specificity were of higher value than AFP in the studies of Pontisso et al. [37].

Increased serum SCCA in patients with liver disease can be considered a valuable marker for early diagnosis of HCC. Especially the SCCA-IgM immune complex, which is highly sensitive. However, since its specificity is quite low, it must be combined with other markers such as serum AFP or DCP to increase its diagnostic value.

3.5 Osteopontin (OPN)

Osteopontin (OPN) is known as a conversion protein and is a glycophosphoprotein associated with integrin, which is overexpressed in many types of malignancies such as lung, breast, and colon cancers [41]. OPN usually manifests in biliary epithelial cells, astrocytes and Kupffer cells, but not in liver cells [42]. However, increased serum OPN expression has been reported in patients with HCC, but not in those with cirrhosis, chronic hepatitis, or healthy controls [43, 44]. In a meta-analysis, the sensitivity and specificity of OPN were 86% for all HCC stages [45]. Shang et al. suggested that serum OPN concentrations at the cut-off level of 91 ng/ml were more sensitive than that of AFP (74% versus 53%) in the diagnosis of HCC. Combining two imprints with an OPN cut-off of 156 ng/ml and an AFP cut-off of 20 ng/ml increased sensitivity and specificity (95% and 96%). The sensitivity and specificity of OPN were 75% and 62% for early HCC, which means the sensitivity was higher than that of AFP, but the specificity lower (46% and 93%). When combined with AFP at the cut-off of 91 ng/ml for OPNs, sensitivity increased to 83% and specificity decreased to 63% [45] (**Table 1**). Based on such findings, OPN can be considered an important marker in HCC diagnosis, especially for tumors in the early stages, and when combined with AFP to significantly increase sensitivity. However, studies with larger sample populations are needed to confirm its relevance.

3.6 Tumor-associated glycoprotein 72 (TAG-72)

Tumor-associated glycoprotein 72 (TAG-72) is a macro-molecular glycoprotein complex, which is rarely expressed in normal tissues, but overexpressed in the majority of human adenocarcinomas, including gastric, colon, and pancreatic cancer. TAG-72 expression is significantly increased in HCC tissues compared to normal liver tissues [46], and it is suspected of promoting tumor invasion and metastasis. A correlation between overexpression of TAG-72 and poor survival in patients with HCC has been observed [46]. This makes TAG-72 a potential prognosis marker for HCC, and anti-TAG-72 monoclonal antibody has been used for tumors clinical detection [47].

3.7 Zinc-α2-glycoprotein (ZAG)

Zinc-α2-glycoprotein (ZAG) is a member of the class I major histocompatibility complex (MHC-I) family. It is considered a new adipokine because of its strong amino acid sequence homology with lipid mobilizing factor (LMF). ZAG is down-regulated in human obesity [48], but it is upregulated in different cancers such as breast, lung and prostate cancers, making it a potential biomarker for these. The serum proteome of the HCC, liver cirrhosis and healthy adult groups have been analyzed and it was found that the ZAG is overexpressed in the HCC patients suggesting a potential biomarker for the early detection of HCC [49].

3.8 Annexin A2

Annexin A2 is a calcium-dependent, phospholipid-binding protein found on the surface of endothelial cells and most epithelial cells [50, 51]. Annexin A2 serum concentrations in patients with HCC were often higher than those with benign liver disease, other malignant tumors, or healthy individuals [52–54]. High annexin A2 levels were observed in 83.2% of early-stage HCC and 78.4% of AFP-negative HCC patients [55]. Annexin A2 sensitivity and specificity were respectively measured at 83.2% and 67.5% in the detection of early-stage HCC, while HCC patients with normal AFP levels were 54.7% and 81.3%, respectively. The diagnostic performance of annexin A2 alone (AUC = 79%) was also greater than for AFP alone (AUC = 73%). As expected, the combination of annexin A2 and AFP further improved the overall diagnostic performance with a sensitivity of 87.4% and a specificity of 68.3%. This makes annexin A2 a potential independent biomarker for detecting early-stage HCC in patients with normal serum AFP.

4. Enzymes and isozymes

4.1 Des-γ-carboxyprothrombin (DCP)

Des-γ-carboxyprothrombin (DCP) or Prothrombin induced by vitamin K absence II (PIVKA II) is a prothrombin molecule which is synthesized in abnormally high amount in HCC. During malignant transformation in liver cells, vitamin K-dependent carboxylase system weakens [56]. In essence, this is a carboxylation defect that leads to increased DCP synthesis [57]. Serum DCP levels in patients with liver cancer have differed from normal individuals [58]. In a comparative study of cases of chronic hepatitis and liver cirrhosis, DCP showed a sensitivity of 72.7% and a specificity of 90.0%, equivalent to AFP [59]. The combination of these two markers improves HCC diagnosis with a sensitivity and a specificity of 74.2% and 87.2%, respectively [60]. Although DCP has proven to have great potential as a biomarker for early diagnosis of HCC, it needs to be verified by further studies, especially in combination with AFP. In a large multicentre study, the sensitivity of DCP was 56% for early HCC diagnosis. Combining DCP with AFP increased the sensitivity from 65–87% 3 months before HCC diagnosis, but the specificity decreased from 84–69% [61].

Although the diagnostic value of DCP has been studied in Asian countries, its assessments in Western countries, especially in Europe, are still limited. A case–control study to evaluate the performance of serum AFP and DCP concentrations for early HCC diagnosis was conducted in France [62]. The cut-off threshold for serum DCP was 42 mAU/ml and 5.5 ng/ml for AFP, resulting in DCP being better than AFP for early diagnosis of HCC with a sensitivity of 77% compared to a 61%

one, and a specificity of 82% compared to a 50% one. The positive forecast value was 76% compared to 51%, and the negative forecast value was 83% compared to 62%. The combination of DCP and AFP improved diagnostic performance. These results further support the value of DCP as a marker for early HCC diagnosis. According to the 2010 recommendations of the Japan Society of Hepatology (JSH), the three biological markers AFP, AFP-L3 and DCP are checked by the state insurance for HCC screening, as a combination of two of the three biomarkers, or all three combined. These three markers help to increase sensitivity without reducing specificity in small liver cancer [63].

4.2 γ-Glutamyl transferase (GGT)

γ-Glutamyl transferase (GGT) is a membrane-binding enzyme, which appears in the development of liver cells during pregnancy, its concentration is high throughout pregnancy and decreases immediately after birth. The total GGT concentration increased in chronic liver diseases, HCC, and some extra-liver cancer diseases [63]. A study by Cui et al. on 90 patients with cirrhosis and 120 patients with HCC showed that the sensitivity of HS-GGT was 74%, irrespective of size, and 43.8% for small tumors (<3 cm) [64] (**Table 1**). The diagnostic value improves when combined with other biomarkers such as AFP, PIVKA II, or AFP-L3. This is a promising sign in the detection of small cancers and can be used in combination with AFP and AFP-L3.

4.3 Matrix metalloproteinases (MMPs)

Matrix metalloproteinase (MMP) is an enzyme belonging to the endopeptidase group, which helps regenerate tissue in various pathogenetic processes including tumor progression, and wound healing [65]. Kuo et al. showed that only cases of HBsAg-positive have high levels of MMP-2 expression [66], but the relationship between other markers of HBV and MMP was not clarified. Positive cases with HBeAg showed a high tendency for portal vein thrombosis along with high manifestations of MMP-7 and MMP-9. MMPs have a synergistic effect on HCC generation, proliferation and invasion, through ways that the study did not elucidate [67]. A significantly higher MMP-9/MMP-2 ratio was found in patients with advanced HCC compared to patients at an early stage [68]. The mRNA of MMP-14, MMP-15 and MMP-2 are highly expressed in most HCC cells suggesting an important role of MMPs in the growth, invasion, and metastasis of tumor cells. Selective inhibitors for these MMPs promise to be an effective mean of preventing the growth and metastasis of HCC [69].

4.4 Glutamine synthetase (GS)

Glutamine synthetase (GS) is an enzyme involved in catalyzing the synthesis of glutamine from glutamate and ammonia, it plays an important role in the function of ammonia metabolism and nitrogen balance of the liver [70]. Research by Haupt et al. demonstrated that GSmRNA increased its tissue and protein expression in the serum of HCC patients [71]. In addition, Osada et al. reported increasing GS expression correlated with cancer progression, suggesting GS can play a role in promoting HCC metastases [72].

4.5 Alpha L fucosidase (AFU)

Alpha L fucosidase (AFU) is a glycosidase responsible for hydrolysing fucoseglycoside bonds of glycoprotein and glycolipids and is found in all mammalian cell lysosomes and is involved in the degenerative reaction of a series of fucoglyco-containing fucoglyco complexes [73]. Serum AFU levels are constantly elevated in cirrhotic patients who tend to progress to HCC. Deugnier et al. found that serum AFU had greater sensitivity and specificity than AFP and that it can be considered a marker for HCC diagnosis. However, the cause of this increased serum AFU activity is still unknown. The most likely explanation is that increased serum AFU activity is a result of an increase in tumor protein synthesis that increases fucoses [74]. Measuring the activity of serum AFU regularly during follow-up of cirrhotic patients provides very useful clinical data in monitoring cirrhosis progression to HCC. Although an increased serum AFU activity was not correlated with tumor size and was common in cases of early HCC, the HCC tumor would appear within a few years in 82% of patients with liver fibrosis if serum AFU activity exceeds 700 nmol/ml/hour. Serum AFU activity increased in 85% of patients at least six months before HCC was detected by a diagnostic imaging method [75]. AFU activity was significantly increased in HCC patients compared with patients with other liver diseases or other cancers. AFU sensitivity is 81.5% and its specificity is 85.4% in HCC diagnosis [76] indicating a promising specific marker for HCC diagnosis.

5. Cytokines

Cytokines are a heterogeneous group of proteins that play roles of mediators in cellular reactions and activities. They are the product mediating and regulating immune processes of immune cells. Some cytokines also act as potential markers for early diagnosis and treatment of HCC.

5.1 Transforming growth factor-β1 (TGF-β1)

Transforming growth factor-β (TGF-β1) is a versatile growth factor associated with proliferation, cell differentiation, embryogenesis, vascular proliferation, invasion and immune activity. One study found that serum TGF-β1 levels increased in the HCC group compared to the group with non-malignant liver disease and the healthy group. With a cut-off of 800 pg./ml, the specificity of TGF-β1 HCC diagnostic serum is above 95%. Taking the same value as the serum AFP at the cut-off of 200 ng/ml, the sensitivity of TGF-β1 is 68%, which is superior to that of AFP (24%). Moreover, in patients with serum AFP within normal limits, increased TGF-β1 levels can be observed in 23% of cases [77]. It has been shown that TGF-β1 and TGF-β1 mRNA can be used as a marker to diagnose and predict HCC due to HBV with a sensitivity and specificity of 89.5% and 94.0% with a cutting level of TGF-β1 > 1.2 g/l [78]. TGF-β1 mediates various biological effects through signal paths and manifestations of TGF-β1 polymorphism may affect tumor susceptibility. The TGF-β1 signaling pathway can be considered as a target for HCC treatment. The subject is currently under study to confirm its role and promises to bring new cancer treatments.

5.2 Vascular endothelial growth factor (VEGF)

Vascular endothelial growth factor (VEGF) acts as an important factor in the process of tumor formation by forming new blood vessel systems that increase in size and promote invasion and metastasis. Studies have shown that angiogenesis is essential in tumor growth, including HCC, which is often characterized by the proliferation of blood vessels [79]. It has been demonstrated that VEGF expression in HCC tissues has a significantly higher incidence of portal vein thrombosis and a lower average survival time than when VEGF expression is not present [80]. In the study of Xiang et al., VEGF was associated with lymph node metastatic characteristics in HCC. In addition, VEGF expression is closely related to relapse and prognosis. Notably, several manifestations of the VEGF receptor are related to some of the clinical characteristics and prognosis of HCC [81]. Inactivation of VEGF165 increases the expression of the *P53* gene that inhibits HCC development, invasion and metastasis.

5.3 Interleukin-8 (IL-8)

Interleukin-8 (IL-8) is a multifunctional CXC chemokine that is involved in the immune response of neutrophils in humans including kinetic phenomena, enzyme release and expression of surface adhesion of molecule. IL-8 also has a direct effect on tumor progression, including the proliferation of vascular endothelial cells and formation of new vessels. In addition, IL-8 increases the likelihood of metastases and new tumor formation in the liver [82]. A study showed that IL-8 serum concentrations increased in HCC patients compared to healthy subjects, it was positively correlated with tumor size (≥5 cm), portal vein thrombosis and advanced stage with lymph node metastases [83]. Therefore, it may be a biological marker that plays a useful role in HCC diagnosis and prognosis.

5.4 Tumor-specific growth factor (TSGF)

Malignant tumors have the ability to synthesize tumor-specific growth factors, releasing them into the capillaries surrounding the tumor and peripheral blood vessels during their development. Therefore, serum TSGF levels may be a marker of tumor survival. In one study, serum TSGF concentrations were used as a diagnostic marker for HCC with 82% sensitivity at 62 UI/ml [84]. Combined with other cancer markers, TSGF may yield higher diagnostic values with increased sensitivity. Theoretically, preeclampsia is highly expressed in many malignant tumors and HCC, but there are currently too few studies evaluating the role of TSGF in other malignancies to consider it as a potential factor. There are other markers, such as serum insulin-like growth factor-II (IGF-II), which can be used as diagnostic or prognostic markers for HCC. A cut-off of 4.1 mg/l of IGF-II obtained results of 63% sensitivity, 90% specificity and 70% accuracy in early HCC diagnosis with small tumor size. Moreover, the combination of IGF-II and AFP (cut-off value of 50 ng/ml) increases sensitivity up to 80% and accuracy up to 88% [85].

5.5 Hepatocyte growth factor (HGF)

Hepatocyte growth factor (HGF) is a multifunctional element produced in many organs in the body, it affects cell division, cell motility, intracellular invasion, and carcinogenesis [86]. In a study in Japan, serum HGF levels are increased significantly in the HCC group compared with cirrhosis, chronic hepatitis and healthy controls groups. With a cutting level of 0.6 ng/ml, its sensitivity can be up to 100% for any AFP or DCP concentration. The serum HGF concentration ≥ 1.0 ng/ml has a shorter shelf life, so it can be used as a prognostic marker for HCC [87]. The authors suggest that HGF causes proliferation and invasion of cancer cells through the expression of c-met receptors. In addition, increased HGF serum levels along with high expression of serum c-met protein after hepatectomy play an important role in predicting tumor recurrence and metastasis. This can be explained by the fact that HGF can increase the production and size of both normal and malignant liver cells after surgery, leading to tumor recurrence [88].

6. Circulating RNAs

6.1 AFP mRNA

AFP mRNA is a highly valuable marker only found in active cancer cells, which might be a sign of tumor metastasis. The non-recurrence time of HCC patients with high AFP mRNA expression after surgery was shorter than the group without this marker expression in liver cells (53% compared to 88% after 1 year; 37% compared to 60% after 2 years) [89]. In the advanced HCC stage, the AFP mRNA expression rate reaches 100%, and also acts as a predictor of recurrence after liver resection. However, the use of this marker in HCC diagnosis remains controversial, possibly due to the fact that it also manifests in many other malignancies and non-cancerous liver diseases [90]. Therefore, it could be used for diagnosis and prognosis when combined with other markers.

6.2 GGT mRNA

Gamma-glutamyl transferase mRNA (GGT mRNA) can be found in the blood and peripheral liver cells of healthy individuals, as well as in patients with benign liver disease, benign liver tumors or HCC. It has 3 types: A, B and C. Type A dominates in normal liver cases, non-cancerous liver diseases, benign tumors and secondary liver cancers, while type C is produced by the yolk during pregnancy. In contrast, type B predominates in HCC [91–93]. During malignant development, expression of GGT mRNA in liver tissues may change from type A to type B [93]. Patients with HCC and high type B expression will have a worse prognosis, with higher odds of a sooner and more serious relapse [94]. Therefore, hepatocellular expression of type B mRNA may be a valuable marker for HCC patients. As in liver tissues, peripheral blood type B expression has also been reported to be significantly higher in HCC patients than in healthy adults [91].

6.3 MicroRNA (miRNA)

MicroRNAs are small non-coding RNAs that inhibit or accelerate the translation process by attenuating or increasing the synthesis of target mRNAs or by binding to additional chains in the UTR region (3′-untranslated region). In recent years, the link between miRNA and tumor development has become a controversial issue. About 500 miRNA genes have been identified and contribute to control a number of cellular processes including proliferation, differentiation and apoptosis. In malignancy, the function of miRNA is determined to be carcinogenic and tumor suppressant [95]. miRNA can regulate many genes at the same time, they control the replication process and determine the characteristics of the cell. The variety in this functional role allows miRNA to be utilized as a diagnostic marker for early detection of cancer, risk assessment, prognosis and as a new therapeutic target.

Yamamoto et al. have used a global miRNA expression profile in mouse liver development and thus shown that miR-500 (miRNA) is a potential biomarker for HCC [95]. Their work showed that miR-500 is significantly associated with the regulation of liver development and thus is related to cirrhosis progression. The serum miR-21 levels were a valuable marker in distinguishing patients with HCC from those with chronic hepatitis with the sensitivity and specificity of 61.1% and 83.3%, respectively. Compared to the healthy group, the sensitivity and specificity were 87.3% and 92.0%, respectively. Both values are higher than serum AFP concentrations, which have been confirmed as a very valuable biological marker for HCC [96]. Serum miR-15b and miR-130b concentrations are relevant miRNA markers that are highly expressed in HCC. miR-130b has 87.7% sensitivity and 81.4% specificity. In contrast, while the sensitivity of miR-15b is high at 98.3%, its specificity is low at 15.3%. Because the sensitivity of these two factors is rather high, it can be used as a valuable marker in HCC screening and early diagnosis with low AFP levels [97].

A group of markers including seven miRNAs (miR-122, miR-192, miR-21, miR-223, miR-26a, miR-27a and miR-801) has been shown to have a great diagnostic performance for HBV related HCC at an early stage [98]. Although its mechanism and signal path are still unknown, the expression of miRNA-29 may increase the susceptibility of cancer cells to apoptosis and reduce the expression of Mcl-1 and Bcl-2. Indeed, it has the ability to inhibit the formation and growth of cancer cells and is a potential marker in HCC prognosis and treatment [99]. MiR-122 is a specific miRNA found only in HCC, which concentration is inversely correlated with cancer growth and likelihood of invasion and metastasis. An analysis of miRNA markers revealed only tumor miR-21 expression and significantly higher serum miR-21 levels in HCC patients compared to those in chronic liver diseases and healthy control groups. Analysis of ROC curve between HCC and control group showed that sensitivity and specificity were 87.3% and 92% respectively, which is higher than that of serum AFP. Therefore, miR-21 is also a promising marker to support early HCC diagnosis [96].

Some of their features and expressions make miRNA particularly attractive as potential biomarkers. First, many miRNAs exhibit high stability and are easily detectable in peripheral blood of HCC patients. Secondly, miRNAs can be identified in urine, which will be a valuable non-invasive biological marker in detecting and managing HCC. The detection of the expression of some miRNAs in the urine (miR-625, miR-532, miR-618, miR-516-5P and miR-650) has been used for early detection of HCC [100]. However, more research is needed regarding miRNA before it can be used to detect HCC at an early stage.

6.4 Long non-coding RNA (lncRNA)

Like other cancers, HCC is characterized by a gradual accumulation of epigenetic changes. Among these changes, lncRNA has been found to play a significant role in the initiation and progression of HCC. Most lncRNAs express the characteristics of each species and the specific characteristics of the tumor. Increased or decreased expression of lncRNA has been found in cancerous tissues. Meanwhile, some lncRNA are found in urine, blood, and other body fluids. Moreover, the use of lncRNA as a marker for cancer pathology is superior to the coding RNA protein, due to the characteristic expression of lncRNA [101]. The sensitivity and specificity of lncRNA for HCC diagnosis found in some recent studies are quite high, while it has been demonstrated that JPX (just proximal to XIST) can have a sensitivity of up to 100% [102]. The 2-lncRNA signal has a high specificity of 90.62% but a low sensitivity of 60.65%, which could make it a potential marker to confirm an HCC diagnosis [103]. Recent findings suggest that lncRNA may be a potential marker for early diagnosis and monitoring of the risk of malignant progression in patients with chronic and highly specific chronic liver disease. These markers may contribute to the definitive HCC diagnosis without the need for histopathological diagnosis (**Table 2**).

miRNA/ LncRNAs	Diagnostic value	AUC	Sensitivity	Specificity	Reference
miR-21	Differentiate HCC from patients with chronic hepatitis		61.1%	83.3%	[16]
miR-21	Differentiate HCC from healthy individuals		87.3%	92.0%	[16]
miR-130b	Differentiate HCC from healthy individuals		87.7%	81.4%	[17]
miR-15b	Differentiate HCC from healthy individuals		98.3%	15.3%	[17]
2-lncRNA	Differentiate HCC from healthy individuals	0.764	60.56%	90.62%	Yu et al. [18]
DANCR	Differentiate HCC from cirrhosis and chronic liver	0.868	83.8%	72.7%	Ma et al. [19]
MALAT1 (plasma)	Differentiate HCC from patients with liver disease	0.66	51.1%	89.3%	Konishi et al. [20]
JPX	Distinguish HCC and control group	0.814	100.0%	52.4%	Ma et al. [21]
UCA1	Distinguish HCC and control group	0,91	91,4%	88,6%	El-Tawdi et al. [22]

Abbreviation: *DANCR, Differentiation Antagonizing Non-protein Coding RNA; MALAT1, metastasis associated lung adenocarcinoma transcript 1; UCA1, urothelial cancer associated 1.*

Table 2.
Diagnostic performance of miRNAs and lncRNAs for HCC.

7. Gene mutations

7.1 Mutations in *TP53* gene

P53 is an important protein in the P53 signaling pathway and mutation or loss of *TP53* gene function leads to abnormal cell growth [104]. Notably, the mutation rate of *TP53* varies by geographic area, reflecting the etiology and epidemiological changes of HCC [105]. Mutations in the *TP53* gene, commonly found in sub-Saharan Africa and Southeast Asia, has the highest incidence of HBV infection and Aflatoxin B1 exposure. In these areas, the most common mutation is TP53 R249S, which is associated with an exposure factor of Aflatoxin B1 [106].

TP53 mutation was identified as one of the common molecular alterations in HCC, of which, the *TP53* R249S mutation in exon 7 was found in HCC patients with a high incidence. Studies suggest that the *TP53* R249S mutation may occur relatively early in areas associated with Aflatoxin exposure and chronic HBV infection [107]. The *TP53* R249S mutation was an important factor in the carcinogenesis of HCC in Brazil, where Aflatoxin exposure is high [108]. In contrast, the *TP53* R249S mutation may not play a role in causing HCC in Egypt, where HCV infection is common [109]. These findings suggest that *TP53* mutations are involved in HCC pathogenesis in individuals with chronic HBV infection, especially in those exposed to high Aflatoxin B1.

Recent reports have shown that *TP53* mutation can be used as a marker to predict HCC in high-risk groups. TP53 mutation has been shown to be associated with significantly higher relapse rates and lower disease-free survival rates [110]. It is also documented that *TP53* mutation rate is about 30% and is associated with additional survival, non-recurrent survival and disease-free survival in HCC patients, with similar results observed in patients infected with HBV and HCV [111, 112]. However, a recent study showed that the *TP53* mutation was only associated with a shorter survival time only in HBV-related HCC, while the R249S mutation was not related to the survival rate in the European patients with HCV-related HCC [113]. Growing evidence suggests that the stability of the *TP53* mutation in tumors is important for its carcinogenic activities, decreasing the expression of the *TP53* mutation that reduces malignant growth of cancer cells. Therefore, the *TP53* mutation, especially at R249S position, can be considered as one of the early markers for HCC diagnosis and is an attractive therapy for cancer treatment.

7.2 hTERT gene mutation

The telomerase reverse transcriptase (hTERT) gene encodes an enzyme that maintains the telomeric DNA length and stabilizes the chromosomes [113]. hTERT is a major determinant of telomerase activity, which plays a key role in protecting cells from apoptosis and transforming into cancerous cells [114]. The reactivation of telomerase activity in cancer may be related to changes that occur during cancer development, including mutations and rearrangements of chromosomes [115].

The frequencies of *hTERT* mutations were observed in about 60% of HCC patients [116] but vary by geographical regions being the most common in Europe (59%) and less common in East Asia (20.7%) [117]. These data indicate that *hTERT* mutation is frequently associated with HCV-related HCC. *hTERT*-promoting mutations have been found with 6% of low-grade dysplasia nodules, 19% of advanced dysplasia nodules, 61% of early HCC and 42% of intermediate and advanced HCC [118]. Another study also found *hTERT* mutation in 57% of patients with chronic hepatitis and in 30% of those with early HCC [119]. Therefore, mutations in the *hTERT* promoter occur early in the course of malignant transformation and persists during tumor development. The regulation and expression of *hTERT* play an important role in the initiation and progression of HCC. *hTERT* mutation is one of the earliest gene mutations in cancer development and is also the most common gene mutation in HCC. Therefore, *hTERT* mutation is one of the most important markers in early diagnosis and may be a promising target for HCC treatment.

7.3 Mutations in ARID1A and ARID2 genes

ARID1A and *ARID2* are two genes in the SWI/SNF complex (SWitch/sucrose non-fermentable) involved in chromosomal reconstruction. The mutation rate of the *ARID1A* and *ARID2* genes found in 10% HCC, depending on the cause. *ARID1A* mutation is associated with alcohol consumption while *ARID2* mutation is often associated with HCV infection [120]. Although the role of these mutations remains unknown, studies have shown that *ARID1A* and *ARID2* genes are associated with the growth of cancer cells through affecting several signaling pathways such as PI3K/AKT, beta-catenin and p53 mutation [121] and are thus potential markers for early HCC detection.

8. DNA methylation

In HCC, methylation can occur in two ways: total methylation and partial methylation. Total methylation affects the structural function of the nucleus by promoting chromosome and genome instability, while partial methylation is associated with tumor suppressor genes [122]. Chronic hepatitis virus infections are the cause of DNA methylation aberrations in cancerous tissues. Although several DNA methyltransferase enzymes such as DNMT1, DNMT3A and DNMT3B have been shown to increase their expression in HCC related to hepatitis viruses, their mechanisms remain controversial and unclear [123].

p16 (CDKN2A), a tumor suppressor gene involved in cell cycle regulation, has been shown to be methylated and is related to clinical parameters in HCC [124]. A study has shown that the methylation levels of *p16* gene increased in tissue samples from cirrhosis to HCC [125]. The methylation level of *p16* gene is also associated with HBV infection, as the level of *p16* methylation is higher in patients with HBV than those without HBV, the *HBx* gene being especially involved in the methylation of the *p16* gene [126, 127]. A study on 64 HCC patients found that 77% of patients had *p16* methylation and that methylation levels were correlated to serum AFP levels [128]. In a meta-analysis on 272 HCC tissue samples, the methylation rate of p16 gene was 58.5%, much higher than those with cirrhosis and chronic hepatitis [129]. Therefore, methylation in the *p16* gene may serve as a promising molecular marker for HCC in patients with HBV infection.

Another potential marker for HCC prognosis is *SOCS1* methylation. *SOCS1* gene plays a role in modulating the JAK/STAT signaling pathway when methylation causes malignant cell proliferation. SOCS1 methylation correlates with tumor size and risk factors for HCC, it is more common in HCV and cirrhotic patients, but less common in HBV-infected groups. A study has shown that the methylation of *SOCS1* gene in peripheral blood accounted for 38% in the HCC group, 20% in the cirrhotic group and 23% in the control group without liver disease. Expression of methylation of *SOCS1* and *RASSF1A* genes in combination with serum AFP increased sensitivity to 86% and specificity to 75% for HCC diagnosis [130]. *SOCS1* methylation is quite common in HCC, and is correlated with a number of clinical parameters and other serum biomarkers like AFP. Therefore, *SOCS1* methylation in combination with serum AFP increases the sensitivity and specificity for early HCC diagnosis.

GSTP1 belongs to the Glutathione S-transferase family, which protects cells against carcinogens, regulates signaling pathways that control cell proliferation and cell death [131]. The methylation in the *GSTP1* gene promoter was observed in prostate cancer, HCC and other malignancies. GSTP1 has been shown to have a high methylation rate in HCC related to HBV or HCV infection. Interestingly, methylation of the *GSTP1* gene in HCC patients was 76.7% and those with high *GSTP1* expression had a shorter survival time [132].

Detecting the methylation status of genes in serum provides a promising method for diagnosis of HCC. A study found aberrant methylation in the *CCND2* gene in 39 out of 70 serum samples of HCC patients and methylation status was associated with a shorter disease-free survival time [133]. Yeo et al. showed that 17 out of 40 (42.5%) plasma samples of HCC patients had methylation in *RASSF1A* gene, and that methylation occurred mainly in patients with tumors ≥4 cm in size [134]. Methylation in *RASSF1A* in the serum of 85 HCC patients and found that 93% had methylation, it is associated with a shorter survival and disease stage [135]. The level of methylation in the *RASSF1A* gene of the HCC group is significantly higher compared to other liver disease groups and thus it is a promising independent marker for early diagnosis and prognosis of HCC [136].

9. Conclusion

A large number of markers have been studied and clinically applied for early diagnosis and monitoring of HCC treatment, of which serum AFP is a widely used with a controversial diagnostic threshold. A number of protein markers such as AFP-L3 and DCP are also being applied to support HCC diagnosis with higher sensitivity and specificity compared to AFP. However, the available marker is neither specific for solely HCC diagnosis nor provides great diagnostic performance for HCC and thus a combination of several serum protein markers can improve the early diagnosis rate. With the development of molecular technology, biomarkers based on miRNA and lncRNA expression, gene mutation (*TP53, hTERT, ARID1A and ARID2*) and DNA methylation have a great potential to improve the rate of HCC diagnosis at an early stage, as well as predicting progression, metastasis and tumor recurrence. In addition, with the development of current cell technology, cancer pathways and the expression of genes specific for HCC tumor may be important markers for early detection and new targets for the treatment of HCC.

Acknowledgements

This study was funded by the Vietnam National Foundation for Science and Technology Development (NAFOSTED; grant number 108.02-2017.15) to Hoang Van Tong. The funder has no role in the study design, data collection and analysis, decision to publish or preparation of the manuscript.

Competing interests

All authors have no conflicts of interest to declare.

Author details

Hoang Van Tong[1,2]*, Pham Van Dung[1], Nguyen Thi Mong Diep[3] and Nguyen Linh Toan[2]

1 Institute of Biomedicine and Pharmacy, Vietnam Military Medical University, Hanoi, Vietnam

2 Department of Pathophysiology, Vietnam Military Medical University, Hanoi, Vietnam

3 Faculty of Natural Sciences, Quy Nhon University, Binh Dinh, Vietnam

*Address all correspondence to: hoangvantong@vmmu.edu.vn

References

[1] Mittal S, El-Serag HB. Epidemiology of hepatocellular carcinoma: Consider the population. J Clin Gastroenterol 2013; 47 Suppl: S2-S6

[2] Torre LA, Bray F, Siegel RL, et al. Global cancer statistics, 2012. CA Cancer J Clin 2015; 65: 87-108

[3] Global Burden of Disease Cancer C, Fitzmaurice C, Allen C, et al. Global, regional, and National Cancer Incidence, mortality, years of life lost, years lived with disability, and disability-adjusted life-years for 32 cancer groups, 1990 to 2015: A Systematic Analysis for the Global Burden of Disease Study. JAMA Oncol 2017; 3: 524-548

[4] Dhanasekaran R, Limaye A, Cabrera R. Hepatocellular carcinoma: Current trends in worldwide epidemiology, risk factors, diagnosis, and therapeutics. Hepat Med 2012; 4: 19-37

[5] Peterson ML, Ma C, Spear BT. Zhx2 and Zbtb20: Novel regulators of postnatal alpha-fetoprotein repression and their potential role in gene reactivation during liver cancer. Semin Cancer Biol 2011; 21: 21-27

[6] IuS T. [Detection of embryo-specific alpha-globulin in the blood serum of a patient with primary liver cancer]. Vopr Med Khim 1964; 10: 90-91

[7] Nagasue N, Inokuchi K, Kobayashi M, et al. Serum alpha-fetoprotein levels after hepatic artery ligation and postoperative chemotherapy: Correlation with clinical status in patients with hepatocellular carcinoma. Cancer 1977; 40: 615-618

[8] Zhou L, Liu J, Luo F. Serum tumor markers for detection of hepatocellular carcinoma. World J Gastroenterol 2006; 12: 1175-1181

[9] Tangkijvanich P, Anukulkarnkusol N, Suwangool P, et al. Clinical characteristics and prognosis of hepatocellular carcinoma: Analysis based on serum alpha-fetoprotein levels. J Clin Gastroenterol 2000; 31: 302-308

[10] Chan SL, Mo F, Johnson PJ, et al. Performance of serum alpha-fetoprotein levels in the diagnosis of hepatocellular carcinoma in patients with a hepatic mass. HPB (Oxford) 2014; 16: 366-372

[11] European Association for Study of Liver EOfRaToC. EASL- EORTC clinical practice guidelines,management of hepatocellular carcinoma. Eur J Cancer 2012; 48: 599-641

[12] Invited Abstract: 19(th) conference of the Asian Pacific Association for the Study of the liver. Hepatol Int 2009; 3: 1-23

[13] Spangenberg HC, Thimme R, Blum HE. Serum markers of hepatocellular carcinoma. Semin Liver Dis 2006; 26: 385-390

[14] Sato Y, Nakata K, Kato Y, et al. Early recognition of hepatocellular carcinoma based on altered profiles of alpha-fetoprotein. N Engl J Med 1993; 328: 1802-1806

[15] Kagebayashi C, Yamaguchi I, Akinaga A, et al. Automated immunoassay system for AFP-L3% using on-chip electrokinetic reaction and separation by affinity electrophoresis. Anal Biochem 2009; 388: 306-311

[16] Oda K, Ido A, Tamai T, et al. Highly sensitive lens culinaris agglutinin-reactive alpha-fetoprotein is useful for early detection of hepatocellular carcinoma in patients with chronic liver disease. Oncol Rep 2011; 26: 1227-1233

[17] Filmus J. The contribution of in vivo manipulation of gene expression to the

understanding of the function of glypicans. Glycoconj J 2002; 19: 319-323

[18] Sung YK, Hwang SY, Park MK, et al. Glypican-3 is overexpressed in human hepatocellular carcinoma. Cancer Sci 2003; 94: 259-262

[19] Filmus J, Capurro M. The role of glypican-3 in the regulation of body size and cancer. Cell Cycle 2008; 7: 2787-2790

[20] Capurro MI, Xiang Y-Y, Lobe C, et al. Glypican-3 promotes the growth of hepatocellular carcinoma by stimulating canonical Wnt signaling. Cancer Research 2005; 65: 6245-6254

[21] Capurro M, Wanless IR, Sherman M, et al. Glypican-3: A novel serum and histochemical marker for hepatocellular carcinoma. Gastroenterology 2003; 125: 89-97

[22] Nakatsura T, Yoshitake Y, Senju S, et al. Glypican-3, overexpressed specifically in human hepatocellular carcinoma, is a novel tumor marker. Biochem Biophys Res Commun 2003; 306: 16-25

[23] Libbrecht L, Severi T, Cassiman D, et al. Glypican-3 expression distinguishes small hepatocellular carcinomas from cirrhosis, dysplastic nodules, and focal nodular hyperplasia-like nodules. Am J Surg Pathol 2006; 30: 1405-1411

[24] Jia X, Liu J, Gao Y, et al. Diagnosis accuracy of serum glypican-3 in patients with hepatocellular carcinoma: A systematic review with meta-analysis. Arch Med Res 2014; 45: 580-588

[25] Joo M, Chi JG, Lee H. Expressions of HSP70 and HSP27 in hepatocellular carcinoma. J Korean Med Sci 2005; 20: 829-834

[26] Luk JM, Lam CT, Siu AF, et al. Proteomic profiling of hepatocellular carcinoma in Chinese cohort reveals heat-shock proteins (Hsp27, Hsp70, GRP78) up-regulation and their associated prognostic values. Proteomics 2006; 6: 1049-1057

[27] Shin E, Ryu HS, Kim SH, et al. The clinicopathological significance of heat shock protein 70 and glutamine synthetase expression in hepatocellular carcinoma. J Hepatobiliary Pancreat Sci 2011; 18: 544-550

[28] Tremosini S, Forner A, Boix L, et al. Prospective validation of an immunohistochemical panel (glypican 3, heat shock protein 70 and glutamine synthetase) in liver biopsies for diagnosis of very early hepatocellular carcinoma. Gut 2012; 61: 1481-1487

[29] Diehl JA, Yang W, Rimerman RA, et al. Hsc70 regulates accumulation of cyclin D1 and cyclin D1-dependent protein kinase. Mol Cell Biol 2003; 23: 1764-1774

[30] Calderwood SK, Khaleque MA, Sawyer DB, et al. Heat shock proteins in cancer: Chaperones of tumorigenesis. Trends Biochem Sci 2006; 31: 164-172

[31] Kladney RD, Bulla GA, Guo L, et al. GP73, a novel Golgi-localized protein upregulated by viral infection. Gene 2000; 249: 53-65

[32] Kladney RD, Cui X, Bulla GA, et al. Expression of GP73, a resident Golgi membrane protein, in viral and nonviral liver disease. Hepatology 2002; 35: 1431-1440

[33] Mao Y, Yang H, Xu H, et al. Golgi protein 73 (GOLPH2) is a valuable serum marker for hepatocellular carcinoma. Gut 2010; 59: 1687-1693

[34] Zhou Y, Yin X, Ying J, et al. Golgi protein 73 versus alpha-fetoprotein as a biomarker for hepatocellular carcinoma: A diagnostic meta-analysis. BMC Cancer 2012; 12: 17

[35] Drake RR, Schwegler EE, Malik G, et al. Lectin capture strategies combined with mass spectrometry for the discovery of serum glycoprotein biomarkers. Mol Cell Proteomics 2006; 5: 1957-1967

[36] Gadducci A, Cosio S, Fanucchi A, et al. The predictive and prognostic value of serum CA 125 half-life during paclitaxel/platinum-based chemotherapy in patients with advanced ovarian carcinoma. Gynecol Oncol 2004; 93: 131-136

[37] Pontisso P, Quarta S, Caberlotto C, et al. Progressive increase of SCCA-IgM immune complexes in cirrhotic patients is associated with development of hepatocellular carcinoma. Int J Cancer 2006; 119: 735-740

[38] Guido M, Roskams T, Pontisso P, et al. Squamous cell carcinoma antigen in human liver carcinogenesis. Journal of Clinical Pathology 2008; 61: 445-447

[39] Beneduce L, Castaldi F, Marino M, et al. Squamous cell carcinoma antigen-immunoglobulin M complexes as novel biomarkers for hepatocellular carcinoma. Cancer 2005; 103: 2558-2565

[40] Pozzan C, Cardin R, Piciocchi M, et al. Diagnostic and prognostic role of SCCA-IgM serum levels in hepatocellular carcinoma (HCC). J Gastroenterol Hepatol 2014; 29: 1637-1644

[41] Shevde LA, Das S, Clark DW, et al. Osteopontin: An effector and an effect of tumor metastasis. Curr Mol Med 2010; 10: 71-81

[42] Kawashima R, Mochida S, Matsui A, et al. Expression of osteopontin in Kupffer cells and hepatic macrophages and stellate cells in rat liver after carbon tetrachloride intoxication: A possible factor for macrophage migration into hepatic necrotic areas. Biochem Biophys Res Commun 1999; 256: 527-531

[43] Abu El Makarem MA, Abdel-Aleem A, Ali A, et al. Diagnostic significance of plasma osteopontin in hepatitis C virus-related hepatocellular carcinoma. Ann Hepatol 2011; 10: 296-305

[44] Shang S, Plymoth A, Ge S, et al. Identification of osteopontin as a novel marker for early hepatocellular carcinoma. Hepatology 2012; 55: 483-490

[45] Wan HG, Xu H, Gu YM, et al. Comparison osteopontin vs AFP for the diagnosis of HCC: A meta-analysis. Clin Res Hepatol Gastroenterol 2014; 38: 706-714

[46] Zhang Y, Deng ZS, Liao MM, et al. Tumor associated glycoprotein-72 is a novel marker for poor survival in hepatocellular carcinoma. Pathol Oncol Res 2012; 18: 911-916

[47] Milenic DE, Brady ED, Garmestani K, et al. Improved efficacy of alpha-particle-targeted radiation therapy: Dual targeting of human epidermal growth factor receptor-2 and tumor-associated glycoprotein 72. Cancer 2010; 116: 1059-1066

[48] Mracek T, Stephens NA, Gao D, et al. Enhanced ZAG production by subcutaneous adipose tissue is linked to weight loss in gastrointestinal cancer patients. Br J Cancer 2011; 104: 441-447

[49] Zhao YJ, Ju Q, Li GC. Tumor markers for hepatocellular carcinoma. Mol Clin Oncol 2013; 1: 593-598

[50] Sharma MC, Sharma M. The role of annexin II in angiogenesis and tumor progression: A potential therapeutic target. Curr Pharm Des 2007; 13: 3568-3575

[51] Lokman NA, Ween MP, Oehler MK, et al. The role of annexin A2 in tumorigenesis and cancer progression. Cancer Microenviron 2011; 4: 199-208

[52] Hollas H, Aukrust I, Grimmer S, et al. Annexin A2 recognises a specific region in the 3'-UTR of its cognate messenger RNA. Biochim Biophys Acta 2006; 1763: 1325-1334

[53] Ji NY, Park MY, Kang YH, et al. Evaluation of annexin II as a potential serum marker for hepatocellular carcinoma using a developed sandwich ELISA method. Int J Mol Med 2009; 24: 765-771

[54] Zhao P, Zhang W, Wang SJ, et al. HAb18G/CD147 promotes cell motility by regulating annexin II-activated RhoA and Rac1 signaling pathways in hepatocellular carcinoma cells. Hepatology 2011; 54: 2012-2024

[55] Sun Y, Gao G, Cai J, et al. Annexin A2 is a discriminative serological candidate in early hepatocellular carcinoma. Carcinogenesis 2013; 34: 595-604

[56] Leerapun A, Suravarapu SV, Bida JP, et al. The utility of Lens culinaris agglutinin-reactive alpha-fetoprotein in the diagnosis of hepatocellular carcinoma: Evaluation in a United States referral population. Clin Gastroenterol Hepatol 2007; 5: 394-402; quiz 267

[57] Naraki T, Kohno N, Saito H, et al. Gamma-Carboxyglutamic acid content of hepatocellular carcinoma-associated des-gamma-carboxy prothrombin. Biochim Biophys Acta 2002; 1586: 287-298

[58] Volk ML, Hernandez JC, Su GL, et al. Risk factors for hepatocellular carcinoma may impair the performance of biomarkers: A comparison of AFP, DCP, and AFP-L3. Cancer Biomark 2007; 3: 79-87

[59] Carr BI, Kanke F, Wise M, et al. Clinical evaluation of lens culinaris agglutinin-reactive alpha-fetoprotein and des-gamma-carboxy prothrombin in histologically proven hepatocellular carcinoma in the United States. Dig Dis Sci 2007; 52: 776-782

[60] Bertino G, Neri S, Bruno CM, et al. Diagnostic and prognostic value of alpha-fetoprotein, des-gamma-carboxy prothrombin and squamous cell carcinoma antigen immunoglobulin M complexes in hepatocellular carcinoma. Minerva Med 2011; 102: 363-371

[61] Lok AS, Sterling RK, Everhart JE, et al. Des-gamma-carboxy prothrombin and alpha-fetoprotein as biomarkers for the early detection of hepatocellular carcinoma. Gastroenterology 2010; 138: 493-502

[62] Pote N, Cauchy F, Albuquerque M, et al. Performance of PIVKA-II for early hepatocellular carcinoma diagnosis and prediction of microvascular invasion. J Hepatol 2015; 62: 848-854

[63] Kudo M, Izumi N, Kokudo N, et al. Management of Hepatocellular Carcinoma in Japan: Consensus-based clinical practice guidelines proposed by the Japan Society of Hepatology (JSH) 2010 updated version. Digestive Diseases 2011; 29: 339-364

[64] Cui R, He J, Zhang F, et al. Diagnostic value of protein induced by vitamin K absence (PIVKAII) and hepatoma-specific band of serum gamma-glutamyl transferase (GGTII) as hepatocellular carcinoma markers complementary to alpha-fetoprotein. Br J Cancer 2003; 88: 1878-1882

[65] Yamamoto K, Murphy G, Troeberg L. Extracellular regulation of metalloproteinases. Matrix Biol 2015; 44-46: 255-263

[66] Kuo LF, Lee CM, Hung CH, et al. High risk of hepatitis B virus reactivation in nucleos(t)ide analogue-induced hepatitis B e antigen seroconverters older than 40 years. Dig Dis Sci 2014; 59: 2580-2587

[67] Ishii M, Mizuguchi T, Kawamoto M, et al. Propensity score analysis demonstrated the prognostic advantage of anatomical liver resection in hepatocellular carcinoma. World J Gastroenterol 2014; 20: 3335-3342

[68] Yeh CB, Hsieh MJ, Hsieh YS, et al. Terminalia catappa exerts Antimetastatic effects on hepatocellular carcinoma through transcriptional inhibition of matrix Metalloproteinase-9 by modulating NF-κB and AP-1 activity. Evid Based Complement Alternat Med 2012; 2012: 595292

[69] Kim KR, Bae JS, Choi HN, et al. The role of serum response factor in hepatocellular carcinoma: An association with matrix metalloproteinase. Oncol Rep 2011; 26: 1567-1572

[70] Brosnan ME, Brosnan JT. Hepatic glutamate metabolism: A tale of 2 hepatocytes. The American Journal of Clinical Nutrition 2009; 90: 857S-861S

[71] Haupt W, Gaunitz F, Gebhardt R. Post-transcriptional inhibition of glutamine synthetase induction in rat liver epithelial cells exerted by conditioned medium from rat hepatocytes. Life Sci 2000; 67: 3191-3198

[72] Osada T, Nagashima I, Tsuno NH, et al. Prognostic significance of glutamine synthetase expression in unifocal advanced hepatocellular carcinoma. J Hepatol 2000; 33: 247-253

[73] Haydon GH, Hayes PC. Screening for hepatocellular carcinoma. Eur J Gastroenterol Hepatol 1996; 8: 856-860

[74] Deugnier Y, David V, Brissot P, et al. Serum alpha-L-fucosidase: A new marker for the diagnosis of primary hepatic carcinoma? Hepatology 1984; 4: 889-892

[75] Ishizuka H, Nakayama T, Matsuoka S, et al. Prediction of the development of hepato-cellular-carcinoma in patients with liver cirrhosis by the serial determinations of serum alpha-L-fucosidase activity. Intern Med 1999; 38: 927-931

[76] Wang JJ, Cao EH. Rapid kinetic rate assay of the serum alpha-L-fucosidase in patients with hepatocellular carcinoma by using a novel substrate. Clin Chim Acta 2004; 347: 103-109

[77] Song BC, Chung YH, Kim JA, et al. Transforming growth factor-beta1 as a useful serologic marker of small hepatocellular carcinoma. Cancer 2002; 94: 175-180

[78] Dong ZZ, Yao DF, Yao M, et al. Clinical impact of plasma TGF-beta1 and circulating TGF-beta1 mRNA in diagnosis of hepatocellular carcinoma. Hepatobiliary Pancreat Dis Int 2008; 7: 288-295

[79] Moon WS, Rhyu KH, Kang MJ, et al. Overexpression of VEGF and angiopoietin 2: A key to high vascularity of hepatocellular carcinoma? Modern Pathology 2003; 16: 552-557

[80] Huang GW, Yang LY, Lu WQ. Expression of hypoxia-inducible factor 1alpha and vascular endothelial growth factor in hepatocellular carcinoma: Impact on neovascularization and survival. World J Gastroenterol 2005; 11: 1705-1708

[81] Zhang L, Wang JN, Tang JM, et al. VEGF is essential for the growth and migration of human hepatocellular carcinoma cells. Mol Biol Rep 2012; 39: 5085-5093

[82] Akiba J, Yano H, Ogasawara S, et al. Expression and function of interleukin-8 in human hepatocellular carcinoma. Int J Oncol 2001; 18: 257-264

[83] Ren Y, Poon RT-P, Tsui H-T, et al. Interleukin-8 serum levels in patients with hepatocellular carcinoma.

Correlations with Clinicopathological Features and Prognosis 2003; 9: 5996-6001

[84] Yin LK, Sun XQ, Mou DZ. Value of combined detection of serum CEA, CA72-4, CA19-9 and TSGF in the diagnosis of gastric cancer. Asian Pac J Cancer Prev 2015; 16: 3867-3870

[85] Tsai JF, Jeng JE, Chuang LY, et al. Serum insulin-like growth factor-II as a serologic marker of small hepatocellular carcinoma. Scand J Gastroenterol 2005; 40: 68-75

[86] Wright LM, Kreikemeier JT, Fimmel CJ. A concise review of serum markers for hepatocellular cancer. Cancer Detect Prev 2007; 31: 35-44

[87] Vejchapipat P, Tangkijvanich P, Theamboonlers A, et al. Association between serum hepatocyte growth factor and survival in untreated hepatocellular carcinoma. J Gastroenterol 2004; 39: 1182-1188

[88] Wu FS, Zheng SS, Wu LJ, et al. [Study on the prognostic value of hepatocyte growth factor and c-met for patients with hepatocellular carcinoma]. Zhonghua Wai Ke Za Zhi 2006; 44: 603-608

[89] Ijichi M, Takayama T, Matsumura M, et al. Alpha-fetoprotein mRNA in the circulation as a predictor of postsurgical recurrence of hepatocellular carcinoma: A prospective study. Hepatology 2002; 35: 853-860

[90] Singhal A, Jayaraman M, Dhanasekaran DN, et al. Molecular and serum markers in hepatocellular carcinoma: Predictive tools for prognosis and recurrence. Crit Rev Oncol Hematol 2012; 82: 116-140

[91] Han GQ, Qin CY, Shu RH. The analysis of gamma-glutamyl transpeptidase gene in different type liver tissues. World J Gastroenterol 2003; 9: 276-280

[92] Han GQ, Qin CY, Ren WH, et al. [Clinical impact of gamma-glutamyl transpeptidase messenger RNA subtypes on early diagnosis of hepatocellular carcinoma]. Ai Zheng 2002; 21: 192-195

[93] Tsutsumi M, Sakamuro D, Takada A, et al. Detection of a unique gamma-glutamyl transpeptidase messenger RNA species closely related to the development of hepatocellular carcinoma in humans: A new candidate for early diagnosis of hepatocellular carcinoma. Hepatology 1996; 23: 1093-1097

[94] Sheen IS, Jeng KS, Tsai YC. Is the expression of gamma-glutamyl transpeptidase messenger RNA an indicator of biological behavior in recurrent hepatocellular carcinoma? World J Gastroenterol 2003; 9: 468-473

[95] Wang J, Sen S. MicroRNA functional network in pancreatic cancer: From biology to biomarkers of disease. J Biosci 2011; 36: 481-491

[96] Tomimaru Y, Eguchi H, Nagano H, et al. Circulating microRNA-21 as a novel biomarker for hepatocellular carcinoma. J Hepatol 2012; 56: 167-175

[97] Liu AM, Yao TJ, Wang W, et al. Circulating miR-15b and miR-130b in serum as potential markers for detecting hepatocellular carcinoma: A retrospective cohort study. BMJ Open 2012; 2: e000825

[98] Zhou J, Yu L, Gao X, et al. Plasma microRNA panel to diagnose hepatitis B virus-related hepatocellular carcinoma. J Clin Oncol 2011; 29: 4781-4788

[99] Xiong Y, Fang JH, Yun JP, et al. Effects of microRNA-29 on apoptosis, tumorigenicity, and prognosis of hepatocellular carcinoma. Hepatology 2010; 51: 836-845

[100] Abdalla MA, Haj-Ahmad Y. Promising candidate urinary MicroRNA biomarkers for the early detection of hepatocellular carcinoma among high-risk hepatitis C virus Egyptian patients. J Cancer 2012; 3: 19-31

[101] Hauptman N, Glavač D. Long non-coding RNA in cancer. Int J Mol Sci 2013; 14: 4655-4669

[102] Ma W, Wang H, Jing W, et al. Downregulation of long non-coding RNAs JPX and XIST is associated with the prognosis of hepatocellular carcinoma. Clin Res Hepatol Gastroenterol 2017; 41: 163-170

[103] Yu J, Han J, Zhang J, et al. The long noncoding RNAs PVT1 and uc002mbe.2 in sera provide a new supplementary method for hepatocellular carcinoma diagnosis. Medicine (Baltimore) 2016; 95: e4436

[104] Wang Z, Jiang Y, Guan D, et al. Critical roles of p53 in epithelial-mesenchymal transition and metastasis of hepatocellular carcinoma cells. PLoS One 2013; 8: e72846

[105] Ierardi E, Rosania R, Zotti M, et al. From chronic liver disorders to hepatocellular carcinoma: Molecular and genetic pathways. World J Gastrointest Oncol 2010; 2: 259-264

[106] Kirk GD, Lesi OA, Mendy M, et al. 249(ser) TP53 mutation in plasma DNA, hepatitis B viral infection, and risk of hepatocellular carcinoma. Oncogene 2005; 24: 5858-5867

[107] Teufel A, Staib F, Kanzler S, et al. Genetics of hepatocellular carcinoma. World J Gastroenterol 2007; 13: 2271-2282

[108] Nogueira JA, Ono-Nita SK, Nita ME, et al. 249 TP53 mutation has high prevalence and is correlated with larger and poorly differentiated HCC in Brazilian patients. BMC Cancer 2009; 9: 204

[109] El-Din HG, Ghafar NA, Saad NE, et al. Relationship between codon 249 mutation in exon 7 of p53 gene and diagnosis of hepatocellular carcinoma. Arch Med Sci 2010; 6: 348-355

[110] Cleary SP, Jeck WR, Zhao X, et al. Identification of driver genes in hepatocellular carcinoma by exome sequencing. Hepatology 2013; 58: 1693-1702

[111] Liu J, Ma Q, Zhang M, et al. Alterations of TP53 are associated with a poor outcome for patients with hepatocellular carcinoma: Evidence from a systematic review and meta-analysis. Eur J Cancer 2012; 48: 2328-2338

[112] Zhan P, Ji YN, Yu LK. TP53 mutation is associated with a poor outcome for patients with hepatocellular carcinoma: Evidence from a meta-analysis. Hepatobiliary Surg Nutr 2013; 2: 260-265

[113] Amaddeo G, Cao Q, Ladeiro Y, et al. Integration of tumour and viral genomic characterizations in HBV-related hepatocellular carcinomas. 2015; 64: 820-829

[114] Bell RJ, Rube HT, Kreig A, et al. Cancer. The transcription factor GABP selectively binds and activates the mutant TERT promoter in cancer. Science 2015; 348: 1036-1039

[115] Akincilar SC, Unal B, Tergaonkar V. Reactivation of telomerase in cancer. Cell Mol Life Sci 2016; 73: 1659-1670

[116] Villanueva A. Hepatocellular Carcinoma. New England Journal of Medicine 2019; 380: 1450-1462

[117] Huang DS, Wang Z, He XJ, et al. Recurrent TERT promoter mutations identified in a large-scale study of multiple tumour types are associated with increased TERT expression and

telomerase activation. Eur J Cancer 2015; 51: 969-976

[118] Nault JC, Calderaro J, Di Tommaso L, et al. Telomerase reverse transcriptase promoter mutation is an early somatic genetic alteration in the transformation of premalignant nodules in hepatocellular carcinoma on cirrhosis. Hepatology 2014; 60: 1983-1992

[119] Yang X, Guo X, Chen Y, et al. Telomerase reverse transcriptase promoter mutations in hepatitis B virus-associated hepatocellular carcinoma. Oncotarget 2016; 7: 27838-27847

[120] Zhu AX, Chen D, He W, et al. Integrative biomarker analyses indicate etiological variations in hepatocellular carcinoma. J Hepatol 2016; 65: 296-304

[121] Abe H, Hayashi A, Kunita A, et al. Altered expression of AT-rich interactive domain 1A in hepatocellular carcinoma. Int J Clin Exp Pathol 2015; 8: 2763-2770

[122] Tischoff I, Tannapfe A. DNA methylation in hepatocellular carcinoma. World J Gastroenterol 2008; 14: 1741-1748

[123] Nagai M, Nakamura A, Makino R, et al. Expression of DNA (5-cytosin)-methyltransferases (DNMTs) in hepatocellular carcinomas. Hepatol Res 2003; 26: 186-191

[124] Esteller M, Corn PG, Baylin SB, et al. A gene hypermethylation profile of human cancer. Cancer Res 2001; 61: 3225-3229

[125] Yu J, Zhang HY, Ma ZZ, et al. Methylation profiling of twenty four genes and the concordant methylation behaviours of nineteen genes that may contribute to hepatocellular carcinogenesis. Cell Res 2003; 13: 319-333

[126] Katoh H, Shibata T, Kokubu A, et al. Epigenetic instability and chromosomal instability in hepatocellular carcinoma. Am J Pathol 2006; 168: 1375-1384

[127] Zhu R, Li BZ, Li H, et al. Association of p16INK4A hypermethylation with hepatitis B virus X protein expression in the early stage of HBV-associated hepatocarcinogenesis. Pathol Int 2007; 57: 328-336

[128] Lin Q, Chen L-b, Tang Y-m, et al. Promoter hypermethylation of p16 gene and DAPK gene in sera from hepatocellular carcinoma (HCC) patients. Chinese Journal of Cancer Research 2005; 17: 250-254

[129] Zang JJ, Xie F, Xu JF, et al. P16 gene hypermethylation and hepatocellular carcinoma: A systematic review and meta-analysis. World J Gastroenterol 2011; 17: 3043-3048

[130] Pasha HF, Mohamed RH, Radwan MI. RASSF1A and SOCS1 genes methylation status as a noninvasive marker for hepatocellular carcinoma. Cancer Biomark 2019; 24: 241-247

[131] Laborde E. Glutathione transferases as mediators of signaling pathways involved in cell proliferation and cell death. Cell Death Differ 2010; 17: 1373-1380

[132] Lee S, Lee HJ, Kim JH, et al. Aberrant CpG island hypermethylation along multistep hepatocarcinogenesis. Am J Pathol 2003; 163: 1371-1378

[133] Tsutsui M, Iizuka N, Moribe T, et al. Methylated cyclin D2 gene circulating in the blood as a prognosis predictor of hepatocellular carcinoma. Clin Chim Acta 2010; 411: 516-520

[134] Yeo W, Wong N, Wong WL, et al. High frequency of promoter hypermethylation of RASSF1A in tumor

and plasma of patients with hepatocellular carcinoma. Liver Int 2005; 25: 266-272

[135] Chan KCA, Lai PBS, Mok TSK, et al. Quantitative analysis of circulating methylated DNA as a biomarker for hepatocellular carcinoma. Clinical Chemistry 2008; 54: 1528-1536

[136] Huang ZH, Hu Y, Hua D, et al. Quantitative analysis of multiple methylated genes in plasma for the diagnosis and prognosis of hepatocellular carcinoma. Exp Mol Pathol 2011; 91: 702-707

Chapter 6

Classification of Hepatocellular Carcinoma Using Machine Learning

Lekshmi Kalinathan, Deepika Sivasankaran, Janet Reshma Jeyasingh, Amritha Sennappa Sudharsan and Hareni Marimuthu

Abstract

Hepatocellular Carcinoma (HCC) proves to be challenging for detection and classification of its stages mainly due to the lack of disparity between cancerous and non cancerous cells. This work focuses on detecting hepatic cancer stages from histopathology data using machine learning techniques. It aims to develop a prototype which helps the pathologists to deliver a report in a quick manner and detect the stage of the cancer cell. Hence we propose a system to identify and classify HCC based on the features obtained by deep learning using pre-trained models such as VGG-16, ResNet-50, DenseNet-121, InceptionV3, InceptionResNet50 and Xception followed by machine learning using support vector machine (SVM) to learn from these features. The accuracy obtained using the system comprised of DenseNet-121 for feature extraction and SVM for classification gives 82% accuracy.

Keywords: Hepatocellular Carcinoma, Feature extraction, Convolution Neural Networks, Prognosis, Machine Learning

1. Introduction

The existing work on Hepatic tumor is concerned with clinical data acquired through blood samples, urine samples and serum test, and non-invasive images like CT, MRI, PET and SPECT. The manual identification of cancer from microscopic biopsy images is subjective in nature and may vary from expert to expert depending on their expertise and other factors which include lack of specific and accurate quantitative measures to classify the biopsy images as normal or cancerous one. Stains such as Hematoxylin and Eosin (H and E stain) are used for better emphasis of the nuclei of liver cells. Based on the amount of stain absorbed by the nuclei, it can be classified into various types since nuclei size increases with the stages of cancer. The stain can also be accumulated on the tissues causing ambiguity to the pathologist. Such ambiguity in the images can be overlooked by an individual. Color normalization is done to highlight the nuclei for visually better features.

IntechOpen

Normalization techniques discussed in the study [1] where the images are classified by their colors using K Means Clustering and JSEG segmentation In this method, the nuclei get segmented as a separate segment. Then it is passed onto the SVM classifier. This technique enables effective segmentation of colored images. Similarly JSEG segmentation technique has two phases: color quantization and spatial segmentation [2]. Color quantization is based on peer group filtering(PGF) and vector quantization to reduce the number of colors in the images. For addressing the drawbacks of JSEG method, contrast map and improved contrast map were obtained. This technique saw a significant improvement in detecting more homogeneous regions than that of JSEG method. Due to the inherent difficulty involved in obtaining liver cell images from the biopsies, Liangqun et al. proposed to use neural networks for feature extraction and SVM for classification [3]. This method aims at providing better efficiency from less number of images.

The findings of the study [4] demonstrated the capability of Convolutional Neural Network (CNN) to recognize distinct features that can detect tumor masses in a histopathological liver tissue image. The author proposed to implement the CNN model for segmentation and classification of different stages of HCC. However, the major drawback of using CNNs for the feature extraction process is that these models need large amounts of data to process. This is a huge challenge for the biomedical field as it is pragmatically difficult to have access to massive data. Moreover, feature learning is pertinent on the size, shape and degree of annotation of images which are not uniform across datasets.

Chen et al. developed a deep convolutional neural network to classify the lung tumor stage and predict the most commonly mutated genes in lung cancer tissue cells [5]. Ehteshami et al. also produced a promising result for the classification of breast tumors using deep learning techniques [6]. The author developed an algorithm to differentiate stroma invasive cancer and stroma from benign biopsies However, the deep learning models were applied to non solid tumors. Thus, it remains uncertain if they can produce the same accuracy when applied to solid tumors.

2. Proposed methodology

The workflow contains 4 modules as follows:

1. Data collection

2. Color normalization

3. Creation of a classifier

Cancer type	Images
Non cancerous	232
Well-differentiated carcinoma	148
Moderately differentiated carcinoma	81
Poorly differentiated	189
TOTAL	687

Table 1.
HCC dataset split-up.

2.1 Data collection

The first phase involved collection of data from Dataset collected from Global Hospital, Perumbakkam, Chennai. In a span of 3 weeks, images were collected from the biopsies of 3 patients. The three types of cancerous images obtained during the data collection phase are well-differentiated, moderately differentiated and poorly differentiated. The total number of images collected is 687 whose split up is given in **Table 1**.

Below are some images from the dataset collected, **Figures 1–4**.

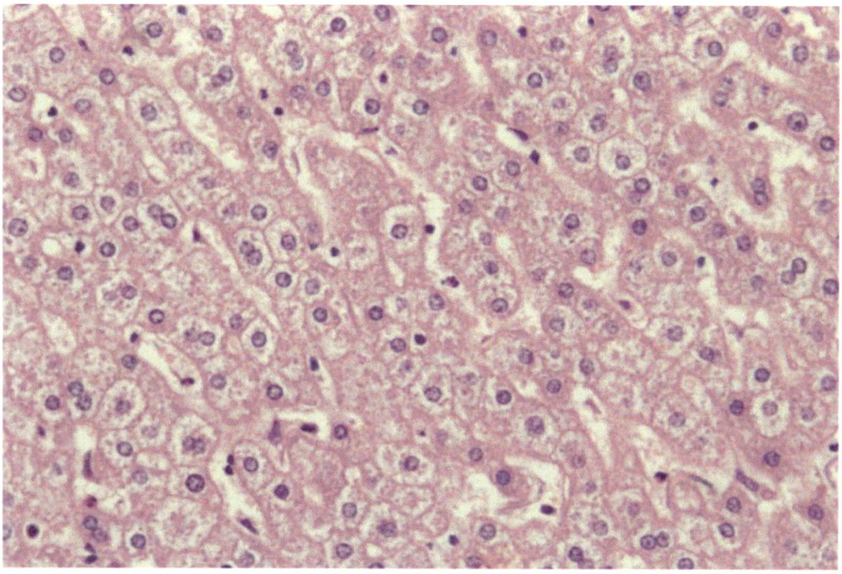

Figure 1.
Non cancerous image.

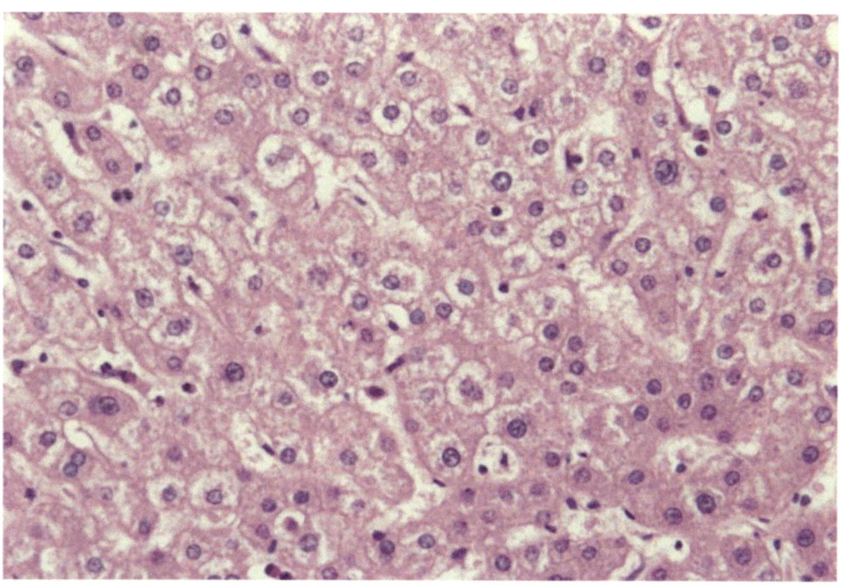

Figure 2.
Well differentiated cancer.

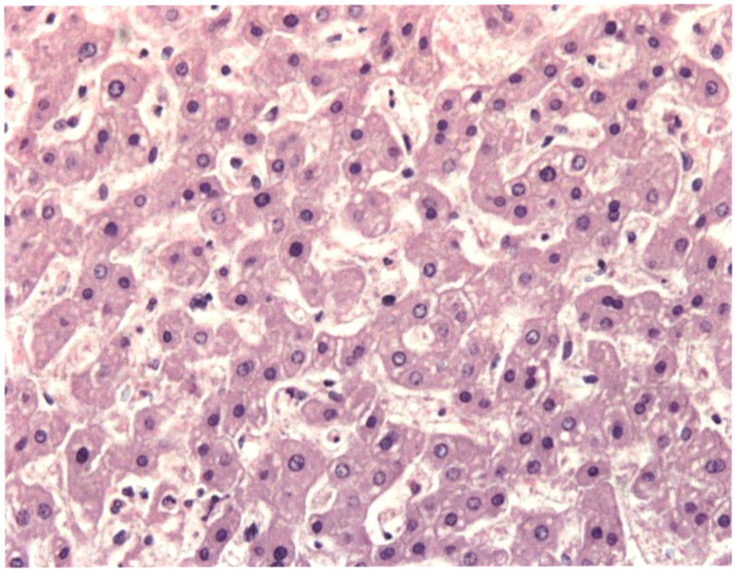

Figure 3.
Moderately differentiated cancer.

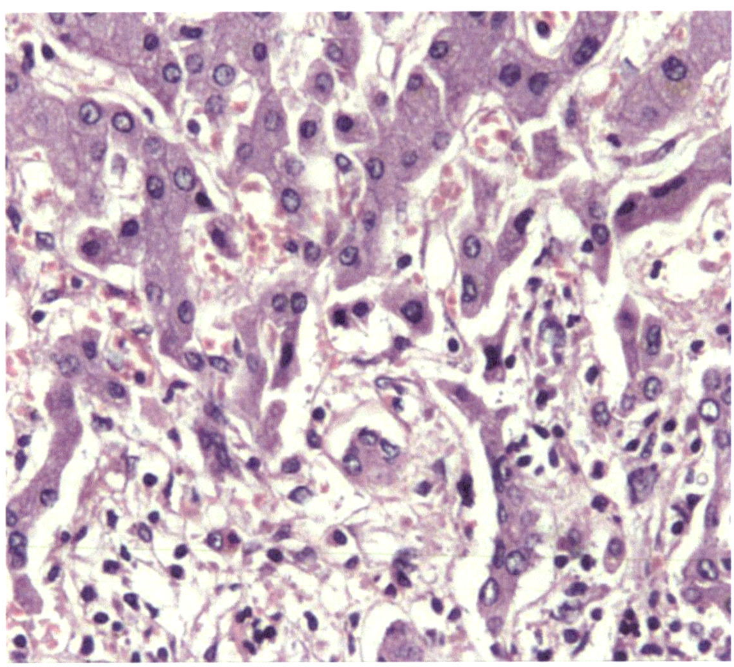

Figure 4.
Poorly differentiated cancer.

2.2 Color normalization

The features of the nuclei include the texture, size and roundness. Applying a stain on these biopsies cause the nuclei to be highlighted due to absorption of the stain. The color difference between the nuclei and the tissues may be visually comparable or less different. Hence, color normalization is done to highlight the nuclei. Highlighting the nuclei makes it easier to extract the features from them.

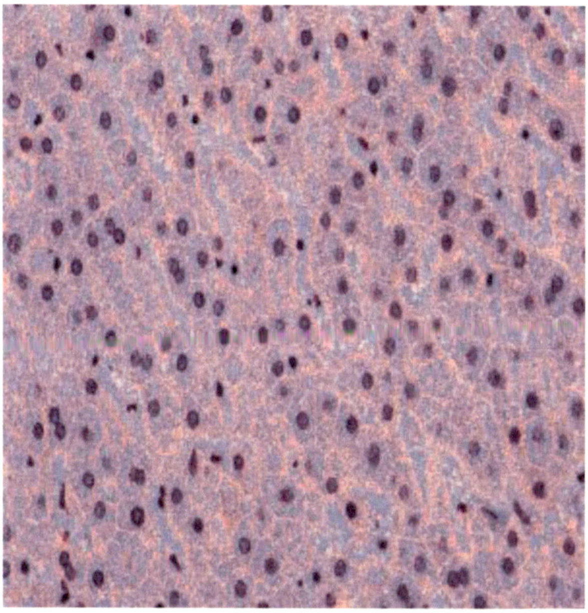

Figure 5.
Normalized non cancerous image.

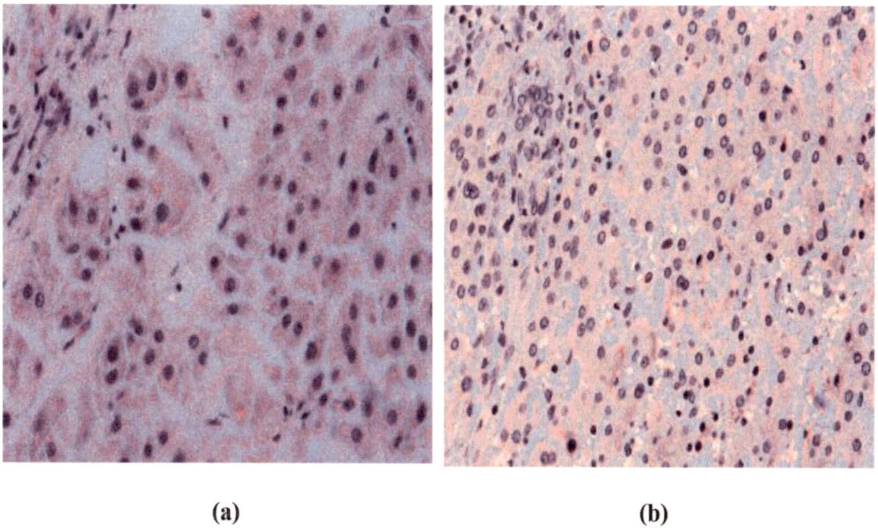

Figure 6.
(a), (b) normalized cancerous images.

The normalization method [3] is exclusive to H and E stain. Normalized images are shown below (**Figures 5** and **6**).

2.3 Creation of a classification system

Using convolution neural networks (CNN) can be less efficient in creating a classifier system mainly due to its requirement of a large dataset to learn from. Using CNN is not a very practical approach as it may not be feasible to collect a dataset containing large numbers of images. Thus an alternative method is proposed where features are extracted from the images using unsupervised deep learning and then a supervised machine learning classifier is used to learn from those features for classification. The advantage of this method is the elimination of overfitting of the class with majority data and the system can work fairly well with less number of images. Using a support vector machine (SVM) the classifier is built and pretrained models such as VGG-16, ResNet50, DenseNet –121, DenseNet –169, DenseNet-201, InceptionV3, InceptionResNet50 and Xception.

3. Performance analysis

To select the best feature extractor from all the pretrained models, metrics such as F1- score and accuracy are considered. Higher accuracies may not be the most efficient and reliable metric always. Hence, F1-score is also considered as it shows individual class performance and is useful when the dataset is highly imbalanced. **Table 2** shows the overall accuracies obtained when all the pretrained models are used.

From **Table 2**, it is found that performance of DenseNet is better than the other deep learning architectures. The performance of the variants of DenseNet is given in **Table 3**. Here it is observed that with the increase in the number of layers of DenseNet from 121 to 201, there is a degradation in the accuracy. Hence, the F1 score is also affected.

S. no	Model	Accuracy (%)
1	Xception	72
2	VGG16	78
3	ResNet50	80
4	InceptionV3	74
4	InceptionResNetV2	45
5	DenseNet	85

Table 2.
Performance of various pretrained models with SVM.

S. no	Model	Accuracy (%)
1	DenseNet –121	82
2	DenseNet –169	84
3	DenseNet –201	81

Table 3.
Performance of DenseNet variants.

S. no	Classifier	Accuracy (%)
1	DenseNet –121 + SVM	82
2	DenseNet –121 + Naive Bayes	70
3	DenseNet –121 + Decision Tree	61

Table 4.
Performance of DenseNet –121 with the classifiers.

Class	Precision	Recall	F1-score	Support
Non cancerous	0.79	0.83	0.81	69
Well-differentiated cancer	0.86	0.81	0.83	37
Moderately differentiated cancer	0.58	0.67	0.62	21
Poorly differentiated cancer	0.97	0.88	0.93	42
Accuracy			0.82	169
Macro average	0.80	0.80	0.80	169
Weighted Average	0.83	0.82	0.82	169

Table 5.
Performance of DenseNet −121 with SVM.

The final pretrained architecture selected for feature extraction is DenseNet −121 to be combined with the machine learning classifiers. Supervised algorithms such as decision tree, SVM, Naive bayes were taken into consideration to find the optimal classifier. The results of the feature extractor and classifier are given in **Table 4**. From **Table 4**, SVM is chosen to be the optimal classifier that works best with DenseNet −121 feature extractor.

DenseNet-121 is chosen due to high f1-score in spite of having less accuracy than DenseNet-169. Performance analysis of DenseNet-121 is given in **Table 5**.

4. Conclusions and future work

From the results obtained, it is observed that this method can provide better accuracy although the dataset is highly imbalanced and when there is a deficit in the dataset. Using convolution neural networks (CNN) can underperform when the dataset is imbalanced and it requires an extensive dataset to learn from. Improvements can be made by obtaining more data. Procuring more images from biopsies and medical data will help improve the system's efficiency and this can be extended as a separate component for the microscope.

Author details

Lekshmi Kalinathan*, Deepika Sivasankaran, Janet Reshma Jeyasingh, Amritha Sennappa Sudharsan and Hareni Marimuthu
Department of Computer Science and Engineering, Sri Sivasubramaniya Nadar College of Engineering, Chennai, India

*Address all correspondence to: lekshmik@ssn.edu.in

References

[1] Himanshu Yadav, Prateek Bansalt and Ramesh Kumar Sunkaria, Color Dependent K-Means Clustering for Color Image Segmentation of Colored Medical Images, 1st International Conference on Next Generation Computing Technologies (NGCT-2015), 2015

[2] Yu-Chou Chang, Dah-Jye Lee, Yong-Gang Wang, Color-Texture Segmentation of Medical Images Based on Local Contrast Information, IEEE Symposium on Computational Intelligence in Bioinformatics and Computational Biology (CIBCB), (2007).

[3] Liangqun Lu and Bernie J. Daigle, Jr. (2020). Prognostic analysis of histopathological images using pre-trained convolutional neural networks: application to hepatocellular carcinoma, PeerJ, doi 10.7717/peerj.8668

[4] Azer, Samy A. (2019) "Deep learning with convolutional neural networks for identification of liver masses and hepatocellular carcinoma: A systematic review." *World journal of gastrointestinal oncology* vol. 11,12: 1218-1230. doi:10.4251/wjgo.v11.i12.1218

[5] Chen, Mingyu & Zhang, Bin & Topatana, Win & Cao, Jiasheng & Zhu, Hepan & Juengpanich, Sarun & Mao, Qijiang & Yu, Hong & Cai, Xiujun. (2020). Classification and mutation prediction based on histopathology H&E images in liver cancer using deep learning. npj Precision Oncology. 4. 14. 10.1038/s41698-020-0120-3.

[6] Ehteshami Bejnordi, B. et al. (2018) Using deep convolutional neural networks to identify and classify tumor-associated stroma in diagnostic breast biopsies. Mod. Pathol. 31, 1502-1512.

Section 3

Treatment of Hepatocellular Carcinoma

Chapter 7

Minimally Invasive Surgery for Hepatocellular Carcinoma; Latest Advances

Alexandros Giakoustidis, Apostolos Koffas, Dimitrios Giakoustidis and Vasileios N. Papadopoulos

Abstract

Surgical resection is the gold standard for hepatocellular carcinoma management for early stages of the disease. With advances in technology and techniques, minimally invasive surgery provides a great number of advantages for these patients during their surgery and for their post-operative care. The selection of patients following a multi-disciplinary approach is of paramount importance. Adding to this, the developments in laparoscopic instruments and training, as well as the promising advantages of robotic surgery along with other forms of technology, increase the pool of patients that can undergo operation safely and with good results worldwide. We review results from great centres worldwide and delineate the accurate multidisciplinary approach for this.

Keywords: laparoscopic, robotic, minimally invasive surgery, hepatocellular carcinoma

1. Introduction

Liver cancer is the 5th most common cancer and the second most frequent cause of cancer-related death globally, with 854,000 new diagnoses and 810,000 deaths per year [1, 2]. Hepatocellular carcinoma (HCC) accounts for approximately 90% of liver cancers and is generally associated with an unfavorable prognosis, with a 5-year overall survival (OS) of 10–15%, mostly due to a delay in establishing an early diagnosis. In case HCC is diagnosed at an earlier stage, the 5-year OS improves and may reach 70%, amid the possibility of curative treatments, such as liver resection (LR), liver transplantation (LT) and ablation [3, 4].

2. Minimally invasive surgery for HCC

2.1 Staging systems and treatment allocation

Once diagnosed, prognostication is pivotal in the management of HCC. Disease staging and classification is intended to assess prognosis and determine treatment candidacy. In patients with HCC, the co-existence of two life-threatening conditions, i.e., cancer and cirrhosis, needs to be tackled with, and further complicates prognostic assessment [5, 6]. The 2018 European Association for the Study of the Liver (EASL) clinical practice guidelines endorsed the Barcelona Clinic Liver Cancer (BCLC) classification [7], as did the recent American Association for the Study of Liver Diseases (AASLD) guidance [3]. According to the BCLC classification system, patients are classified into five stages (0, A, B, C and D) according to pre-established prognostic variables. These variables comprise tumor characteristics (size, number, vascular invasion, lymph node involvement, distant metastases), liver function (bilirubin, portal hypertension, liver function preservation) and patient's health status (ECOG).

2.2 Liver resection

Determining eligibility for LR involves assessment of the tumor burden; assessment of liver function; the extent of hepatectomy and the expected volume of the future liver remnant; and the presence of portal hypertension and other co-morbidities. Liver function is objectively estimated by the Child-Pugh score and patients with Child-Pugh B or C are deemed at a high risk of liver failure following LR, even after a minor resection. More recently, the model for end-stage liver disease (MELD) score was integrated into the EASL guidelines for treatment allocation [7, 8]. The absence of cirrhosis allows for larger and more complex resections, and is associated with viable postoperative mortality and morbidity, even after major hepatic resection, with a 5-year OS of 50% [9–13]. Conversely, clinically significant portal hypertension (CSPH), defined as HVPG >10 mmHg, is a well-established predictor of liver decompensation and death after LR [14–18].

Surgery represents the backbone of HCC treatment, resulting in the best outcomes in appropriately-selected candidates. LR and LT represent the first-line treatment in individuals with early-stage tumors on an intention-to-cure perspective. In particular, the latest EASL guidance recommends LR in cases of a resectable solitary nodule without macrovascular invasion and extrahepatic spread, regardless of size [7, 19]. The AASLD guidelines advocate LR in patients with Child-Pugh A compensated cirrhosis and resectable HCC, i.e., solitary tumor <5 cm with or without vascular invasion, or multifocal tumor <5 cm [3]. Finally, the Asian Pacific Association for the Study of the Liver (APASL) recommends that all tumors without extrahepatic spread may be considered for LR, regardless of vascular invasion, number and size of lesions [4].

2.3 A laparoscopic approach

The advent of laparoscopic techniques transformed the treatment landscape of HCC. In spite of the relative paucity of prospective randomized studies, the laparoscopic approach appears to convey similar oncological outcomes with respect to conventional surgery [20]. Laparoscopic LR allows the preservation of the abdominal wall, minimizes peritoneal trauma, and is associated with fewer complications in comparison with open surgery, including both overall and liver-related complications, as also shown in a recent meta-analysis including 6,812 patients. Additionally, no differences in operative time, blood loss, intraoperative complications, hospital stay, and morbidity were found in laparoscopic LR for cirrhotics in comparison with non-cirrhotics [21–28]. Several studies demonstrated that minimally-invasive surgical techniques in patients with cirrhosis are associated with reduced risk of post-operative hepatic decompensation and liver failure [29–31]. Interestingly, this technique also appears safe in the elderly, even for a major hepatectomy, and is associated with improved outcomes [32–36]. One should bear in mind though that laparoscopic hepatectomy should be carried out in specialist centres and following appropriate training and education of all team members involved. The importance of this factor is highlighted as the keys to successful LR include technical mastering of laparoscopic hepatic portal occlusion which can be more challenging than in laparotomy, and the lack of operational feel and need for rapid reactive mode as well as accurate hemostasis.

In light of the above, EASL 2018 clinical practice guidelines recommend laparoscopic LR for HCC resection in expert centres and for selected surgical candidates [7]. Similarly, the AASLD also recognizes the advantages of laparoscopic techniques in selected scenarios [3]. EASL recommends [7] that tumor size and location should determine optimal surgical approach. In particular, laparoscopic-robotic LR for HCC may be considered for tumors located in superficial peripheral positions of the liver; and is associated with optimal survival outcomes, low complication rate and reduced inpatient time. Minimally-invasive LR can be an effective option in very early (≤2 cm) and early HCC. Ablation represents still the treatment modality of choice for this disease stage, owing to the higher cost-effectiveness [16] and to milder liver function impact. However, several studies report that patients treated with minimally-invasive LR for such tumors, mainly located in superficial or antero-lateral positions, suffer less adverse outcomes and shorter hospitalization, in comparison with conventional open techniques, while achieving competitive oncologic results with respect to ablation [37–40].

Limited resections conducted via laparoscopic LR may also be considered for curative resection in selected patients with HCC with a borderline liver profile (i.e., Child Pugh B7, moderate portal hypertension and/or bilirubin around 2 mg/dl), especially in specialized centres [7]. A study reported that patients with Child-Pugh A and Child-Pugh B/C cirrhosis who underwent laparoscopic LR had a similar perioperative course [26]. Laparoscopic LR has also been explored as an option for patients with CSPH. A recent study by Lim *et al* assessed the short-term outcomes in patients with and without CSPH [41]. Although broadening eligibility criteria for minimally-invasive techniques would increase the rate LR, morbidity and hospital stay would be a significant concern for patients with CSPH. In light of the above, LT remains the gold standard in cases of HCC and advanced liver disease. Nevertheless, the laparoscopic approach may be beneficial prior to LT for HCC, with significantly reduced de-listing and death after LT when prior LR was performed laparoscopically [42]. Whether laparoscopic LR should also be considered in patients with HCC and CSPH not eligible for LT, will need to be addressed with further studies. Lastly, the safety and feasibility of laparoscopic major hepatectomy has been reported after sequential transarterial chemoembolization (TACE), which is classically associated with increased surgical difficulty [43]. Additionally, laparoscopic LR can be applied in living donor liver transplantation (LDLT) in centres with extensive experience in both laparoscopic LR and open LDLT.

2.4 Robotic liver surgery

Similar to laparoscopic LR, robotic LR is also emerging as an interesting minimally-invasive surgical technique, demonstrating a relative safe profile and allowing for an easier access to hepatic segments not amenable to laparoscopic approach, such as posterior sectionectomies and resection of tumors located in superior segments 4a and 8 [44]. The development of minimally invasive surgical techniques for liver tumors is in general limited by the characteristics of the liver itself, such as its texture, abundant blood supply, an increased number of structural variations of blood vessels and bile ducts.

A recent literature review including 10 studies on robotic liver resection for HCC (with a total of 302 patients) reported disease-free (DFS) and OS at 2 years of 72–84% and 94–98%, respectively [44]. It has also been proposed that a robotic approach may also improve the access to the abdomen in cases of recurrent disease with potential requirement of LT, expanding the opportunities of both down-staging and bridging strategies [45]. The broad use of the robotic approach, however, is limited due to several factors, most importantly the cost of the robotic surgical devices compared to laparoscopic equipment. Several analyses on costs of robotic surgery have been reported, with controversial findings regarding the balance between costs and benefits [46–51]. With regard to instrumentation, the lack of an efficient robotic transection device such as the Ultasonographic Aspirator (UA) is the most important limitation of robotic liver surgery. Another limitation would be the spatial distance between the operating and robotic platform and its considerable size, making undocking and gaining access to the patient particularly challenging in emergency scenarios [52, 53]. Lastly, a non-negligible obstacle of robotic surgery is the operative time, that is in the majority longer in comparison with other surgical approaches. In view of the above, robotic LR needs to be better evaluated before being integrated into routine clinical practice and therapeutic algorithms. On the other hand, however, robotic LR can overcome certain traditional laparoscopic liver resection limitations like the inflexible fixation of the operating instruments as well as visual result [54]. The Robotic System appears superior in regard to these limitations and there are constant developments in the field as per instruments applied crucial to LR. At present, the Da Vinci Robotic surgical assistant system is in use in several centres for both benign and malignant liver diseases with similar indications applied as per the laparoscopic LR, and in certain cases demonstrating a more advantageous nature [55].

2.5 Cost of minimally invasive surgery

The results so far comparing robotic to laparoscopic and open LR are conflicting as per the cost effect to the institution hosting them. A single institution retrospective study from the University of Washington compared cost data for 71 robotic LR to 88 open procedures and reported that although there were higher perioperative costs for the robotic procedures, the postoperative costs and subsequent direct hospital costs were lower when compared with open procedures, attributing this possibly to a 2-day shorter hospital stay on average after robotic procedures [56]. On the other hand other studies have demonstrated a higher cost for robotic LR when compared to both laparoscopic and open procedures although in some the trend of less hospital stay was in favor of the robotic procedures [57–59].

2.6 Emerging technologies

Recent advances in liver surgery from a technological aspect include near-infrared fluorescent (NIF) imaging applied intra-operatively. NIF imaging has been set in use in several laparoscopic and robotic camera systems enabling the identification of various dyes, such as indocyanine green, injected preoperatively. Indocyanine green is a green dye that is preferentially metabolized by hepatocytes and excreted in the biliary tree and it lights up the biliary tree. Its use has been utilized for robotic and laparoscopic assisted cholecystectomy. It has also been more recently applied for a more accurate parenchymal dissection following vascular control by identifying perfused from poorly perfused hepatic parenchyma [60].

Future advances of robotic liver surgery include the application of preoperative planning with virtual reality (VR) models and real-time augmented reality (AR) intra- operative endoscopic overlays to assist with surgical navigation on *da Vinci* ® surgical systems. Computer-based three-dimensional (3D) reconstructions of liver tumors have been shown to benefit the accuracy of tumor localization and precision of operative planning for liver surgery [61, 62]. Intraoperative Ultrasound is routinely used for real-time identification of liver tumors both in open and minimally invasive LR. However, with AR being developed to overlay accurate 3D reconstruction data onto the operative field itself, it can potentially eliminate the need to divert the attention from the operative field and to translate the 2D images into a 3D construct.

3. Conclusions

With the constant evolution of technology, it would be without a doubt that surgery techniques in terms of access and instrument implementation would evolve as well. Laparoscopic liver surgery appears to have gained considerable ground especially in centres where liver surgery and laparoscopic expertise co-exist. The robotic approach is still quite variable between institutions, as well as between countries and continents. Thus one can only anticipate for advances in minimally invasive surgery to continue as long as there are specialized liver centres aiming to increase patient volume undergoing surgery and decrease hospital stay, complications rates and in general offer the best possible liver service.

Conflict of interest

"The authors declare no conflict of interest."

Author details

Alexandros Giakoustidis[1]*, Apostolos Koffas[2], Dimitrios Giakoustidis[1] and Vasileios N. Papadopoulos[1]

1 Faculty of Medical Sciences, A' Department of Surgery, General Hospital Papageorgiou, School of Medicine, Aristotle University Thessaloniki, Thessaloniki, Greece

2 Department of Gastroenterology, General University Hospital of Larisa, Larisa, Greece

*Address all correspondence to: alexgiakoustidis@gmail.com

References

[1] Akinyemiju T, Abera S, Ahmed M, Alam N, Alemayohu MA, Allen C, et al. The burden of primary liver cancer and underlying etiologies from 1990 to 2015 at the global, regional, and national level. JAMA Oncol 2017;3:1683-1691.

[2] Fact Sheets by Population-Globocan-IARC n.d. http://globocan.iarc.fr/Pages/fact_sheets_population.aspx (accessed December 18, 2017)

[3] Marrero JA, Kulik LM, Sirlin CB, Zhu AX, Finn RS, Abecassis MM, et al. Diagnosis, staging, and management of hepatocellular carcinoma: 2018 practice guidance by the American Association for the Study of Liver Diseases. Hepatology 2018;68(2):723-750.

[4] Omata M, Cheng AL, Kokudo N, Kudo M, Lee JM, Jia J, et al. Asia-Pacific clinical practice guidelines on the management of hepatocellular carcinoma: a 2017 update. Hepatol Int 2017;11(4):317-370.

[5] Setiawan VW, Wilkens LR, Lu SC, Hernandez BY, Le Marchand L, Henderson BE. Association of coffee intake with reduced incidence of liver cancer and death from chronic liver disease in the US multiethnic cohort. Gastroenterology 2015;148:118-25; quiz e15.

[6] Sorrentino P, Tarantino L, D'Angelo S, Terracciano L, Ferbo U, Bracigliano A, et al. Validation of an extension of the international non-invasive criteria for the diagnosis of hepatocellular carcinoma to the characterization of macroscopic portal vein thrombosis. J Gastroenterol Hepatol 2011;26:669-677.

[7] European Association for the Study of the Liver. EASL Clinical Practice Guidelines: Management of hepatocellular carcinoma. J Hepatol . 2018 Jul;69(1):182-236. doi: 10.1016/j.jhep.2018.03.019.

[8] Vitale A, Burra P, Frigo AC, Trevisani F, Farinati F, Spolverato G, et al. Survival benefit of liver resection for patients with hepatocellular carcinoma across different Barcelona Clinic Liver Cancer stages: a multicentre study. J Hepatol 2015;62(3):617-624.

[9] Smoot RL, Nagorney DM, Chandan VS, Que FG, Schleck CD, Harmsen WS, et al. Resection of hepatocellular carcinoma in patients without cirrhosis. Br J Surg 2011;98(5):697-703.

[10] Thelen A, Benckert C, Tautenhahn HM, Hau HM, Bartels M, Linnemann J, et al. Liver resection for hepatocellular carcinoma in patients without cirrhosis. Br J Surg 2013;100(1):130-137.

[11] Lewis RH, Glazer ES, Bittenbinder DM, O'Brien T, Deneve JL, Shibata D, et al. Outcomes following resection of hepatocellular carcinoma in the absence of cirrhosis. J Gastrointest Cancer 2019;50(4):808-815.

[12] Lang H, Sotiropoulos GC, Dömland M, Frühauf NR, Paul A, Hüsing J, et al. Liver resection for hepatocellular carcinoma in non-cirrhotic liver without underlying viral hepatitis. Br J Surg 2005;92(2):198-202.

[13] Llovet JM, Fuster J, Bruix J. Intention-to-treat analysis of surgical treatment for early hepatocellular carcinoma: resection versus transplantation. Hepatology 1999;30(6):1434-1440

[14] de Franchis R, Faculty BV. Revising consensus in portal hypertension: report of the Baveno V consensus workshop on methodology of diagnosis and therapy in portal hypertension. J Hepatol 2010;53(4):762-768.

[15] Ishizawa T, Hasegawa K, Aoki T, Takahashi M, Inoue Y, Sano K, et al.

Neither multiple tumors nor portal hypertension are surgical contraindications for hepatocellular carcinoma. Gastroenterology 2008;134(7):1908-1916.

[16] Cucchetti A, Piscaglia F, Cescon M, Ercolani G, Terzi E, Bolondi L, et al. Conditional survival after hepatic resection for hepatocellular carcinoma in cirrhotic patients. Clin Cancer Res 2012;18(16):4397-4405.

[17] Roayaie S, Jibara G, Tabrizian P, Park J-W, Yang J, Yan L, et al. The role of hepatic resection in the treatment of hepatocellular cancer. Hepatology 2015;62(2):440-451.

[18] Berzigotti A, Reig M, Abraldes JG, Bosch J, Bruix J. Portal hypertension and the outcome of surgery for hepatocellular carcinoma in compensated cirrhosis: a systematic review and meta-analysis. Hepatology 2015;61:526-536.

[19] European Association for the Study of the Liver, European Organisation for Research and Treatment of Cancer. EASL-EORTC clinical practice guidelines: management of hepatocellular carcinoma. J Hepatol 2012;56(4):908-943.

[20] Goumard C, Farges O, Laurent A, Cherqui D, Soubrane O, Gayet B, et al. An update on laparoscopic liver resection: the French Hepato-Bilio-Pancreatic Surgery Association statement. J Visc Surg 2015;152(2):107-112.

[21] Cherqui D, Laurent A, Tayar C, Chang S, Van Nhieu JT, Loriau J, et al. Laparoscopic liver resection for peripheral hepatocellular carcinoma in patients with chronic liver disease: midterm results and perspectives. Ann Surg 2006;243(4):499-506.

[22] Sarpel U, Hefti MM, Wisnievsky JP, Roayaie S, Schwartz ME, Labow DM. Outcome for patients treated with laparoscopic versus open resection of hepatocellular carcinoma: case-matched analysis. Ann Surg Oncol 2009;16(6):1572-1577.

[23] Nguyen KT, Marsh JW, Tsung A, Steel JJL, Gamblin TC, Geller DA. Comparative benefits of laparoscopic vs open hepatic resection: a critical appraisal. Arch Surg 2011;146(3):348-356.

[24] Kasai M, Cipriani F, Gayet B, Aldrighetti L, Ratti F, Sarmiento JM, et al. Laparoscopic versus open major hepatectomy: a systematic review and meta-analysis of individual patient data. Surgery 2018;163(5):985-995.

[25] Di Sandro S, Danieli M, Ferla F, Lauterio A, De Carlis R, Benuzzi L, et al. The current role of laparoscopic resection for HCC: a systematic review of past ten years. Transl Gastroenterol Hepatol 2018;3:68.

[26] Morise Z, Sugioka A, Kawabe N, Umemoto S, Nagata H, Ohshima H, et al. Pure laparoscopic hepatectomy for hepatocellular carcinoma patients with severe liver cirrhosis. Asian J Endosc Surg 2011;4(3):143-146.

[27] Xiangfei M, Yinzhe X, Yingwei P, Shichun L, Weidong D. Open versus laparoscopic hepatic resection for hepatocellular carcinoma: a systematic review and meta-analysis. Surg Endosc 2019;33(8):2396-2418.

[28] Abu Hilal M, Aldrighetti L, Dagher I, Edwin B, Troisi RI, Alikhanov R, et al. The Southampton consensus guidelines for laparoscopic liver surgery: from indication to implementation. Ann Surg 2018;268(1):11-18.

[29] Roayaie S, Obeidat K, Sposito C, Mariani L, Bhoori S, Pellegrinelli A, et al. Resection of hepatocellular cancer ≤2 cm: Results from two Western centers. Hepatology 2013;57:1426-1435.

[30] Han H-S, Shehta A, Ahn S, Yoon Y-S, Cho JY, Choi Y. Laparoscopic vs. open liver resection for hepatocellular carcinoma: Case – matched study with propensity score matching. J Hepatol 2015;63:643-650.

[31] Sposito C, Battiston C, Facciorusso A, Mazzola M, Muscara C, Scotti M, et al. Propensity score analysis of outcomes following laparoscopic or open liver resection for hepatocellular carcinoma. Br J Surg 2016;103:871-880.

[32] Amato B, Aprea G, De Rosa D, Milone M, di Domenico L, Amato M, et al. Laparoscopic hepatectomy for HCC in elderly patients: risks and feasibility. Aging Clin Exp Res 2017;29(Suppl 1):179-183.

[33] Nomi T, Hirokawa F, Kaibori M, Ueno M, Tanaka S, Hokuto D, et al. Laparoscopic versus open liver resection for hepatocellular carcinoma in elderly patients: a multi-centre propensity score-based analysis. Surg Endosc 2020;34(2):658-666.

[34] Yu X, Yan YC, Chen G, Yu H. The efficacy and safety of totally laparoscopic hepatectomy for non-cirrhotic hepatocellular carcinoma in the elderly. BMC Surg 2018;18(1):118.

[35] Andert A, Lodewick T, Ulmer TF, Schmeding M, Schöning W, Neumann U, et al. Liver resection in the elderly: a retrospective cohort study of 460 patients - feasible and safe. Int J Surg 2016;28:126-130.

[36] Cauchy F, Fuks D, Nomi T, Dokmak S, Scatton O, Schwarz L, et al. Benefits of laparoscopy in elderly patients requiring major liver resection. J Am Coll Surg 2016;222(2):174-184.e10.

[37] Soubrane O, Goumard C, Laurent A, Tranchart H, Truant S, Gayet B, et al. Laparoscopic resection of hepatocellular carcinoma: a French survey in 351 patients. HPB 2014;16:357-365.

[38] Parks KR, Kuo Y-H, Davis JM, O' Brien B, Hagopian EJ. Laparoscopic vs. open liver resection: a meta-analysis of long-term outcome. HPB (Oxford) 2014;16:109-18.

[39] Morise Z, Ciria R, Cherqui D, Chen K-H, Belli G, Wakabayashi G. Can we expand the indications for laparoscopic liver resection? A systematic review and meta-analysis of laparoscopic liver resection for patients with hepatocellular carcinoma and chronic liver disease. J Hepatobiliary Pancreat Sci 2015;22:342-352.

[40] Takahara T, Wakabayashi G, Beppu T, Aihara A, Hasegawa K, Gotohda N, et al. Long-term and perioperative outcomes of laparoscopic vs. open liver resection for hepatocellular carcinoma with propensity score matching: a multi-institutional Japanese study. J Hepatobiliary Pancreat Sci 2015;22:721-727.

[41] Lim C, Osseis M, Lahat E, Doussot A, Sotirov D, Hemery F, et al. Safety of laparoscopic hepatectomy in patients with hepatocellular carcinoma and portal hypertension: interim analysis of an open prospective study. Surg Endosc 2019;33(3):811-820.

[42] Levi Sandri GB, Lai Q, Ravaioli M, DI Sandro S, Balzano E, Pagano D, et al. The role of salvage transplantation in patients initially treated with open vs minimally invasive liver surgery: an intention-to-treat analysis. Liver Transpl 2020;26(5):878-887.

[43] Goumard C, Komatsu S, Brustia R, Fartoux L, Soubrane O, Scatton O. Technical feasibility and safety of laparoscopic right hepatectomy for hepatocellular carcinoma following sequential TACE-PVE: a comparative study. Surg Endosc 2017;31(5):2340-2349.

[44] Magistri P, Tarantino G, Assirati G, Olivieri T, Catellani B, Guerrini GP, et al.

Robotic liver resection for hepatocellular carcinoma: a systematic review. Int J Med Robot 2019;15(4):e2004.

[45] Magistri P, Olivieri T, Assirati G, Guerrini GP, Ballarin R, Tarantino G, et al. Robotic Liver Resection Expands the Opportunities of Bridging Before Liver Transplantation. Liver Transplant Off Publ Am Assoc Study Liver Dis Int Liver Transplant Soc. 2019 Jul;25(7): 1110-2.

[46] Giulianotti PC, Coratti A, Sbrana F, Addeo P, Bianco FM, Buchs NC, et al. Robotic liver surgery: results for 70 resections. Surgery 2011;149(1) :29-39.

[47] Lai ECH, Yang GPC, Tang CN. Robot-assisted laparoscopic liver resection for hepatocellular carcinoma: short-term outcome. Am J Surg 2013;205(6):697-702.

[48] Chen P-D, Wu C-Y, Hu R-H, Chou W-H, Lai H-S, Liang J-T, et al. Robotic versus open hepatectomy for hepatocellular carcinoma: a matched comparison. Ann Surg Oncol 2017;24(4):1021-1028.

[49] Magistri P, Tarantino G, Guidetti C, Assirati G, Olivieri T, Ballarin R, et al. Laparoscopic versus robotic surgery for hepatocellular carcinoma: the first 46 consecutive cases. J Surg Res 2017;217:92-99.

[50] Mejia A, Cheng SS, Vivian E, Shah J, Oduor H, Archarya P. Minimally invasive liver resection in the era of robotics: analysis of 214 cases. Surg Endosc. 2020;34(1):339-48.

[51] Cortolillo N, Patel C, Parreco J, Kaza S, Castillo A. Nationwide outcomes and costs of laparoscopic and robotic vs. open hepatectomy. J Robot Surg. 2019;13(4):557-65.

[52] Di Benedetto F, Magistri P, Halazun KJ. Use of robotics in liver donor right hepatectomy. Hepatobiliary Surg Nutr. 2018;7(3):231-2.

[53] Miller C. Preparing for the inevitable: The death of a living liver donor. Liver Transplant. Off Publ Am Assoc Study Liver Dis Int Liver Transplant Soc. 2014;20 Suppl 2:S47-51.

[54] Hu L, Yao L, Li X, Jin P, Yang K, Guo T. Effectiveness and safety of robotic-assisted versus laparoscopic hepatectomy for liver neoplasms: a meta-analysis of retrospective studies. *Asian J Surg* 2018;41:401-16

[55] Gonzalez-Ciccarelli LF, Quadri P, Daskalaki D, Milone L, Gangemi A, Giulianotti PC. Robotic approach to hepatobiliary surgery. *Chirurg* 2017;88:19-28.

[56] Sham JG, Richards MK, Seo YD, Pillarisetty VG, Yeung RS, Park JO. Efficacy and cost of robotic hepatectomy: is the robot cost-prohibitive? J Robot Surg. 2016;10(4):307-313.

[57] Ji WB, Wang HG, Zhao ZM, Duan WD, Lu F, Dong JH. Robotic-assisted laparoscopic anatomic hepatectomy in China: initial experience. Ann Surg. 2011;253(2):342-348

[58] Yu YD, Kim KH, Jung DH, et al. Robotic versus laparoscopic liver resection: a comparative study from a single center. Langen- becks Arch Surg. 2014;399(8):1039-1045

[59] Beard RE, Tsung A. Minimally Invasive Approaches for Surgical Management of Primary Liver Cancers Cancer Control. 2017 Jul-Sep;24(3):1073274817729234.

[60] Labadie K, Sullivan K.M. and O. Park J. Surgical Resection in HCC. Liver Cancer http://dx.doi.org/10.5772/intechopen.81345

[61] Lamadé W, Glombitza G, Fischer L, et al. The impact of 3-dimensional reconstructions on operation planning

in liver surgery. Archives of Surgery. 2000;**135**(11):1256-1261

[62] Bangeas P, Tsioukas V, Papadopoulos VN, Tsoulfas G. Role of innovative 3D printing models in the management of hepatobiliary malignancies. J Hepatol 2019 Jul 27;11(7):574-585. doi: 10.4254/wjh.v11.i7.574.

Chapter 8

Laparoscopic Liver Resection for Hepatocellular Carcinoma

Melina Vlami, Nikolaos Arkadopoulos and Ioannis Hatzaras

Abstract

Hepatocellular carcinoma (HCC), remains one of the most common causes of cancer-related death globally. HCC typically arises in the setting of chronic liver disease and cirrhosis and as such, treatment must be balanced between the biology of the tumor, underlying liver function and performance status of the patient. Hepatic resection is the procedure of choice in patients with high-performance status who harbor a solitary mass (regardless of size). Before the first laparoscopic hepatectomy (LH) was described as early as 1991, open hepatectomy (OH) was the only choice for surgical treatment of liver tumors. LH indications were initially based solely on tumor location, size, and type and was only used for partial resection of the anterolateral segments. Since then, LH has been shown to share the benefits of other laparoscopic procedures, such as earlier recovery and discharge, and reduced postoperative pain; these are obtained with no differences in oncologic outcomes compared to open resection. Specific to liver resection, LH can limit the volume of intraoperative blood loss, shorten portal clamp time and decrease overall and liver-specific complications. This chapter will offer an overview of standard steps are in pursuing laparoscopic liver resection, be it for a minor segmentectomy or a lobectomy.

Keywords: hepatocellular carcinoma, resection, laparoscopic, technique

1. Introduction

Despite advances in medical, surgical and locoregional therapies, hepatocellular carcinoma (HCC), the most common primary liver cancer, remains one of the most common causes of cancer-related death globally. Hepatocellular carcinoma is the fifth most common frequently occurring cancer in men, the ninth in women and is the second leading cause of death from cancer worldwide. It is estimated that by 2025 more than 1 million individuals will be affected by liver cancer annually.

HCC typically arises in the setting of chronic liver disease and cirrhosis. In fact, the rate of disease occurrence depends upon the complex interplay between the host, disease and environmental factors. This type of liver cancer contributes to up to 40% of all patient deaths in cirrhosis, making it the single most common cause of death in this patient population. The most prominent and well researched risk factors for HCC are Hepatitis B and C infections, accounting for 50% of all cases. Furthermore, there is a clear geographical distribution in the epidemiology of hepatocellular carcinoma, with the highest incidence seen in developing countries with high rates of chronic hepatitis B and aflatoxin exposure. In contrast the lowest incidence rates are seen in some European countries that also have a lower incidence of the before mentioned risk factors. Interestingly, increasing Hepatitis B vaccination, effective Hepatitis C treatment, reducing levels of aflatoxin exposure are now shifting the global epidemiology of HCC. Metabolic disorders, including Non-Alcoholic Steatohepatitis (NASH) and diabetes mellitus, along with obesity and insulin resistance, are now emerging as direct causative factors of HCC, particularly in the West. These evolving patterns of demographic and epidemiologic characteristics bear interesting implications in the diagnosis and management of patients with HCC [1–4].

2. Management

Cirrhosis patients should be followed within surveillance programs, that aim for early detection of suspicious nodules and effective treatment. Diagnosis of HCC is achieved with imaging and corroborated with an increased tumor marker alpha-fetoprotein blood (AFP) testing. Percutaneous biopsy is seldomly required for diagnosis.

HCC treatment in the setting of liver cirrhosis must be balanced between the biology of the tumor, and host characteristics such as the underlying liver function, presence or not of portal hypertension and ECOG status of the patient. When evaluating a patient for resection, the functional liver remnant must be carefully assessed and its adequate vascular inflow and outflow ascertained, along with biliary drainage. In the event of marginal functional liver remnant, portal vein embolization should be entertained to decrease the possibility of post-operative liver failure.

The most common staging systems for HCC include the Barcelona Clinic Liver Cancer (BCLC), Cancer of the Liver Italian Program (CLIP), and pathologic tumor-node-metastasis (pTNM). In clinical practice, there is no ideal system that can be applicable to every patient in predicting survival [5].

3. The BCLC system

The Barcelona Clinic Liver Cancer (BCLC) staging system is widely used since its inception and remains the most validated and reliable system for prognostication, due to its treatment recommendations based on stage and its ability to offer predictions on patient survival. The BCLC staging system uses variables addressing tumor stage, liver functional status, physical status and cancer-related symptoms. Subsequently, the BCLC staging system can link the stages described with a treatment algorithm.

The initial authors of the BCLC staging system created a position of safety algorithm that proposes:

- Surgical resection for early HCC (i.e. stages 0 and A)

- Transarterial chemoembolization (TACE) or chemotherapy for patients with intermediate to advanced HCC – Stages B and C

- Palliative/symptomatic-only supportive treatment for patients with end-stage disease – Stage D

The combination of tumor specific staging criteria along with host specific information regarding severity of cirrhosis and symptoms have gained the BCLC staging system wide adoption by clinicians around the world. Criticisms of the BCLC staging system focus on the outdated studies the guidelines were based on and the available surgical and intensive care techniques that were available at the time these were first reported.

In fact, using modern approaches to hepatectomy and enhanced postoperative care, several authors were able to demonstrate improved perioperative outcomes and long-term survival for well selected BCLC B and in some cases BCLC C patients managed operatively. These successes point to a trend in pushing the limits of the original more conservative guidelines, thereby offering a better survival to those patients deemed to be good candidates for resection. This endeavor however has to be taken cautiously, and patients that offered resection outside class A should be managed at high volume centers and at minimum be discussed at a multispecialty tumor board. With more and more BCLC staging system patients being considered for hepatectomy, the BCLC system should be revised to reflect modern liver surgery safety standards, and BCLC stages B should not be considered as absolute contraindications to surgery [6–10].

3.1 Tumor-node-metastasis staging system

According to this system, the most important prognostic factors is the extent or vascular invasion (T1 without, T2 with) within the tumor. Another important prognosticator accounted for in the T portion of the TNM staging system is number of tumors (T3) and direct invasion of other organs (T4). Lymph nodes are only seldomly affected with a histologic diagnosis of HCC, therefore only rarely we observe a N1 status on these patients. Naturally, metastatic disease is denoted as M1 [11].

Although the BCLC staging system has been found to be applicable for all stages of HCC limitations of all of the other systems have been identified. For example, the AJCC (TNM) staging system has limited usefulness since a large portion of HCC patients do not undergo surgery. The most comprehensive comparison between HCC prognostic scores has recently been published by Marrero et al., who analyzed a population homogeneously including all HCC disease strata and drew a retrospective comparison between seven HCC staging systems on a prospectively enrolled cohort: the BCLC system proved to offer the best prognostic score [12].

4. Liver function assessment

An initial assessment of hepatic function involves liver function testing including measurement of serum levels of bilirubin, aspartate aminotransferase (AST), alanine transaminase (ALT), alkaline phosphatase (ALP), measurement of prothrombin time (PT) expressed as international normalized ratio (INR), albumin, and platelet count (surrogate for portal hypertension). Other recommended tests include complete blood count (CBC), blood urea nitrogen (BUN), and creatinine to assess kidney function; creatinine is also an established prognostic marker in patients with liver disease. Further assessment of hepatic functional reserve prior to hepatic resection in patients with cirrhosis may be performed with different tools such as US and MRI elastography (which may provide and quantify the degree of cirrhosis-related fibrosis), and seldomly non-focal liver biopsy, and transjugular liver biopsy with pressure measurements.

The Child-Pugh classification has been traditionally used for the assessment of hepatic functional reserve in patients with cirrhosis. The Child-Pugh score incorporates laboratory measurements (i.e., serum albumin, bilirubin, PT) as well as more subjective clinical assessments of encephalopathy and ascites. It provides a general estimate of the liver function by classifying patients as having compensated (class A) or decompensated (classes B and C) cirrhosis. Advantages of the Child-Pugh score include ease of performance and the inclusion of non-laboratory, clinical parameters.

An important additional assessment of liver function not included in the Child-Pugh score is an evaluation of signs of clinically significant portal hypertension (i.e., esophagogastric varices, splenomegaly, splenorenal shunts and recanalization of the umbilical vein, thrombocytopenia). Evidence of portal hypertension may be evident on axial imaginsg (CT/MRI). Esophageal varices may be evaluated using esophagogastroduodenoscopy (EGD) or contrast-enhanced cross – sectional imaging.

The Model for End-Stage Liver Disease (MELD) is another system for the evaluation of hepatic reserve. MELD is a mathematical model based on regression analysis which employees a numerical scale ranging from 6 (best) to 40 (worst) for individuals 12 years or older. It is derived using three laboratory values (serum bilirubin, creatinine, and INR) and was originally devised to provide an assessment of mortality for patients undergoing transjugular intrahepatic portosystemic shunts (TIPS), but has been therefore incorporated as an algorithm of gauging suitability for liver transplants [13].

Which HCC patient is a candidate for resection?

Patients being considered for resection must have a high-performance status and be medically fit for what is a major operation. In general hepatic resection is the procedure of choice as a potentially curative option in patients with good liver function (generally Child-Pugh Class A without – or with mild – portal hypertension), who harbor a solitary mass (regardless of size) albeit, without major vascular invasion. In addition, the future liver remnant should be measured at minimum 20% in patients without cirrhosis and at least 40% with Child-Pugh Class A cirrhosis. Lastly, the future liver remnant should be projected to have adequate vascular and biliary inflow/outflow. Hepatic resection is controversial in patients with limited but multifocal disease and in those where tumors are seen to invade major vessels [13].

5. Partial hepatectomy

Surgical removal of a portion of a patient's liver (partial hepatectomy) is beneficial in removing the tumor that it harbors and thereby limiting its growth and spread to other organs. Partial hepatectomy for well-selected patients with HCC can nowadays be performed with low operative morbidity (<25%) and mortality (≤2–5%). Results of large retrospective studies have shown 5-year survival rates for patients with preserved liver function and early-stage HCC of approximately 70%.

Since liver resection for patients with HCC includes removal of functional liver parenchyma in the setting of underlying liver disease, careful patient selection, based on patient characteristics as well as characteristics of the liver and the tumor(s), is essential. Beyond functional liver remnant volume and adequacy of vascular inflow & outflow, technical considerations related to tumor and liver anatomy, must be taken into account before a patient is determined to have potentially resectable disease.

Resection is recommended only in the setting of preserved liver function. The Child-Pugh score provides an estimate of liver function, although it has been suggested that it is more useful as a tool to rule out patients for liver resection (i.e., serving as a means to identify patients with substantially decompensated liver disease). An evaluation of the presence of significant portal hypertension is also an important part of the surgical assessment.

6. Operative approach: open vs. laparoscopic hepatectomy

Before the first laparoscopic hepatectomy (LH) was described as early as 1991, open hepatectomy (OH) was the only choice for surgical treatment of liver tumors. LH indications were initially based solely on tumor location, size, and type and was only used for partial resection of the anterolateral segments.

Several studies have been conducted comparing laparoscopic liver resection (LLR) versus open liver resection (OLR) for hepatocellular carcinoma (HCC), however, the optimal therapeutic approach has not been established [10, 14–20].

A 2019 systematic review and meta-analysis by the Department of Hepatobiliary Surgery of Bengbu Medical College analyzed 17 studies comparing OH and LH. This metanalysis included 2004 patients and showed the following findings: For short-term outcomes, LH was associated with less blood loss, lower blood transfusion rates, reduced occurrence of postoperative complications, wider surgical margin, shorter postoperative hospital stay, and declined rate of mortality (all $P < 0.05$). However, there was no significant difference in operation time ($P = 0.67$) between the two groups, whereas tumor size was larger in OH ($P = 0.004$). As for long-term outcomes, 1-, 3-, 5-year OS and 1-year DFS were higher in LH group (all $P < 0.05$). Nevertheless, there were no significant differences in 3- and 5-year DFS ($P = 0.23$ and 0.83, respectively) [18].

Another 2018 European systematic review and meta-analysis of individual patient data by Meidai Kasai et al. also compared outcomes of LH and OH. A total of 917 patients were divided into the laparoscopic (427) and open (490) groups from 8 selected studies. Interestingly, the hospital stay was significantly shorter, and the total morbidity was lower in the laparoscopic group. When classified by severity, the incidence of postoperative minor complications was lower in the LH group, however, that of major complications was not significantly different. The operative time was longer in the laparoscopic group; however, intraoperative blood loss, perioperative mortality, and blood transfusions were comparable between the two groups. The overall survival in the patients with colorectal liver metastases and hepatocellular carcinoma was not significantly different between the two groups in this metaanalysis [20].

It is clear that LLR has the same benefits as other laparoscopic procedures, such as earlier, recovery and discharge, and reduced postoperative pain. It is also important to underline the many benefits of the laparoscopic approach are obtained while there are no differences in oncologic outcomes compared to OLR. Furthermore, the studies showed the specific advantages of LLR: lower volume of blood loss, shorter portal clamp time and less overall and liver-specific complications, for selected patients and within the technical capabilities of each experienced center. LLR also allows for better visibility and manipulation in a small operative field under some conditions, such as repeat hepatectomy with adhesions. Laparoscopic surgery makes subsequent abdominal operations easier by reducing adhesions. It was reported that the salvage transplantation after previous LLR is associated with reductions of operation time, blood loss, and transfusion requirements, compared to that after OLR. Therefore, it is advantageous not only in reducing future adhesions but also in decreasing the need for adhesiolysis in repeat abdominal exploration.

The safety and feasibility of LLR and its short-term benefits for the patients with HCC and CLD have also been well demonstrated. Reduction of surgery-induced stress by LLR, especially in the patients with HCC and CLD, decreases the risk of refractory ascites due to the preservation of venous and lymphatic collateral flows. In result, this reduces the risk of water or electrolyte imbalances and hypoproteinemia that could lead to liver failure.

Although currently there is no established adjuvant therapy for patients with hepatocellular carcinoma who undergo resection, patients do recover fully faster after laparoscopic hepatectomy. As such, when future effective adjuvant modalities emerge, patients who undergo laparoscopic resection will be fully recovered and ready to receive these much sooner than patients who undergo an open resection. This has been shown in patients with colorectal liver metastasis who undergo laparoscopic liver resection to have a prognostic benefit compared to patients who undergo an open resection.

7. Technical considerations

In general, "peripheral" liver segments can be resected laparoscopically much easier than "central". This applies to the left lateral segment (II & III) and to segments V & VI). Segments adjacent to the diaphragm (segments II, VII, VIII), are more challenging to access and safely resect laparoscopically. A thoracoscopic approach could be considered in these situations, but this is accompanied by the challenges of entering the pleural space and lack of quick hepatic hilum access, should one be needed intraoperatively. In addition a formal hepatic lobectomy is more challenging laparoscopically than it is open. It is therefore intuitive for a novice laparoscopic surgeon to start performing the easier, peripheral, resections first, and build a routine in mobilizing the liver, addressing problems, controlling hemorrhage etc., before embarking in bigger resections. The reported learning curve is 50 cases before a surgeon can take on more challenging cases, including laparoscopic lobectomy. It should be emphasized that during the first 50 cases, conversion rate can be as high as 50%, which is never worrisome and should never be considered a sign of failure. In almost all case, conversion is a sign of surgical maturity on behalf of the surgeon.

In is important to underline that the key initial steps are standard in pursuing laparoscopic liver resection, be it for a minor segmentectomy or a lobectomy. Set up, important for all surgical operations, is of paramount significance when it comes to LLR. The wrong setup can render a straightforward case into a very difficult one, necessitating needless conversion to open exploration. During LLR there is no surgical hand in the abdomen to gently but swiftly retract the liver and enable its mobilization, and/or tamponade a bleeding vessel. Surgical ingenuity has led to utilization of gravity to assist in retracting and mobilization, or the opposite in the event of hemorrhage during LLR.

We present herein a step by step laparoscopic approach through a video which highlights key points including surgical set up, placement of trocars, full mobilization of a liver lobe, facilitating access and resection of lesions in subdiaphragmatic hepatic segments through a minimally invasive peritoneal approach.

8. Technique

The video presented herein concerns the laparoscopic resection of a 2 cm liver mass in segment 7. The patient had a solid mass but in Computed Tomography and Magnetic Resonance imaging, and was FDG avid on PET CT. The patient, an otherwise healthy 51-year-old woman, with no past medical or surgical history. Of note, the patient provided consent to use the recorded video of her operation while protecting her privacy and maintaining her anonymity. In this video, we summarize key steps/technical tips with laparoscopic liver resections from our experience with minimally invasive hepatectomies, and highlight the challenges of subdiaphragmatic liver lesion resections. As mentioned, several key maneuvers are highlighted which apply to laparoscopic liver resection, of all segments.

One of the most important key elements of laparoscopic liver resection especially for resection of the right lobe, is positioning the patient in a full left lateral decubitus position, with the patient's trunk at 90-degree angle to the operating room table and the right upper extremity position securely over the patient's right chest. Drawing from the experience of laparoscopic adrenalectomies, the full left lateral position allows for easier, lateral access to the right lobe of the liver. "Jackknifing" the table opens up the working space at the far right of the abdominal musculature even more.

This approach is taking advantage of the weight of the liver itself, which is rotated medially by gravity as mobilization progresses, and obviates the need for an additional port for a liver retractor. An arm rest for the patient's right upper extremity should be employed to position it at a comfortable position over and above the upper right chest. Appropriate padding should be placed under the left axilla and at all pressure points of the trunk. The patient's abdomen, particularly the right upper quadrant at a minimum, should be left unobstructed for laparoscopic port placement but also for a quick laparotomy (through a generous right subcostal incision), should the need arise intraoperatively. The patient's body should be secured on the operating table in a fashion that will enable steep Trendelenburg and reverse Trendelenburg positioning, as well as rotation of the table to the right and left without patient slipping. We favor a belt around the patient's hip as well as stop latches at the lower spine and suprapubic areas. Intravenous fluid administration should be kept to a minimum until parenchymal transection, as is true for all liver resections.

Initially, just three 5 mm ports are placed, as shown in image 1, one for a high definition 5 mm camera and two for the laparoscopic instruments. Insufflation of the abdomen is instituted at a pressure of 12 mm Hg, with the ability to increase the intra-abdominal pressure up to 20 mm Hg should venous or low-pressure parenchymal bleeding is encountered. Depending on the most beneficial camera view and angle of approach, one of the 5 mm working ports is converted into a 12 mm port, once the desirable degree of hepatic mobilization is obtained. The upsized port can accommodate a vascular cartridge-loaded stapler or the laparoscopic ultrasound probe for intraoperative sonographic examination of the parenchyma.

Mobilization of the right lobe can proceed working laterally to medially and freeing up the retroperitoneal attachments and the right triangular ligament of the right lobe as shown in the video, https://www.dropbox.com/s/v247mnbo385shnt/hatzaras%20lap%20hepatectomy%20S7%202.mp4?dl=0. Gravity works to the surgeon's benefit, medializing the lobe as the dissection proceeds. Dividing fully the right triangular ligament is facilitated by additional gentle liver retraction with the right hand instrument, while a vessel-sealing device is yielded with the left hand. The right adrenal quickly comes into view, and care should be used to avoid injuring the fragile gland or its small feeding vessels (e.g. superior adrenal artery and vein). Caution is especially important in the case of a large tumor in the right lobe of the liver, which has been chronically pressing against the right adrenal gland, fusing the right adrenal with the liver capsule, and causing local venous hypertension in the small venous branches; these should be dissected carefully and clipped individually. Care should also be paid to avoiding injuring the diaphragm, which if entered, would lead to pneumothorax; if this was to occur, it can be repaired laparoscopically with heavy absorbable suture, over a suction device that will empty the air from the ipsilateral hemithorax.

Although not shown in this video, this positioning and initial hepatic mobilization allows for the inferior vena cava (IVC) to be fully exposed, if this lateral to medial dissection is continued more medially. The small direct branches from posterior of the right lobe to the IVC can be dissected, clipped and divided as needed. The IVC ligament may also be fully dissected, a vessel loop passed around it and a vascular cartridge-loaded stapler used to transect it safely. Lastly the inferior surface of the right hepatic vein can be encountered and skeletonized, and if the bare area superiorly is fully mobilized, the right hepatic vein can be encircled with a vessel loop and ligated with a vascular stapler.

To avoid the necessity of inflow control at the hilum, and outflow control at the hepatic veins, we frequently use microwave ablation to demarcate the target area of resection before transection of the parenchyma (key move#4). We aim for a 1 cm wide by 3 or 4 cm deep thermal ablation zone, which provides a safe, nearly bloodless transection zone. Alternatively, if the goal is to achieve a completely laparoscopic right hemihepatectomy, the surgeon should perform a cholecystectomy; then by using intraoperative laparoscopic ultrasound to identify the right portal bundle immediately superior and posterior the gallbladder fossa. If clearly identified, the operative surgeon can use a Glissonian approach, perform two shallow hepatotomies, each approximately half an inch long and 1 inch apart, in such a way to accommodate a vascular stapler which will ligate intrahepatically the right portal structures. Excellent demarcation of the right lobe will be seen after successful completion of this maneuver.

Once mobilization is completed we laparoscopically place "liver handles", two number one braided sutures though and through the parenchyma of the intended specimen in a figure-of eight fashion (key move#5), ensuring to avoid the tumor itself. These "liver handles" are brought through the abdominal wall from a separate lateral stab incision using a suture passer and we secure them with a hemostatic clamp. This maneuver allows easy, gentle extracorporeal intraoperative manipulation of the liver area to be resected. An alternative option of achieving this retraction in lateral lesions is to place a vessel loop around the fully mobilized right lobe, and exteriorize it from the abdominal cavity with a suture passer through a medial separate stab incision; this allows gentle upward retraction of the right liver lobe, the soon to-be-resected portion falls to the right, "opening the book" for the surgeon to deploy the vessel-sealing device and the vascular staplers. We typically use the Harmonic scalpel (Ethicon/Johnson & Johnson, Somerville, NJ) to transect the superficial portion of the parenchyma, followed by "vascular staplers" for the deeper portion. The 12 mm Hg intra-abdominal pressure in combination with the microwave ablation transection treatment renders the transection field relatively bloodless, a clear benefit of laparoscopic hepatectomy, obviating the need for transfusion. After resection and irrigation, we place a hemostatic agent on the cut surface of the liver. The combination of energy transection and vascular stapling allows the pace of the operation to be brisk, and it is typically completed in under 3 hours. The specimen can be removed through a 5–8 cm incision usually in the Pfannenstiel position. With these maneuvers, LLR can achieve the same outcome as the open approach, in the same time, with the same if not lower risk of transfusion, alas, with a much speedier recovery.

9. Conclusion

In the last two decades, liver surgery has become a much safer surgical procedure to be offered to patients with hepatic malignancies, including Hepatocellular Carcinoma. The laparoscopic approach to liver resection has evolved in parallel. Despite a steep learning curve, LLR can achieve excellent outcomes for well selected patients with Hepatocellular Carcinoma.

Author details

Melina Vlami, Nikolaos Arkadopoulos and Ioannis Hatzaras*
Department of Surgery, National and Kapodistrian University of Athens, Athens, Greece

*Address all correspondence to: ihatzaras@gmail.com

References

[1] Llovet JM, Kelley RK, Villanueva A, Singal AG, Pikarsky E, Roayaie S, et al. Hepatocellular carcinoma. Nature Reviews Disease Primers. 2021;7(1):6. DOI: 10.1038/s41572-020-00240-3

[2] Hartke J, Johnson M, Ghabril M. The diagnosis and treatment of hepatocellular carcinoma. Seminars in Diagnostic Pathology. 2017;**34**(2):153-159. DOI: 10.1053/j.semdp.2016.12.011

[3] Wallace MC, Preen D, Jeffrey GP, Adams LA. The evolving epidemiology of hepatocellular carcinoma: A global perspective. Expert Review of Gastroenterology & Hepatology. 2015;**9**(6):765-779. DOI: 10.1586/17474124.2015.1028363

[4] Budny A, Kozłowski P, Kamińska M, Jankiewicz M, Kolak A, Budny B, et al. Epidemiologia i czynniki ryzyka rozwoju raka wątrobowokomórkowego [Epidemiology and risk factors of hepatocellular carcinoma]. Polski Merkuriusz Lekarski. 2017;**43**(255): 133-139

[5] Tellapuri S, Sutphin PD, Beg MS, Singal AG, Kalva SP. Staging systems of hepatocellular carcinoma: A review. Indian Journal of Gastroenterology. 2018;**37**(6):481-491. DOI: 10.1007/s12664-018-0915-0

[6] Cillo U, Vitale A, Grigoletto F, Farinati F, Brolese A, Zanus G, et al. Prospective validation of the Barcelona clinic liver Cancer staging system. Journal of Hepatology. 2006;**44**(4):723-731. DOI: 10.1016/j.jhep.2005.12.015

[7] Li JW, Goh BG, Chang PE, Tan CK. Barcelona clinic liver cancer outperforms Hong Kong liver cancer staging of hepatocellular carcinoma in multiethnic Asians: Real-world perspective. World Journal of Gastroenterology. 2017;**23**(22):4054-4063. DOI: 10.3748/wjg.v23.i22.4054

[8] Llovet JM, Fuster J, Bruix J. Barcelona-clínic liver cancer group. The Barcelona approach: Diagnosis, staging, and treatment of hepatocellular carcinoma. Liver Transplantation. 2004;**10**(2 Suppl. 1):S115-S120. DOI: 10.1002/lt.20034

[9] Moris D, Felekouras E. Ignore reality but not the consequences of its ignorance: Broaden guidelines in surgery of hepatocellular carcinoma. Hepatology. 2017;**65**:1772-1773

[10] Naar L, Hatzaras I. Liver resection for hepatocellular carcinoma and the Barcelona clinic liver Cancer criteria: Is it time to push the limits? Annals of Surgical Oncology. 2020;**27**:2122-2124

[11] Selçuk H. Prognostic factors and staging systems in hepatocellular carcinoma. Experimental and Clinical Transplantation. 2017;**15**(Suppl. 2): 45-49. DOI: 10.6002/ect.TOND16.L11

[12] Llovet JM, Brú C, Bruix J. Prognosis of hepatocellular carcinoma: The BCLC staging classification. Seminars in Liver Disease. 1999;**19**(3):329-338. DOI: 10.1055/s-2007-1007122

[13] Hatzaras I, Bischof DA, Fahy B, Cosgrove D, Pawlik TM. Treatment options and surveillance strategies after therapy for hepatocellular carcinoma. Annals of Surgical Oncology. 2014; **21**(3):758-766. DOI: 10.1245/s10434-013-3254-5

[14] Morise Z. Laparoscopic liver resection for the patients with hepatocellular carcinoma and chronic liver disease. Translational Gastroenterology and Hepatology. 2018;**3**:41. DOI: 10.21037/tgh.2018.07.01

[15] Jiang S, Wang Z, Ou M, Pang Q, Fan D, Cui P. Laparoscopic versus open hepatectomy in short- and long-term outcomes of the hepatocellular

carcinoma patients with cirrhosis: A systematic review and Meta-analysis. Journal of Laparoendoscopic & Advanced Surgical Techniques. Part A. 2019;**29**(5):643-654. DOI: 10.1089/lap.2018.0588

[16] Xiangfei M, Yinzhe X, Yingwei P, Shichun L, Weidong D. Open versus laparoscopic hepatic resection for hepatocellular carcinoma: A systematic review and meta-analysis. Surgical Endoscopy. 2019;**33**(8):2396-2418. DOI: 10.1007/s00464-019-06781-3

[17] Yoshida H, Taniai N, Yoshioka M, Hirakata A, Kawano Y, Shimizu T, et al. Current status of laparoscopic hepatectomy. Journal of Nippon Medical School. 2019;**86**(4):201-206. DOI: 10.1272/jnms.JNMS.2019_86-411

[18] Morise Z. Developments and perspectives of laparoscopic liver resection in the treatment of hepatocellular carcinoma. Surgery Today. 2019;**49**(8):649-655. DOI: 10.1007/s00595-019-1765-9

[19] Zheng H, Huang SG, Qin SM, Xiang F. Comparison of laparoscopic versus open liver resection for lesions located in posterosuperior segments: A meta-analysis of short-term and oncological outcomes. Surgical Endoscopy. 2019;**33**(12):3910-3918. DOI: 10.1007/s00464-019-07071-8

[20] Kasai M, Cipriani F, Gayet B, Aldrighetti L, Ratti F, Sarmiento JM, et al. Laparoscopic versus open major hepatectomy: A systematic review and meta-analysis of individual patient data. Surgery. 2018;**163**(5):985-995. DOI: 10.1016/j.surg.2018.01.020

Chapter 9

Treatment of Advanced Hepatocellular Carcinoma

Mahmoud Aryan, Ellery Altshuler, Xia Qian and Wei Zhang

Abstract

Hepatocellular Carcinoma (HCC) is the fifth most common cancer and represents the fourth most common cause of cancer related death worldwide. Treatment of HCC is dictated based upon cancer stage, with the most universally accepted staging system being the Barcelona Clinic Liver Cancer (BCLC) staging system. This system takes into account tumor burden, active liver function, and patient performance status. BCLC stage C HCC is deemed advanced disease, which is often characterized by preserved liver function (Child-Pugh A or B) with potential portal invasion, extrahepatic spread, cancer related symptoms, or decreased performance status. Sorafenib has been the standard treatment for advanced HCC over the past decade; however, its use is limited by low response rates, decreased tolerance, and limited survival benefit. Researchers and clinicians have been investigating effective treatment modalities for HCC over the past several years with a focus on systemic regimens, locoregional therapy, and invasive approaches. In this systemic review, we discuss the management of advanced HCC as well as the ongoing research on various treatment opportunities for these patients.

Keywords: hepatocellular carcinoma, advanced stage, systemic therapy, locoregional therapy

1. Introduction

Primary liver cancer represents an enduring global threat as the fifth most common cancer worldwide and the second highest global cause of cancer-related mortality [1]. The most common form of liver cancer is hepatocellular carcinoma (HCC), which makes up over 90% of primary hepatic malignancies and independently represents the fourth most common cause of cancer-related death worldwide [2, 3]. Hepatotropic viruses such as hepatitis B virus (HBV), hepatitis C virus (HCV), and hepatitis D virus (HDV) are the most common causes of HCC, accounting for at least 80% of cases. HCC is also prevalent in individuals with underlying cirrhosis with other risk factors being alcohol use, non-alcoholic fatty liver disease (NAFLD), diabetes mellitus, obesity, aflatoxin exposure, hereditary hemochromatosis, tobacco use, oral contraceptive use, and other inherited metabolic disorders including tyrosinemia and glycogen storage disease type 1 (Von Gierke disease) [4–7].

The American Association for the Study of Liver Disease (AASLD) recommends that adults with cirrhosis undergo screening for HCC given the overall observed mortality benefit. Surveillance consists of abdominal ultrasonography every six months either with or without alpha fetoprotein (AFP) measurement. Patients who have a lesion ≥ 1 cm or AFP measurement ≥ 20 ng/mL are recommended to undergo further diagnostic evaluation with multiphasic computed tomography (CT) scan or magnetic resonance imaging (MRI) of the abdomen [8, 9]. In some instances, HCC can be diagnosed radiographically via LI-RADS criteria (LR-5 is diagnostic), which consists of imaging findings of washout, enhancing capsule, and threshold growth in addition to overall size diameter increase over the course of months [10]. In instances in which lesions are indeterminate or cannot be diagnosed radiographically, patients typically undergo either biopsy or close interval repeat imaging [8].

Solid tumor oncological staging is usually based on the tumor (T), node (N), and metastasis (M) classification system. This system does not take into account the degree of liver dysfunction or patient performance status and is less useful for predicting the course of HCC [9]. The Barcelona Clinic Liver Cancer (BCLC) staging system is the most universally accepted staging system for HCC as it takes into account tumor burden, liver functional status, and patient performance status. In the BCLC system, patients are classified into different stages, including very early (BCLC stage 0), early (BCLC stage A), intermediate (BCLC stage B), advanced (BCLC stage C), and terminal (BCLC stage D). Very early to early-stage HCC (BCLC stage 0 or A) cancers are treated with curative intent through resection, ablation, or even liver transplant (LT); overall survival is as high as 75% at 5 years. The standard of care for patients with intermediate stage HCC (BCLC stage B) is transarterial chemoembolization (TACE) or transarterial radioembolization (TARE). Patients with advanced HCC (BCLC stage C) often present with cancer-related symptoms but usually have moderately preserved liver function (Child-Pugh A or B). These patients receive systemic therapy, though other treatment modalities are under investigation. BCLC stage D HCC is considered terminal and is usually managed with best supportive care [11, 12].

Unfortunately, over 80% of HCC are diagnosed at the advanced stage (BCLC stage C or D). Therapy options such as TACE and tumor resection are often not appropriate in these patients, and 5-year survival is as low as 18% [13, 14]. Researchers and physicians have been investigating potential effective treatment options in these patients in the past decade and have made great advances. In this systemic review, we summarize the latest strategies and upcoming methods of managing advanced (BCLC stage C) HCC.

2. First line systemic therapy

HCC has been historically considered a chemotherapy-resistant tumor. Most chemotherapy agents require hepatic metabolism and cannot be used in the setting of severely impaired liver function [15]. Overall survival is often dictated by underlying hepatic function rather than extensive tumor burden. Despite these challenges, researchers have applied targeted immunotherapy for advanced HCC treatment and, at least in certain clinical scenarios, have found benefit [16].

2.1 Atezolizumab + Bevacizumab combination therapy

Multi-agent combination therapy with atezolizumab and bevacizumab has recently replaced sorafenib as first line treatment for advanced HCC. Atezolizumab and bevacizumab are monoclonal antibodies that target program death ligand 1 (PD-L1) and vascular endothelial growth factor (VEGF), respectively [17, 18]. When used together, these medications inhibit both T cell apoptosis and angiogenesis. The combination of these medications was compared to sorafenib in patients with treatment naïve advanced HCC in the IMbrave150 trial. The trial showed that patients treated with atezolizumab and bevacizumab had significantly improved overall survival (OS) and progression free survival (PFS) when compared to those treated with sorafenib [17]. Adverse events occurred at similar rates among the two groups, with the most common adverse effects in patients given atezolizumab with bevacizumab being hypertension and proteinuria. Following systemic review of nine randomized control trials, the American Society of Clinical Oncology (ASCO) has deemed combined atezolizumab/bevacizumab as the first line treatment for advanced HCC applicable to those with Child-Pugh A liver disease, Eastern Cooperative Oncology Group Performance Status (ECOG PS) no higher than one and treated esophageal varices (EV) [18]. Recent updates from Finn and colleagues on the IMbrave150 trial reported that median OS was 19.2 months in those taking atezolizumab and bevacizumab vs. 13.4 months in those taking sorafenib (HR, 0.66 [95% CI, 0.52, 0.85]; P=0.0009). At 18 months, those treated with atezolizumab and bevacizumab had an OS of 52% while patients on sorafenib has an OS of 40%. Atezolizumab and bevacizumab combination therapy has demonstrated the longest OS in a front-line phase III clinical study for advanced HCC to date and remains the standard of care for treatment-naïve, advanced HCC [19].

2.2 Sorafenib

Tyrosine protein kinase inhibitors (TKIs) had been at the forefront of advanced HCC treatment for quite some time. The first TKI approved by the Food and Drug Administration (FDA) for treatment of advanced HCC was sorafenib, which was first approved for treatment of unresectable HCC in 2007 (**Table 1**). This TKI targets VEGF, platelet derived growth factor (PDGF), and others molecular pathways to inhibit angiogenesis [20]. The Sorafenib Hepatocellular Carcinoma Assessment Randomized Protocol (SHARP) study was the first multi-center, placebo-controlled, phase III clinical trial in untreated, Child-Pugh A advanced HCC patients, and demonstrated a 2.8-month overall survival (OS) in those treated with sorafenib versus placebo (10.7 vs. 2.9 months) [21]. Further clinical trials and subset analysis showed that sorafenib provides survival benefit in patients with HCC not amendable to loco-regional therapy, though the benefit appears to be greater for patients

Regimen	ASCO recommendations	Criteria for use
Atezolizumab + Bevacizumab	First-line	ECOG PS ≤ 1, Child-Pugh A, following EV treatment
Sorafenib	First-line	When there are contraindications to Atezolizumab – Bevacizumab therapy
Lenvatinib	First-line	
Nivolumab	First-line or Second-line	
Cabozantinib	Second-line or Third-line	
Regorafenib	Second-line	Those who failed Sorafenib
Ramucirumab	Second-line	AFP ≥ 400
Pembrolizumab	Second-line	
Nivolumab + Ipilimumab	No recommendations	

Table 1.
American Society of Clinical Oncology (ASCO) recommendations for systemic therapy in advanced (BCLC stage C) HCC [18].

with Child Pugh A cirrhosis than Child Pugh B cirrhosis [22]. Cheng et al. performed a randomized, double-blind, placebo control trial of sorafenib in the Asian Pacific region in patients with advanced HCC. Following six weeks of therapy, patients treated with sorafenib had significantly higher median OS (6.5 months vs. 4.2 months; [HR] 0.68 [95% CI 0.50–0.93]; $p=0.014$) and time to progression (2.8 months vs. 1.4 months; HR 0.57 [0.42–0.79]; $p=0.0005$) [23]. Despite the clinical benefits of sorafenib, many patients are unable to tolerate the significant side-effects, which include diarrhea, hand and feet skin irritation, weight-loss, and electrolyte derangements [21, 24, 25]. With its OS benefits and effects on disease progression, sorafenib remains a first-line option for advanced HCC [18].

2.3 Lenvatinib

Following the success of Sorafenib, several other TKIs were developed as potential treatment options in advanced HCC patients. Lenvatinib is a TKI that targets multiple pathways within angiogenesis including VEGF receptors, fibroblast growth factor (FGF) receptors, platelet derived growth factor (PDGF) alpha as well as RET and KIT [26]. An open-label, multicenter, phase III clinical trial known as the REFLECT trial showed lenvatinib to be non-inferior to sorafenib in advanced HCC patients with respect to OS. In the same trial, patients treated with lenvatinib had a higher incidence of hypertension, decreased appetite, and weight loss, while those treated with sorafenib had a higher incidence of hand-foot skin reaction (HFSR) and diarrhea. Patients treated with lenvatinib had significantly better progression-free survival (PFS) (7.4 months vs. 3.7 months, $p < 0.001$), time to progression (8.9 months vs. 3.7 months, $p < 0.001$), and objective response rate (24.1% vs. 9.2%, $p < 0.001$) [25, 27]. Vogel et al. analyzed prognostic factors of the REFLECT trial and reported that baseline liver function tests such as albumin-bilirubin grade and Child-Pugh score were predictive of OS. These markers may be used to monitor overall safety and efficacy of lenvatinib treatment. Regardless of baseline liver function, lenvatinib led to longer OS than sorafenib [28]. Given this data, the ASCO now considers lenvatinib a reasonable first-line treatment option for advanced HCC [18].

Ongoing studies are being conducted on the use of lenvatinib alongside nivolumab, an anti-PD-1 monoclonal antibody often used as second line therapy for HCC, in patients with unresectable, advanced HCC. Early results from the phase 1b trial of this open label study show that lenvatinib combined with nivolumab is well tolerated in BCLC stage C HCC with multiple patients demonstrating partial or complete response [29].

3. Second line systemic therapy

3.1 Cabozantinib

Other agents have been investigated for advanced HCC for patients with disease resistant to first-line therapy. Cabozantinib is a TKI that targets mesenchymal-epithelial transition (MET) factor to disrupt hepatocyte growth factor pathway, a pathway that is often important for HCC oncogenesis [30]. A phase III clinical study known as the CELESTIAL trial showed that for patients who had suffered disease progression while on sorafenib, cabozantinib led to longer OS and PFS than placebo [31–33]. Although adverse effects such as diarrhea, HFSR, hypertension, nausea, and decreased appetite, were found to be twice as high in the cabozantinib group than in the placebo group, the effects were generally mild and considered manageable [31–33]. Given its clinical benefit, the ASCO has classified cabozantinib as a second-line therapy for advanced HCC [18].

3.2 Regorafenib

Regorafenib is another TKI that has been utilized as a second-line agent in advanced HCC [18, 34, 35]. The RESORCE trial along with other studies support the use of regorafenib in treatment-resistant advanced HCC with active investigations focusing on applying the use of regorafenib in combination with other medications against advanced HCC [36]. When comparing cabozantinib and regorafenib as second line therapy in patients who had failed sorafenib therapy, the side effect profile of these medications was similar (with only increased incidence of diarrhea in patients taking Regorafenib), and both therapies provided similar benefits in regard to OS and PFS [37].

3.3 Apatinib

The latest TKI to show efficacy in advanced HCC is a VEGF receptor inhibitor called apatinib. This medication had been implemented in patients with hepatitis B infection in the past. Li et al. performed a multi-center, double blind, randomized phase III control trial in China in patients with advanced HCC refractory to at least one systemic agent [38]. The median OS was significantly higher in those treated with apatinib compared to placebo (8.7 months vs. 6.8 months, $p < 0.05$). The most common adverse effects of apatinib were hypertension, thrombocytopenia, and HFSR [38].

3.4 Nivolumab

Clinicians have also applied the use immunomodulatory checkpoint inhibitors as treatment for advanced HCC. Nivolumab is an immunoglobulin (IgG) 4 antibody that targets program death 1 (PD-1) on the surface of T cells to promote the anti-tumor properties of T cells [39]. Clinical trials have shown nivolumab to be a safe treatment option for advanced HCC with non-comparison studies showing durable and effective clinical response to treatment [40]. Multicenter phase III clinical trials comparing nivolumab to sorafenib are currently underway [41, 42]. Interim results of the CheckMate 459 trial, a randomized, multicenter phase III study, have shown no significant difference in median OS between nivolumab and sorafenib; however, the objective response rate was as high as 15% in those taking nivolumab vs. 7% in those taking sorafenib [41, 42]. Additionally, nivolumab was associated with superior health-related quality of life with patients reporting fewer side effects [43].

3.5 Pembrolizumab

Pembrolizumab is another monoclonal antibody directed against PD-1 that has been used as therapy for patients with advanced HCC [44]. The KEYNOTE trials were conducted to evaluate the efficacy of pembrolizumab and were expanded to compare the use of pembrolizumab following disease progression while on sorafenib to best supportive care. Despite pembrolizumab reducing the risk of death by 22%, there was no significant difference in OS between the two groups [44, 45]. Continued research is ongoing regarding the use of this anti-PD-1 agent for advanced HCC treatment.

3.6 Ramucirumab

Ramucirumab is a monoclonal antibody directed against vascular endothelial growth factor receptor 2 (VEGFR-2) that is approved for advanced HCC therapy in patients with alpha-fetoprotein (AFP) levels ≥400 ng/mL. Ramucirumab was initially compared versus placebo in a double-blind, multicenter, randomized control phase III trial known as REACH-1; unfortunately, there was no statistically significant difference in OS for those given ramucirumab or placebo in those who had failed first line sorafenib therapy [46]. Following subgroup analysis of the REACH-1 trial, the REACH-2 trial showed that ramucirumab had a statistically significant survival benefit compared to placebo in patients with AFP ≥400 ng/mL [47, 48]. The side-effect profile of ramucirumab is mild, with only reported increased frequency of hypertension and proteinuria, making it a second-line therapy for advanced HCC by the ASCO for patients with AFP ≥400 ng/mL [18, 46, 47]. Given its specific target population, ramucirumab is not routinely used in HCC patients with AFP <400 ng/mL.

3.7 Ipilimumab

Ipilimumab is a monoclonal antibody that targets cytotoxic T-lymphocyte-associated protein 4 (CTLA-4) to downregulate immune function. The Checkmate 040 trial assessed the use of ipilimumab alongside nivolumab for advanced HCC patients and demonstrated combination therapy to have an object response rate twice as high as nivolumab monotherapy (31% vs. 14%) This combination therapy was also well tolerated with an acceptable side effect profile when compared to similar systemic therapy [49, 50].

The Checkmate 040 trial was expanded to investigate triple combination therapy consisting of nivolumab, ipilimumab, and cabozantinib altogether [51]. When compared to the combination of just nivolumab and ipilimumab, those on triple therapy had a longer period of progression-free survival (6.8 months vs. 5.5 months). Treatment related adverse events were higher in those taking triple therapy with a discontinuation rate of 20% in the triple therapy group and 3% in the double therapy group [51].

4. Locoregional therapy

Therapies in the form of embolization fall under the category of locoregional therapy and are typically contraindicated in patients with advanced HCC with underlying vascular invasion, extrahepatic spread, or poor performance status. However, some patients with advanced HCC classified as BCLC stage C have benefited from locoregional therapies [52].

4.1 TACE

Advanced HCC patients with tumor invasion off a branch of the portal vein or limited extrahepatic disease involvement have been trialed with TACE therapy [53]. TACE consists of injecting an emulsified chemotherapeutic agent into the hepatic artery flowing towards the underlying tumor, followed by embolization of the vessel to contain the drug and localize cell death within the malignancy [52, 53]. TACE has historically been more successful in localized disease without extrahepatic or diffuse vascular involvement and serves as the first-line treatment for intermediate (BCLC stage B) HCC. Consensus regarding the overall clinical utility of TACE in advanced HCC when compared to systemic therapy remains under discussion [54]. Certain studies have shown TACE to be clinically safe and feasible in select advanced HCC patients with good collateral blood flow, and a meta-analysis reported TACE to be associated with higher treatment responses in advanced HCC when compared to other more conservative treatment approaches [54]. However, a retrospective analysis by Pinter and colleagues demonstrated no significant difference in OS between patients treated with TACE versus sorafenib, with Child-Pugh class predicting OS in these patients [55]. Meanwhile, Choi et al., reported through retrospective analysis that TACE in addition to sorafenib is associated with significantly increased time to progression when compared to sorafenib therapy alone, though no difference was seen with regard to OS [56]. Other retrospective studies including the TACTICS trial also found that combining TACE with sorafenib in advanced HCC improved progression-free survival when compared to sorafenib therapy alone [57–61].

4.2 Y-90 trans-arterial radio-embolization

Y-90 trans-arterial radio-embolization (TARE) is a therapy modality by which the isotope yttrium90 is delivered in in small vector beads to malignancy areas through branches of the hepatic artery [62]. TARE has been applied to treatment of advanced HCC in tumors that invade discrete segmental areas of the liver. Additionally, TARE has been shown to decrease overall portal vein tumor thrombus load [62]. Recent data indicates that when comparing the efficacy of TARE vs. sorafenib in advanced HCC patients, those who underwent TARE had a significantly higher tumor response rate, though there was no significant difference in OS [63]. Studies have also been conducted on combining TARE with systemic therapy in advanced HCC. No clear benefit was seen when combining TARE with sorafenib [64]; however, there have been case reports or series of positive outcomes in combining TARE with different systemic modalities [65, 66].

Most recently, a multicenter, single-arm, retrospective study conducted at three separate medical centers called the LEGACY study assessed the clinical efficacy of TARE therapy in unrespectable HCC [67]. Chemoembolization served as a primary treatment for 72.2% of the cohort with advanced disease. The three-year OS rate for the entire cohort was 86.6% with 62.2% of patients experiencing a duration of response of greater than six months [67]. This study led to the FDA approval of TheraSphere Y-90 Glass Microsphere for treatment of advanced HCC [68].

Garin et al. conducted research on the dosimetry of TARE therapy through a randomized, multicenter, open-label phase II trial known as DOSISPHERE-01 [69]. Patients received either a standard dose of Y-90 to the perfused lobe or a personalized dose of Y-90 targeted to the index lesion. Results showed that personalized dosimetry significantly improved response rates when compared to standard dosimetry in cases of locally advanced HCC (71% vs. 35%, $p < 0.01$) [69].

4.3 Hepatic artery infusion chemotherapy

Hepatic artery infusion chemotherapy (HAIC) has been used in the treatment of advanced HCC to directly delivery high concentrations of chemotherapeutic agents [70]. Studies on advanced HCC lesions that were unresectable, refractory to TACE, or associated with portal vein thrombus (PVT) have demonstrated positive responses to HAIC within patient cohorts. Groups in Korea and Japan have implemented HAIC with agents including cisplatin, 5-fluororuacil (5-FU), and pegylated interferon α-2b [70]. A randomized trial comparing interferon therapy coupled with 5-FU HAIC to sole interferon therapy in advanced HCC patients showed a significantly higher response rate (45.6% vs. 24.6%, $p < 0.05$) and longer median progression free survival (6.5 months vs. 3.3 months, $p=0.0048$) in the patients who received HAIC [71]. In their study comparing HAIC and sorafenib in advanced HCC patients, Song and colleagues reported that the median overall survival was significantly longer in the patients who received HAIC (OS: 7.1 months vs. 5.5 months, $p < 0.05$) [72].

5. Surgery

As medical and surgical expertise continue to improve, surgery is no longer contraindicated in some advanced HCC patients [73]. Surgical resection of advanced HCC, either in the form of hepatectomy or en-bloc resection, has been revisited as a potentially efficacious way of increasing OS. Data has shown that the overall median survival time in advanced HCC patients with PVT who undergo surgical resection to be between 8 and 22 months, with OS between 21.7% to 69.6% at one year [74]. Given the high incidence of post-operative recurrence, multi-disciplinary approach to surgical planning on a case-by-case basis is needed [74, 75]. Liang and colleagues performed a meta-analysis and found that patients who underwent surgical resection of advanced HCC with PVT had longer OS than those who were treated with TACE therapy [76].

The combination of systemic therapy with surgical resection has also been applied to advanced HCC patients. Takeyama et al. studied the use of sorafenib as a potential neo-adjuvant therapy prior to surgical resection. Patients who underwent surgical resection following treatment with sorafenib had a significantly increased three-year survival than patients who underwent therapy with sorafenib alone [77]. Incorporating surgical resection with other treatment modalities including TACE and radiofrequency ablation have also promoted positive prognostic outcomes in select patients [74, 75]. Overall, the indication for surgical therapy in advanced HCC patients with or without PVT requires a multi-disciplinary approach and may entail utilizing systemic or locoregional therapy during treatment planning.

6. Future directions

Several systemic agents have been trialed for treatment of advanced HCC over the past decade. As newer agents are approved for use in advanced HCC, combined treatment options remain intriguing topics for investigation. Gosain et al. have hypothesized that sorafenib and pembrolizumab may have synergistic effects and are currently conducting a trial to evaluate the efficacy of these drugs when used in combination [78]. Given the favorable response rates of nivolumab that were seen in the Checkmate 040 trial, Welling et al. are conducting a phase II, randomized control of nivolumab combined with HuMax-IL8 and cabiralizumab (an anti-CSF1R antibody) in advanced HCC patients. HuMax-IL8 (now known as BMS-986253) is a novel, fully human monoclonal antibody that inhibits interleukin-8 (IL-8) [79]. Combining locoregional with systemic therapy is also under investigation [80]. Among multiple studies being conducted, the EMERALD-1 trial is a randomized, double-blind, placebo-controlled phase III study assessing anti-PD-1 agent durvalumab alongside TACE therapy with or without bevacizumab [81].

Alternative molecular targets are also being evaluated. El-Khouiery et al. are currently working on an advanced HCC phase I trial of humanized agonist IgG2 monoclonal antibodies to a specific tumor necrosis factor receptor known as OX40. Underlying safety and pharmacodynamic dose-dependent response are now being investigated [82]. Another phase I trial currently underway involves a small activating RNA (saRNA) known as MTL-CEBPA that targets transcription factor C/EBP-α, which is involved in hepatic homeostasis and cell-cycle control. The preliminary results showed that it is relatively safety and can have potential synergistic efficacy with tyrosine kinase inhibitors in HCC [83]. Like new combinations of locoregional-systemic combinations and new uses of systemic agents, novel molecular-targeting agents offer hope for improved outcomes in advanced HCC.

Author details

Mahmoud Aryan[1], Ellery Altshuler[2], Xia Qian[3] and Wei Zhang[3]*

1 Department of Internal Medicine, University of Alabama at Birmingham, Birmingham, AL, USA

2 Department of Internal Medicine, University of Florida, Gainesville, FL, USA

3 Division of Gastroenterology and Hepatology, University of Florida, Gainesville, FL, USA

*Address all correspondence to: doczwqx@gmail.com; wei.zhang@medicine.ufl.edu

References

[1] Bray F, Ferlay J, Soerjomataram I, Siegel RL, Torre LA, Jemal A. Global cancer statistics 2018: GLOBOCAN estimates of incidence and mortality worldwide for 36 cancers in 185 countries. CA Cancer J Clin 2018; 68: 394-424.

[2] European Association for the Study of the Liver. Electronic address eee, European Association for the Study of the L. EASL Clinical Practice Guidelines: Management of hepatocellular carcinoma. J Hepatol 2018; 69: 182-236.

[3] Yang JD, Hainaut P, Gores GJ, Amadou A, Plymoth A, Roberts LR. A global view of hepatocellular carcinoma: Trends, risk, prevention and management. Nat Rev Gastroenterol Hepatol 2019; 16: 589-604.

[4] Ghouri YA, Mian I, Rowe JH. Review of hepatocellular carcinoma: Epidemiology, etiology, and carcinogenesis. J Carcinog 2017; 16: 1.

[5] Ringelhan M, Pfister D, O'Connor T, Pikarsky E, Heikenwalder M. The immunology of hepatocellular carcinoma. Nat Immunol 2018; 19: 222-232.

[6] Kulik L, El-Serag HB. Epidemiology and Management of Hepatocellular Carcinoma. Gastroenterology 2019; 156: 477-491 e471.

[7] Forner A, Llovet JM, Bruix J. Hepatocellular carcinoma. Lancet 2012; 379: 1245-1255.

[8] Lim J, Singal AG. Surveillance and diagnosis of hepatocellular carcinoma. Clin Liver Dis (Hoboken) 2019; 13: 2-5.

[9] Marrero JA, Kulik LM, Sirlin CB, Zhu AX, Finn RS, Abecassis MM et al. Diagnosis, staging, and Management of Hepatocellular Carcinoma: 2018 practice guidance by the American Association for the Study of Liver Diseases. Hepatology 2018; 68: 723-750.

[10] Chernyak V, Fowler KJ, Kamaya A, Kielar AZ, Elsayes KM, Bashir MR et al. Liver imaging reporting and data system (LI-RADS) version 2018: Imaging of hepatocellular carcinoma in At-risk patients. Radiology 2018; 289: 816-830.

[11] Bruix J, Reig M, Sherman M. Evidence-based diagnosis, staging, and treatment of patients with hepatocellular carcinoma. Gastroenterology 2016; 150: 835-853.

[12] Ayuso C, Rimola J, Vilana R, Burrel M, Darnell A, Garcia-Criado A et al. Diagnosis and staging of hepatocellular carcinoma (HCC): Current guidelines. Eur J Radiol 2018; 101: 72-81.

[13] Bobolts LR. Hepatocellular carcinoma: Considerations for managed care professionals. Am J Manag Care 2020; 26: S220-S226.

[14] Li D, Sedano S, Allen R, Gong J, Cho M, Sharma S. Current treatment landscape for advanced hepatocellular carcinoma: Patient outcomes and the impact on quality of life. Cancers (Basel) 2019; 11.

[15] Eatrides J, Wang E, Kothari N, Kim R. Role of systemic therapy and future directions for hepatocellular carcinoma. Cancer Control 2017; 24: 1073274817729243.

[16] Sonbol MB, Riaz IB, Naqvi SAA, Almquist DR, Mina S, Almasri J et al. Systemic therapy and sequencing options in advanced hepatocellular carcinoma: A systematic review and network meta-analysis. JAMA Oncol 2020; 6: e204930.

[17] Finn RS, Qin S, Ikeda M, Galle PR, Ducreux M, Kim TY et al. Atezolizumab

plus Bevacizumab in Unresectable Hepatocellular Carcinoma. N Engl J Med 2020; 382: 1894-1905.

[18] Gordan JD, Kennedy EB, Abou-Alfa GK, Beg MS, Brower ST, Gade TP et al. Systemic therapy for advanced hepatocellular carcinoma: ASCO guideline. J Clin Oncol 2020; 38: 4317-4345.

[19] Finn RS QS, Ikeda M, Galle PR, Ducreux M, Kim TY et al. IMbrave150: Updated overall survival (OS) data from a global, randomized, open-label phase III study of atezolizumab (atezo) + bevacizumab (bev) versus sorafenib (sor) in patients (pts) with unresectable hepatocellular carcinoma (HCC). J Clin Oncol 2021; 39(3_suppl): 267.

[20] Sarcognato S, Garcia-Lezana T, Villanueva A. Mechanisms of action of drugs effective in hepatocellular carcinoma. Clin Liver Dis (Hoboken) 2019; 14: 62-65.

[21] Llovet JM, Ricci S, Mazzaferro V, Hilgard P, Gane E, Blanc JF et al. Sorafenib in advanced hepatocellular carcinoma. N Engl J Med 2008; 359: 378-390.

[22] Vogel A, Saborowski A. Current strategies for the treatment of intermediate and advanced hepatocellular carcinoma. Cancer Treat Rev 2020; 82: 101946.

[23] Cheng AL, Kang YK, Chen Z, Tsao CJ, Qin S, Kim JS et al. Efficacy and safety of sorafenib in patients in the Asia-Pacific region with advanced hepatocellular carcinoma: A phase III randomised, double-blind, placebo-controlled trial. Lancet Oncol 2009; 10: 25-34.

[24] Keating GM. Sorafenib: A review in hepatocellular carcinoma. Target Oncol 2017; 12: 243-253.

[25] Raoul JL, Kudo M, Finn RS, Edeline J, Reig M, Galle PR. Systemic therapy for intermediate and advanced hepatocellular carcinoma: Sorafenib and beyond. Cancer Treat Rev 2018; 68: 16-24.

[26] Matsuki M, Hoshi T, Yamamoto Y, Ikemori-Kawada M, Minoshima Y, Funahashi Y et al. Lenvatinib inhibits angiogenesis and tumor fibroblast growth factor signaling pathways in human hepatocellular carcinoma models. Cancer Med 2018; 7: 2641-2653.

[27] Kudo M, Finn RS, Qin S, Han KH, Ikeda K, Piscaglia F et al. Lenvatinib versus sorafenib in first-line treatment of patients with unresectable hepatocellular carcinoma: A randomised phase 3 non-inferiority trial. Lancet 2018; 391: 1163-1173.

[28] Vogel A, Frenette, C., Sung, M. W., Daniele, B., Baron, A. D., Chan, S. L. et al. Baseline liver function and outcomes in the phase III REFLECT study in patients with unresectable hepatocellular carcinoma (uHCC). J Clin Oncol 2020; 38(4-suppl): 524.

[29] Kudo M, Ikeda, M., Motomura, K., Okusaka, T., Kato, N., Dutcus, C. E., et al. A phase Ib study of lenvatinib (LEN) plus nivolumab (NIV) in patients (pts) with unresectable hepatocellular carcinoma (uHCC): Study 117. J Clin Oncol 2020; 38(4_suppl).

[30] ML BP, Miksad RA. Cabozantinib in the treatment of hepatocellular carcinoma. Future Oncol 2017; 13: 1915-1929.

[31] Abou-Alfa GK, Meyer T, Cheng AL, El-Khoueiry AB, Rimassa L, Ryoo BY et al. Cabozantinib in patients with advanced and progressing hepato cellular carcinoma. N Engl J Med 2018; 379: 54-63.

[32] Deeks ED. Cabozantinib: A review in advanced hepatocellular carcinoma. Target Oncol 2019; 14: 107-113.

[33] Xiang Q, Chen W, Ren M, Wang J, Zhang H, Deng DY et al. Cabozantinib suppresses tumor growth and metastasis in hepatocellular carcinoma by a dual blockade of VEGFR2 and MET. Clin Cancer Res 2014; 20: 2959-2970.

[34] Personeni N, Pressiani T, Santoro A, Rimassa L. Regorafenib in hepatocellular carcinoma: Latest evidence and clinical implications. Drugs Context 2018; 7: 212533.

[35] Heo YA, Syed YY. Regorafenib: A Review in Hepatocellular Carcinoma. Drugs 2018; 78: 951-958.

[36] Bruix J, Qin S, Merle P, Granito A, Huang YH, Bodoky G et al. Regorafenib for patients with hepatocellular carcinoma who progressed on sorafenib treatment (RESORCE): A randomised, double-blind, placebo-controlled, phase 3 trial. Lancet 2017; 389: 56-66.

[37] Kelley RK, Mollon P, Blanc JF, Daniele B, Yau T, Cheng AL et al. Comparative efficacy of Cabozantinib and Regorafenib for advanced hepatocellular carcinoma. Adv Ther 2020; 37: 2678-2695.

[38] Li Q, Qin, S., Gu, S., Chen, X., Lin, L., Wang, Z., et al. Apatinib as second-line therapy in Chinese patients with advanced hepatocellular carcinoma: A randomized, placebo-controlled, double-blind, phase III study. J Clin Oncol 2020; 38(15_suppl): 4507.

[39] Finkelmeier F, Czauderna C, Perkhofer L, Ettrich TJ, Trojan J, Weinmann A et al. Feasibility and safety of nivolumab in advanced hepatocellular carcinoma: Real-life experience from three German centers. J Cancer Res Clin Oncol 2019; 145: 253-259.

[40] El-Khoueiry AB, Sangro B, Yau T, Crocenzi TS, Kudo M, Hsu C et al. Nivolumab in patients with advanced hepatocellular carcinoma (CheckMate 040): An open-label, non-comparative, phase 1/2 dose escalation and expansion trial. Lancet 2017; 389: 2492-2502.

[41] Yau T, Kang, Y. K., Kim, T. Y., El-Khoueiry, A. B., Santoro, A., Sangro, B., et al. CheckMate 459: A randomized, multi-center phase III study of nivolumab (NIVO) vs sorafenib (SOR) as first-line (1L) treatment in patients (pts) with advanced hepatocellular carcinoma (aHCC). Ann Oncol 2019; 30(5-suppl): 874-875.

[42] Sangro B, Park, J., Finn, R., Cheng, A., Mathurin, P., Edeline, J., et al. LBA-3 CheckMate 459: Long-term (minimum follow-up 33.6 months) survival outcomes with nivolumab versus sorafenib as first-line treatment in patients with advanced hepatocellular carcinoma. Ann Oncol 2020; 31 (3-suppl): 241-242.

[43] Edeline J, Yau, T., Park, J. W., Kudo, M., Han, K. H., Mathurin, P., et al. CheckMate 459: Health-related quality of life (HRQoL) in a randomized, multicenter phase III study of nivolumab (NIVO) versus sorafenib (SOR) as first-line (1L) treatment in patients (pts) with advanced hepatocellular carcinoma (aHCC). J Clin Oncol 2020; 38(4_suppl): 483.

[44] Finn RS, Ryoo, B. Y., Merle, P., Kudo, M., Bouattour, M., Lim, H. Y., et al. Results of KEYNOTE-240: phase 3 study of pembrolizumab (Pembro) vs best supportive care (BSC) for second line therapy in advanced hepatocellular carcinoma (HCC). J Clin Oncol 2019; 37(15_suppl): 4004.

[45] Finn RS, Ryoo BY, Merle P, Kudo M, Bouattour M, Lim HY et al. Pembrolizumab As second-line therapy in patients with advanced hepatocellular carcinoma in KEYNOTE-240: A randomized, double-blind, phase III trial. J Clin Oncol 2020; 38: 193-202.

[46] Zhu AX, Park JO, Ryoo BY, Yen CJ, Poon R, Pastorelli D et al. Ramucirumab

versus placebo as second-line treatment in patients with advanced hepatocellular carcinoma following first-line therapy with sorafenib (REACH): A randomised, double-blind, multicentre, phase 3 trial. Lancet Oncol 2015; 16: 859-870.

[47] Zhu AX, Kang YK, Yen CJ, Finn RS, Galle PR, Llovet JM et al. Ramucirumab after sorafenib in patients with advanced hepatocellular carcinoma and increased alpha-fetoprotein concentrations (REACH-2): A randomised, double-blind, placebo-controlled, phase 3 trial. Lancet Oncol 2019; 20: 282-296.

[48] Syed YY. Ramucirumab: A review in hepatocellular carcinoma. Drugs 2020; 80: 315-322.

[49] Yau T, Kang YK, Kim TY, El-Khoueiry AB, Santoro A, Sangro B et al. Efficacy and safety of Nivolumab plus Ipilimumab in patients with advanced hepatocellular carcinoma previously treated with Sorafenib: The CheckMate 040 randomized clinical trial. JAMA Oncol 2020; 6: e204564.

[50] Parikh ND, Marshall A, Betts KA, Song J, Zhao J, Yuan M et al. Network meta-analysis of nivolumab plus ipilimumab in the second-line setting for advanced hepatocellular carcinoma. J Comp Eff Res 2021; 10: 343-352.

[51] Yau T, Kang, Y. K., Kim, T. Y., El-Khoueiry, A. B., Santoro, A., Sangro, B., et al. Nivolumab (NIVO) plus ipilimumab (IPI) combination therapy in patients (Pts) with advanced hepatocellular carcinoma (aHCC): Long-term results from CheckMate 040. J Clin Oncol 2021; 39(3_suppl): 269.

[52] Raoul JL, Forner A, Bolondi L, Cheung TT, Kloeckner R, de Baere T. Updated use of TACE for hepatocellular carcinoma treatment: How and when to use it based on clinical evidence. Cancer Treat Rev 2019; 72: 28-36.

[53] Crocetti L, Bargellini I, Cioni R. Loco-regional treatment of HCC: Current status. Clin Radiol 2017; 72: 626-635.

[54] Luo J, Guo RP, Lai EC, Zhang YJ, Lau WY, Chen MS et al. Transarterial chemoembolization for unresectable hepatocellular carcinoma with portal vein tumor thrombosis: A prospective comparative study. Ann Surg Oncol 2011; 18: 413-420.

[55] Pinter M, Hucke F, Graziadei I, Vogel W, Maieron A, Konigsberg R et al. Advanced-stage hepatocellular carcinoma: transarterial chemoembolization versus sorafenib. Radiology 2012; 263: 590-599.

[56] Choi GH, Shim JH, Kim MJ, Ryu MH, Ryoo BY, Kang YK et al. Sorafenib alone versus sorafenib combined with transarterial chemoembolization for advanced-stage hepatocellular carcinoma: Results of propensity score analyses. Radiology 2013; 269: 603-611.

[57] Kudo M, Ueshima K, Ikeda M, Torimura T, Tanabe N, Aikata H et al. Randomised, multicentre prospective trial of transarterial chemoembolisation (TACE) plus sorafenib as compared with TACE alone in patients with hepatocellular carcinoma: TACTICS trial. Gut 2020; 69: 1492-1501.

[58] Kudo M, Ueshima, K., Ikeda, M., Torimura, T., Aikata, H., Izumi, N., et al. TACTICS: Final overall survival (OS) data from a randomized, open label, multicenter, phase II trial of transcatheter arterial chemoembolization (TACE) therapy in combination with sorafenib as compared with TACE alone in patients (pts) with hepatocellular carcinoma (HCC). J Clin Oncol 2021; 39(3_supp): 270.

[59] Zhang X, Wang K, Wang M, Yang G, Ye X, Wu M et al. Transarterial

chemoembolization (TACE) combined with sorafenib versus TACE for hepatocellular carcinoma with portal vein tumor thrombus: A systematic review and meta-analysis. Oncotarget 2017; 8: 29416-29427.

[60] Varghese J, Kedarisetty C, Venkataraman J, Srinivasan V, Deepashree T, Uthappa M et al. Combination of TACE and Sorafenib improves outcomes in BCLC stages B/C of hepatocellular carcinoma: A single Centre experience. Ann Hepatol 2017; 16: 247-254.

[61] Qu XD, Chen CS, Wang JH, Yan ZP, Chen JM, Gong GQ et al. The efficacy of TACE combined sorafenib in advanced stages hepatocellullar carcinoma. BMC Cancer 2012; 12: 263.

[62] Somma F, Stoia V, Serra N, D'Angelo R, Gatta G, Fiore F. Yttrium-90 trans-arterial radioembolization in advanced-stage HCC: The impact of portal vein thrombosis on survival. PLoS One 2019; 14: e0216935.

[63] Chow PKH, Gandhi M, Tan SB, Khin MW, Khasbazar A, Ong J et al. SIRveNIB: Selective internal radiation therapy versus Sorafenib in Asia-Pacific patients with hepatocellular carcinoma. J Clin Oncol 2018; 36: 1913-1921.

[64] Kulik L, Vouche M, Koppe S, Lewandowski RJ, Mulcahy MF, Ganger D et al. Prospective randomized pilot study of Y90+/−sorafenib as bridge to transplantation in hepatocellular carcinoma. J Hepatol 2014; 61: 309-317.

[65] Zhan C, Ruohoniemi D, Shanbhogue KP, Wei J, Welling TH, Gu P et al. Safety of combined Yttrium-90 Radioembolization and immune checkpoint inhibitor immunotherapy for hepatocellular carcinoma. J Vasc Interv Radiol 2020; 31: 25-34.

[66] Wehrenberg-Klee E, Goyal L, Dugan M, Zhu AX, Ganguli S. Y-90 Radioembolization combined with a PD-1 inhibitor for advanced hepatocellular carcinoma. Cardiovasc Intervent Radiol 2018; 41: 1799-1802.

[67] Salem R, Johnson GE, Kim E, Riaz A, Bishay V, Boucher E et al. Yttrium-90 Radioembolization for the Treatment of Solitary, Unresectable Hepatocellular Carcinoma: The LEGACY Study. Hepatology 2021.

[68] FDA. https://www.fda.gov/medical-devices/recently-approved-devices/theraspheretm-p200029, 2021.

[69] Garin E, Tselikas L, Guiu B, Chalaye J, Edeline J, de Baere T et al. Personalised versus standard dosimetry approach of selective internal radiation therapy in patients with locally advanced hepatocellular carcinoma (DOSISPHERE-01): A randomised, multicentre, open-label phase 2 trial. Lancet Gastroenterol Hepatol 2021; 6: 17-29.

[70] Song MJ. Hepatic artery infusion chemotherapy for advanced hepatocellular carcinoma. World J Gastroenterol 2015; 21: 3843-3849.

[71] Yamashita T, Arai K, Sunagozaka H, Ueda T, Terashima T, Yamashita T et al. Randomized, phase II study comparing interferon combined with hepatic arterial infusion of fluorouracil plus cisplatin and fluorouracil alone in patients with advanced hepatocellular carcinoma. Oncology 2011; 81: 281-290.

[72] Song DS, Song MJ, Bae SH, Chung WJ, Jang JY, Kim YS et al. A comparative study between sorafenib and hepatic arterial infusion chemotherapy for advanced hepatocellular carcinoma with portal vein tumor thrombosis. J Gastroenterol 2015; 50: 445-454.

[73] Zhu J, Yin T, Xu Y, Lu XJ. Therapeutics for advanced hepatocellular carcinoma: Recent

advances, current dilemma, and future directions. J Cell Physiol 2019; 234: 12122-12132.

[74] Sakamoto K, Nagano H. Surgical treatment for advanced hepatocellular carcinoma with portal vein tumor thrombus. Hepatol Res 2017; 47: 957-962.

[75] Sakamoto K, Nagano H. Outcomes of surgery for hepatocellular carcinoma with tumor thrombus in the inferior vena cava or right atrium. Surg Today 2018; 48: 819-824.

[76] Liang L, Chen TH, Li C, Xing H, Han J, Wang MD et al. A systematic review comparing outcomes of surgical resection and non-surgical treatments for patients with hepatocellular carcinoma and portal vein tumor thrombus. HPB (Oxford) 2018; 20: 1119-1129.

[77] Takeyama H, Beppu T, Higashi T, Kaida T, Arima K, Taki K et al. Impact of surgical treatment after sorafenib therapy for advanced hepatocellular carcinoma. Surg Today 2018; 48: 431-438.

[78] Gosain R, Mukherjee, S., Lee, S. S., Miller, A., Minderman, H., Maguire, O., et al. Phase Ib/II study of sorafenib (SOR) and pembrolizumab (PEM) in advanced hepatocellular cancer (HCC). J Clin Oncol 2020; 38(4_suppl): 594.

[79] Welling T, Beri, N., Siolas, D., Cohen, D. J., Becker, D. J., Zhong, H., et al. A phase II, randomized, controlled trial of nivolumab in combination with BMS-986253 or cabiralizumab in advanced hepatocellular carcinoma (HCC) patients. J Clin Oncol 2020; 38(4_suppl): 598.

[80] Farsad K, Nabavizadeh N, Kardosh A, Jou JH, Naugler WE, Kolbeck KJ. Combined locoregional and systemic therapy for advanced hepatocellular carcinoma: Finally, the future is obscure. Ann Transl Med 2020; 8: 1700.

[81] Sangro B, Kudo, M., Qin, S., Ren, Z., Chan, S., Joseph, E., et al. P-347 A phase 3, randomized, double-blind, placebo-controlled study of transarterial chemoembolization combined with durvalumab or durvalumab plus bevacizumab therapy in patients with locoregional hepatocellular carcinoma: EMERALD-1. Ann Onc 2020; 31(3_supp): 202-203.

[82] El-Khoueiry AB, Spano, J. P., Angevin, E., Doi, T., Bullock, A. J., Harris, W. P., et al. Analysis of OX40 agonist antibody (PF-04518600) in patients with hepatocellular carcinoma. J Clin Oncol 2020; 38(4_suppl): 523.

[83] Sarker D, Plummer R, Meyer T, Sodergren MH, Basu B, Chee CE et al. MTL-CEBPA, a small activating RNA therapeutic Upregulating C/EBP-alpha, in patients with advanced liver cancer: A first-in-human, Multicenter, open-label, phase I trial. Clin Cancer Res 2020; 26: 3936-3946.

Chapter 10

Research Frontier of Accurate Diagnosis and Treatment Guided by Molecular Typing of Hepatocellular Carcinoma

Haicaho Zhao, Changzhou Chen and Jiefeng He

Abstract

Liver cancer will continue to be a major disease threatening the lives and health of our people in the next few decades. In recent years, with the development of early diagnosis and treatment of liver cancer, precise liver resection, and the development of targeted and immunotherapeutic drugs, the survival rate of liver cancer patients has been improved. Nevertheless, due to the high heterogeneity of liver cancer, patients with liver cancer in the same clinical stage still have great differences in response to treatment and prognosis. New staging and classification indicators are urgently needed to facilitate accurate diagnosis and treatment of liver cancer, so as to further improve the survival rate of patients. The continuous progress and development of multi-omics technology, single-cell technology, tumor molecular visualization technology and medical artificial intelligence, etc., make the molecular classification of liver cancer more and more approaching the true nature of tumor biological characteristics, thus contributing to the accurate diagnosis and treatment of liver cancer.

Keywords: hepatocellular carcinoma, tumor heterogeneity, molecular typing, diagnosis, treatment

1. Introduction

Liver cancer is a major disease that seriously threatens the lives and health of our people. In recent years, the clinical diagnosis and treatment of liver cancer and innovative research have made remarkable progress. Nevertheless, due to the high heterogeneity of liver cancer, patients with liver cancer of the same clinical stage still have great differences in response to treatment and prognosis. There is an urgent need for new staging and classification indicators to facilitate accurate diagnosis and treatment of liver cancer, so as to further improve the survival rate of patients.

Liver cancer is considered to be one of the most heterogeneous tumors [1]. Due to the high heterogeneity of liver cancer, no "cancer-dependent genes" related to liver cancer have been found so far, which makes the therapeutic effect of molecular targeted therapy of liver cancer very small and lacks theoretical basis [2]. The heterogeneity of liver cancer includes inter-tumor heterogeneity and intra-tumor heterogeneity, both of which are distinguished from each other and closely related.

Among them, there are both genetic heterogeneity and microenvironment heterogeneity. Tumor heterogeneity indicates the insufficiency of "genetic characteristics and microenvironmental information obtained from a single biopsy", which has important theoretical value and clinical significance for studying the development history of individual liver cancer, overcoming drug resistance, and achieving individual precise treatment. The continuous progress and development of multi-omics technology, single-cell technology, tumor molecular visualization technology, and medical artificial intelligence have brought the molecular classification of liver cancer closer to the true nature of tumor biological characteristics, thereby helping the implementation and health of accurate diagnosis and treatment of liver cancer China's strategic planning.

2. Molecular typing based on transcriptome

With the progress of gene chips and second-generation sequencing technology, it is possible to analyze tumor gene expression changes without bias at the whole genome level, and the molecular typing of liver cancer first started from the exploration of transcriptomics. The gene microarray analysis of primary and metastatic HCC showed that the gene expression signature of primary HCCs with accompanying metastasis was very similar to that of their corresponding metastases, implying that genes favoring metastasis progression were initiated in the primary tumors. The constructed 153 gene expression markers could divide HCC into metastatic and non-metastatic types with a prediction accuracy of 78% [3]. At present, a number of studies have divided liver cancer into proliferative and non-proliferative types through transcriptomics methods, with the two molecular types each accounting for 50% [4–10]. The proliferative type is characterized by activation of PI3K-Akt–mTOR, Ras-MAPK, MET, and other cell proliferation-related signaling pathways, which are usually associated with HBV infection, and are driven by TP53 inactivation, FGF19, and/or CCND1 amplification, and has a poor prognosis. The non-proliferative type is more heterogeneous and is usually associated with alcoholic liver disease and HCV infection, with a relatively good prognosis. The proliferative type can be further divided into Hoshida S1 and S2 subtypes [4]. Strong enrichment of the WNT signature in subclass S1 compared with S2 or S3, suggesting preferential WNT activation in S1 tumors. Hoshida S2 tumors were strongly enriched in signatures of EpCAM、AFP and IGF2 positivity. The non-proliferative Hoshida S3 subtype is still heterogeneous, including the classical Wnt pathway activation subtype mediated by CTNNB1 mutation [5]. The Cancer Genome Atlas (TCGA) analyzed 363 hepatocellular carcinoma cases by whole-exome sequencing and DNA copy number analyses, DNA methylation, RNA, miRNA, and proteomic expression also. Integrative molecular HCC subtyping incorporating unsupervised clustering of five data platforms identified three subtypes:iClust1 ~ 3. Then iClust1 consisted predominantly of Hoshida S2 patients whereas iClust 2 subtype corresponds to Hoshida S3 subtype (CTNNB1 mutant subtype), and iClust 3 subtype corresponds to TP53 mutation and Hoshida S1 subtype [7]. These transcriptome-based molecular typing revealed the intrinsic molecular characteristics of liver cancer and had potential clinical significance.

3. Molecular typing based on tumor microenvironment

The immunoinflammatory microenvironment is the seventh characteristic of tumors [11]. Hepatocellular carcinoma is a typical immunoinflammatory and microenvironment-related tumor. Imbalance of immune-inflammatory response in the microenvironment is one of the key mechanisms for the occurrence and development of liver cancer [12, 13]. It has been discovered that the prognosis model of HCC constructed by integrating microenvironmental immune response, angiogenesis, and interstitial reaction can accurately predict the recurrence and metastasis of patients after surgery, highlighting the importance of stromal biology in HCC progression [14]. Based on immune-related gene expression level in the tumor microenvironment, HCC can be divided into the type of immune activation, the depletion of immune and immune exemption, various accounts for 10% ~ 25%, including immune activation type high expression of adaptive immune-related genes, immune depletion type high expression of TGF-β mediated immune suppression and T cell depletion related genes, immune exemption type is characterized by lack of T cells and CTNNB1 mutations [8]. According to the situation of immune cell infiltration, it can be divided into three subtypes: Immune-high, Immune-mid, and Immune-low. The Immune-high subtype was characterized by increased B−/plasma-cell and T cell infiltration, and the Immune-high subtype and B-cell infiltration were identified as independent positive prognostic factors. Low immune subtypes with a high Treg/CD4 ratio had the worst prognosis [15]. Further research found that: Comprehensive liver cancer immune microenvironment score (CD3, CD27, CD68, CD103, PD1) and tumor size, degree of differentiation, the prognosis model constructed by GGT is significantly better than the traditional clinical staging, and patients can be divided into high, medium, and Low-risk 3 groups [16]. Immune microenvironment typing has a certain clinical guiding value. For example, patients with Immune exemption type characterized by CTNNB1 mutations do not respond to programmed death-receptor-1(PD-1) / programmed death-ligand 1(PD-L1) inhibitors due to the lack of T cell infiltration. In addition, β-catenin activation conferred resistance to anti–PD-1 therapy in murine models [17]. There is no doubt that microenvironmental immune cells are highly plastic and heterogeneous. The results of single-cell sequencing showed that there were 11 T cell subsets with different functional phenotypes in the HCC microenvironment. It is necessary to further elucidate the microenvironmental characteristics and regulatory mechanisms of each subtype [18]. In addition, the liver itself is the most common metastatic organ for liver cancer, and the interaction between liver cells and immune cells creates a "metastasis-promoting microenvironment." The results of a number of studies have shown that the microenvironment of the adjacent liver tissue or tumor junction area plays an important role in the invasion and metastasis of liver cancer [19, 20]. Studies have shown that 17 inflammatory cytokine gene expression markers such as CSF1 can divide the adjacent tissues into metastasis-promoting microenvironment type and anti-metastatic microenvironment type, among which metastasis-promoting microenvironment type has high expression of Th2 cytokines and low expression of Th1 Cytokine as a feature [21]. Hoshida *et al.* [22] analyzed the expression profile of adjacent tissues of liver cancer and found that gene expression markers composed of 186 genes related to liver function and inflammation can divide liver cancer into good prognosis and poor prognosis. The poor prognosis is characterized by late recurrence, suggesting that the gene markers in the adjacent tissues may be related to the new liver cancer.

The presence of multifocal tumors, developed either from intrahepatic metastasis (IM) or multicentric occurrence (MO), is a distinct feature of hepatocellular carcinoma (HCC). The results of the study show that there are significant differences between IM and MO tumors, and their immune microenvironment also shows temporal and spatial heterogeneity: IM has fewer T lymphocytes and abundant M2 macrophage infiltration, while MO has higher Suppressive immune checkpoints, which also resulted in immune editing mainly occurring in MO rather than IM.

Similar to the mutation profile, the neoantigens and TCR components shared in tumors are higher in IM patients, but very few in MO. In addition, the loss of HLA heterozygosity occurs in 17% of multifocal liver cancers, which prevents a large number of predicted neoantigens from being effectively presented to the immune system and reduces the actual mutation load, especially in IM patients [23].

Immune inflammatory cells in the tumor microenvironment are not only an important prognostic factor but also determine their response to specific treatment methods, especially tumor immunotherapy. With the advancement of flow cytometry, immunostaining, and biological information technology, we can identify and classify the microenvironmental immune cell population with unprecedented precision. Immune inflammatory cells in the liver cancer microenvironment have significant inter-tumor heterogeneity and intra-tumor tissue heterogeneity in terms of density, location distribution, phenotype, and functional status; while the migration and differentiation of immune cells in tissues have temporal and spatial differences Qualitatively, liver cancer cells use this characteristic of immune cells to dynamically domesticate and edit them, leading to local immunosuppression, suggesting the plasticity of the liver cancer microenvironment [24–26].

4. Molecular typing based on proteome

Proteins are the direct executors of life activities and proteomics is one of the effective methods to search for molecular markers. The molecular characteristics of 110 cases of early hepatocellular carcinoma were analyzed and compared by proteomics [27]. The heterogeneity of early hepatocellular carcinoma was divided into the subtypes S-I, S-II, and S-III, each of which has a different clinical outcome. TGF-β and other tumor proliferation-related proteins were highly expressed in the S-III subtype, which was consistent with the Hoshida S1 subtype, and the prognosis was poor. S-II and S-I subtypes were characterized by high expression of Wnt and CTNNB1, consistent with Hoshida S2 and S3 subtypes. Proteomics is also an effective way to find drug targets. At present, the direct targets of liver cancer-targeted drugs with multi-kinase inhibitors and immunotherapy with immune checkpoint inhibitors are all proteins. S-III, which is characterized by disrupted cholesterol homeostasis, is associated with the lowest overall rate of survival and the greatest risk of a poor prognosis after first-line surgery. The knockdown of sterol O-acyltransferase 1 (SOAT1)-high expression of which is a signature specific to the S-III subtype-alters the distribution of cellular cholesterol, and effectively suppresses the proliferation and migration of hepatocellular carcinoma. Finally, on the basis of a patient-derived tumor xenograft mouse model of hepatocellular carcinoma, that treatment with avasimibe, an inhibitor of SOAT1, markedly reduced the size of tumors that had high levels of SOAT1 expression, which indicates that SOATI may become a new target of S-III subtype, namely Hoshida S1 subtype liver cancer [27]. Gene mutation induced by aristolochic acid is a characteristic pathogenic factor in China and even in Asia except for viral hepatitis B [28]. The mutation "fingerprint" of aristolochic acid is significantly positively correlated with tumor mutation burden, tumor neoantigen burden, CD8+ T cell infiltration, and immune microenvironment tolerance, suggesting these patients may benefit from immunotherapy [18]. On the other hand, the microenvironment of CTNNB1 mutation patients is immuno-privileged and may not benefit from immunotherapy. Further multi-omics analysis of liver cancer found that CTNNB1 mutation is related to the phosphorylation of serine 36 in ALDOA (fructose-1,6-bisphosphate aldolase) [29]. ALDOA phosphorylation promotes tumor cell proliferation by promoting anaerobic glycolysis and knocking down ALDOA significantly inhibits tumor proliferation. Therefore, ALDOA may be an important potential therapeutic target for CTNNB1 mutant liver cancer.

5. Molecular typing based on metabolic characteristics

Cell metabolism is downstream of gene regulation and protein action network, reflecting the terminal information of life activities. The liver is the largest metabolic organ of the human body, and metabolic reprogramming undoubtedly plays an important role in the occurrence and development of liver cancer [30]. Multi-omics research results show that glycolysis and fatty acid metabolism are up-regulated in liver cancer tissues, while liver-specific metabolic pathways are down-regulated in liver cancer tissues, such as gluconeogenesis, detoxification, bile acid metabolism, and urea-ammonia metabolism [23]. The combined markers of glycine cholic acid and phenylpropionate tryptophan identified based on metabonomics technology can accurately diagnose liver cancer 1 year in advance [31]. The high heterogeneity of the liver cancer mutation spectrum and expression spectrum will inevitably lead to the heterogeneity of its metabolome level. By constructing a genome-scale metabolic network model, liver cancer can be divided into iHCC type 1 to 3. iHCC1 showed the highest fluxes in the metabolism of amino acids, cofactors and coenzymes, pyruvate, fatty acid oxidation, carnitine shuttle, steroids, TCA, and oxidative phosphorylation. iHCC2 exhibited specific features including lower fatty acid biosynthesis and high glutamine metabolism, and β-catenin–associated up-regulated fatty acid oxidation. Finally, iHCC3 tumors were associated with multiple features of malignant tumors, including hypoxic behavior, epithelial-to-mesenchymal transition, higher fluxes in fatty acid biosynthesis, and a strong Warburg effect [32]. Whether tumor metabolic reprogramming is the initiating factor of cancer or the accompanying result of cancer, there is still much controversy. Preliminary research results show that amino acid metabolism-related genes such as proline synthase PYCR1 play an important role in the occurrence and development of liver cancer [33].

6. Conclusion

In recent years, many breakthroughs have been made in the treatment of liver cancer. Following sorafenib, lenvatinib, regorafenib, cabozantinib and combination therapies centered on immune checkpoints have come out to promote the progress of liver cancer drug treatment. However, due to the high heterogeneity of liver cancer, the overall effectiveness of the above drugs is still limited. Accurate molecular classification of liver cancer not only contributes to the decision-making of individualized diagnosis and treatment of liver cancer, and personalized drug treatment, but also greatly deepens clinicians' understanding of the complexity and heterogeneity of liver cancer, so as to formulate a more accurate and effective treatment strategy. The new molecular typing system should be closely integrated with clinical-pathological information, which can not only reflect changes at the molecular level but also have guiding significance for clinical diagnosis and personalized treatment or predicting prognosis. The author believes that with the progress and development of multi-omics technology, single-cell technology, tumor molecular visualization technology, and medical artificial intelligence, the molecular classification of liver cancer will become closer and closer to the essence of tumor biological characteristics, and ultimately achieve disease precision treatment.

Author details

Haicaho Zhao[1]*, Changzhou Chen[2,3] and Jiefeng He[1]

1 Shanxi Bethune Hospital, Shanxi Academy of Medical Sciences, Tongji Shanxi Hospital, Third Hospital of Shanxi Medical University, Taiyuan, China

2 Department of Liver Surgery and Transplantation, Liver Cancer Institute, Zhongshan Hospital, Fudan University, Shanghai, China

3 Key Laboratory of Carcinogenesis and Cancer Invasion, Fudan University, Shanghai, China

*Address all correspondence to: zhaohaichao00@163.com

References

[1] Li L, Wang H. Heterogeneity of liver cancer and personalized therapy [J]. Cancer Leu, 2016, 379(2):191-197.

[2] Rmaileh AA, Solaimuthu B, Tanna M, et al. Large-Scale Differential Gene Expression Transcriptomic Analysis Identifies a Metabolic Signature Shared by All Cancer Cells. Biomolecules. 2020;10(5):701

[3] Ye QH, Qin LX, Forgues M, et al. Predicting hepatitis B virus-positive metastatic hepatocellular carcinomas using gene expression profiling and supervised machine learning. Nat Med. 2003;9(4):416-423. doi:10.1038/nm843

[4] Hoshida Y, Nijman SM, Kobayashi M, et al. Integrative transcriptome analysis reveals common molecular subclasses of human hepatocellular carcinoma. Cancer Res. 2009;69(18):7385-7392. doi:10.1158/0008-5472.CAN-09-1089.

[5] Chiang DY, Villanueva A, Hoshida Y, et al. Focal gains of VEGFA and molecular classification of hepatocellular carcinoma. Cancer Res. 2008;68(16):6779-6788. doi:10.1158/0008-5472.CAN-08-0742

[6] Lee JS, Chu IS, Heo J, et al. Classification and prediction of survival in hepatocellular carcinoma by gene expression profiling. Hepatology. 2004;40(3):667-676. doi:10.1002/hep.20375

[7] Cancer Genome Atlas Research Network. Electronic address: wheeler@bcm.edu; Cancer Genome Atlas Research Network. Comprehensive and Integrative Genomic Characterization of Hepatocellular Carcinoma. *Cell*. 2017;169(7):1327-1341.e23. doi:10.1016/j.cell.2017.05.046

[8] Sia D, Jiao Y, Martinez-Quetglas I, et al. Identification of an Immune-specific Class of Hepatocellular Carcinoma, Based on Molecular Features. *Gastroenterology*. 2017;153(3):812-826. doi:10.1053/j.gastro.2017.06.007

[9] Boyault S, Rickman DS, de Reyniès A, et al. Transcriptome classification of HCC is related to gene alterations and to new therapeutic targets. Hepatology. 2007;45(1):42-52. doi:10.1002/hep.21467

[10] Shimada S, Mogushi K, Akiyama Y, et al. Comprehensive molecular and immunological characterization of hepatocellular carcinoma. EBio Medicine. 2019;40:457-470. doi:10.1016/j.ebiom.2018.12.058

[11] Hanahan D, Weinberg RA. Hallmarks of cancer: the next generation. Cell. 2011;144(5):646-674. doi:10.1016/j.cell.2011.02.013

[12] Lee JW, Stone ML, Porrett PM, et al. Hepatocytes direct the formation of a pro-metastatic niche in the liver. Nature. 2019;567(7747):249-252. doi:10.1038/s41586-019-1004-y

[13] Ringelhan M, Pfister D, O'Connor T, Pikarsky E, Heikenwalder M. The immunology of hepatocellular carcinoma. Nat Immunol. 2018;19(3):222-232. doi:10.1038/s41590-018-0044-z

[14] Gao Q, Wang XY, Qiu SJ, et al. Tumor stroma reaction-related gene signature predicts clinical outcome in human hepatocellular carcinoma. Cancer Sci. 2011;102(8):1522-1531. doi:10.1111/j.1349-7006.2011.01981.x

[15] Kurebayashi Y, Ojima H, Tsujikawa H, et al. Landscape of immune microenvironment in hepatocellular carcinoma and its additional impact on histological and molecular classification. Hepatology. 2018;68(3):1025-1041. doi:10.1002/hep.29904

[16] Tian MX, Liu WR, Wang H, et al. Tissue-infiltrating lymphocytes signature predicts survival in patients with early/intermediate stage hepatocellular carcinoma. BMC Med. 2019;17(1):106. Published 2019 Jun 5. doi:10.1186/s12916-019-1341-6

[17] Ruiz de Galarreta M, Bresnahan E, Molina-Sánchez P, et al. β-Catenin Activation Promotes Immune Escape and Resistance to Anti-PD-1 Therapy in Hepatocellular Carcinoma. Cancer Discov. 2019;9(8):1124-1141. doi:10.1158/2159-8290.CD-19-0074

[18] Zheng C, Zheng L, Yoo JK, et al. Landscape of Infiltrating T Cells in Liver Cancer Revealed by Single-Cell Sequencing. Cell. 2017;169(7):1342-1356.e16. doi:10.1016/j.cell.2017.05.035

[19] Kuang DM, Zhao Q, Wu Y, et al. Peritumoral neutrophils link inflammatory response to disease progression by fostering angiogenesis in hepatocellular carcinoma. J Hepatol. 2011;54(5):948-955. doi:10.1016/j.jhep.2010.08.041

[20] Liu LZ, Zhang Z, Zheng BH, et al. CCL15 Recruits Suppressive Monocytes to Facilitate Immune Escape and Disease Progression in Hepatocellular Carcinoma. Hepatology. 2019;69(1):143-159. doi:10.1002/hep.30134

[21] Budhu A, Forgues M, Ye QH, et al. Prediction of venous metastases, recurrence, and prognosis in hepatocellular carcinoma based on a unique immune response signature of the liver microenvironment. Cancer Cell. 2006;10(2):99-111. doi:10.1016/j.ccr.2006.06.016

[22] Hoshida Y, Villanueva A, Kobayashi M, et al. Gene expression in fixed tissues and outcome in hepatocellular carcinoma. N Engl J Med. 2008;359(19):1995-2004. doi:10.1056/NEJMoa0804525

[23] Dong LQ, Peng LH, Ma LJ, et al. Heterogeneous immunogenomic features and distinct escape mechanisms in multifocal hepatocellular carcinoma. J Hepatol. 2020;72(5):896-908. doi:10.1016/j.jhep.2019.12.014

[24] Gu FM, Li QL, Gao Q, et al. IL-17 induces AKT-dependent IL-6/JAK2/STAT3 activation and tumor progression in hepatocellular carcinoma. Mol Cancer. 2011;10:150. Published 2011 Dec 15. doi:10.1186/1476-4598-10-150

[25] Gao Q, Wang XY, Qiu SJ, et al. Overexpression of PD-L1 significantly associates with tumor aggressiveness and postoperative recurrence in human hepatocellular carcinoma. Clin Cancer Res. 2009;15(3):971-979. doi:10.1158/1078-0432.CCR-08-1608

[26] Gao Q, Qiu SJ, Fan J, et al. Intratumoral balance of regulatory and cytotoxic T cells is associated with prognosis of hepatocellular carcinoma after resection. J Clin Oncol. 2007;25(18):2586-2593. doi:10.1200/JCO.2006.09.4565

[27] Jiang Y, Sun A, Zhao Y, et al. Proteomics identifies new therapeutic targets of early-stage hepatocellular carcinoma. Nature. 2019;567(7747):257-261. doi:10.1038/s41586-019-0987-8

[28] Ng AWT, Poon SL, Huang MN, et al. Aristolochic acids and their derivatives are widely implicated in liver cancers in Taiwan and throughout Asia. Sci Transl Med. 2017;9(412):eaan6446. doi:10.1126/scitranslmed.aan6446

[29] Gao Q, Zhu H, Dong L, et al. Integrated Proteogenomic Characterization of HBV-Related Hepatocellular Carcinoma [published correction appears in Cell. 2019 Nov 14;179(5):1240]. Cell. 2019;179(2):561-577.e22. doi:10.1016/j.cell.2019.08.052

[30] Satriano L, Lewinska M, Rodrigues PM, Banales JM, Andersen JB.

Metabolic rearrangements in primary liver cancers: cause and consequences. Nat Rev Gastroenterol Hepatol. 2019;16(12):748-766. doi:10.1038/s41575-019-0217-8

[31] Luo P, Yin P, Hua R, et al. A Large-scale, multicenter serum metabolite biomarker identification study for the early detection of hepatocellular carcinoma. Hepatology. 2018;67(2):662-675. doi:10.1002/hep.29561

[32] Bidkhori G, Benfeitas R, Klevstig M, et al. Metabolic network-based stratification of hepatocellular carcinoma reveals three distinct tumor subtypes. Proc Natl Acad Sci U S A. 2018;115(50):E11874-E11883. doi:10.1073/pnas.1807305115

[33] Ding Z, Ericksen RE, Escande-Beillard N, Lee QY, Loh A, Denil S, Steckel M, Haegebarth A, Wai Ho TS, Chow P, Toh HC, Reversade B, Gruenewald S, Han W. Metabolic pathway analyses identify proline biosynthesis pathway as a promoter of liver tumorigenesis. J Hepatol. 2020 Apr;72(4):725-735. doi: 10.1016/j.jhep.2019.10.026.

Chapter 11

Surgical Therapy of Hepatocellular Carcinoma: State of the Art Liver Resection

Spyridon Davakis, Michail Vailas, Alexandros Kozadinos, Panagiotis Sakarellos, Anastasia Karampa, Dimitrios Korkolis, Georgios Glantzounis, Alexandros Papalampros and Evangelos Felekouras

Abstract

Hepatocellular carcinoma (HCC) represents the third most common cause of cancer-related death, showing incremental growth rates throughout the last decades. HCC requires multidisciplinary approach in a group of patients suffering from underlying chronic liver disease, usually in the setting of cirrhosis. The mainstay of treatment in resectable cases is surgery, with anatomic and non-anatomic liver resections widely implemented, as well as liver transplantation in well-selected individuals. Nowadays, there is a variety of liver parenchyma transection devices used by hepatobiliary surgeons in specialized centers, which has significantly improved postoperative outcomes in HCC patients. Therefore, hepatectomy is considered safe and feasible and should be the main therapeutic option for HCC patients, candidates for resection. Liver resection utilizing cavitron ultrasonic aspirator in combination with bipolar radiofrequency ablation is safe and effective for the treatment of HCC with favorable clinical and oncological outcomes.

Keywords: Hepatocellular Carcinoma, cirrhosis, surgical treatment, liver resection, technique, outcomes

1. Introduction

The evolution and development of the surgical techniques utilized during liver resection for Hepatocellular Carcinoma (HCC) are largely an account of the efforts to minimize bleeding during liver parenchymal transection. There is a close relation between blood loss and unfavorable outcomes during liver resection. The modern era liver transection techniques are based on notable advances in solid organ imaging (Computed Tomography, Magnetic Resonance Imaging, Ultrasound), vastly improved anesthetic management, enhanced knowledge of segmental liver anatomy as described by Couinaud [1], refined surgical techniques with notable appreciation of the functional reserve of the liver remnant, as well as the liver regeneration process [2].

Major hepatectomies had been associated with mortality rates of up to 20% during 1990's, and excessive bleeding was an important and common cause of operative mortality [3]. However, liver resection can now be accomplished with mortality rates of less than 2% in most specialized hepato-pancreato-biliary (HPB) centers [4].

While better patient selection and improved assessment of functional liver remnant are important factors [5], reduced blood loss and the diminishing need for blood transfusion have been additional reasons for improved peri-operative outcome [6]. Other advances in operative technique, including improved delineation of the optimal transection plane with intra-operative ultrasound [7] and the benefit of intermittent inflow occlusion, have also contributed to a reduction in blood loss during major liver resections [8].

The technique of parenchymal transection in hepatic resection has been a topic of great debate for decades worldwide. Finger fraction and clamp-crush techniques have been presented more than fifty years ago and have established as standard approach for liver transection. Significant technological improvements over the past thirty years have led to utilization and adoption of specific surgical instruments and devices for liver transection, such as radiofrequency ablation (RF), ultrasonic cavitron aspirators (Cusa), bipolar sealers (Aquamantis), bipolar energy devices (Ligasure), ultrasonic dissectors (Harmonic), water jet and Tissue link, amongst others [5, 9, 10].

2. Prehistory of liver surgery (1886–1950)

Liver surgery has been a huge chapter in modern surgery and more groundbreaking evolution is still yet to come. Its meaningful to review the beginning of hepatic resections that were reported in the 19th century and follow the journey up to modern times and the techniques that are used today.

The first hepatic operation was done and reported back in 1886 by Lius. He achieved the first partial hepatectomy to a patient with a hepatic adenoma. Reportedly, the use of sharp instruments and Paquelins cautery were utilized for this operation. Unfortunately, post -op hemorrhage was uncontrollable, and the patient died. It is interesting to note that even back in the 19th century, the use of cautery by liquid means was prominent [11].

Following the pioneer of hepatic surgery, Bruns (1888- metastatic liver cancer) and von Eiselberg (1893-hemangioma) attempted hepatectomies. Furthermore, Keen described in 1899 a liver wedge resection in 3 of his patients [12]. In 1891 Lucke achieved the first successful left lobar liver carcinoma excision [13]. In 1908 a very famous physician, whose technique is predominantly used around the world today in hepatic operations, Doctor Pringle, performed abdominal operation in 4 patients with hepatic bleeding of traumatic cause. He managed to control the hemorrhage by clamping the hepatic vein and artery. Only 1 patient survived after this maneuver [14].

In 1911 Wendel reported the first successful right hepatectomy in a 44-year-old woman. He followed the instructions of Cantlie's functional anatomy in detail. Primarily hilar dissection and ligation of right hepatic artery and right hepatic duct was achieved, and furthermore dissection through the quite avascular plane described by Cantlie was performed. Only a year later, Lin applied a new technique. The goal was to resect and destroy liver parenchyma with minimal damage to vessels. This concept will be followed over the years up to present times. The use of the "finger fracture method" served such purpose by resecting parenchyma and leaving vessels undamaged and ready for ligation [15].

As years passed by, it is more evident that 5 historic factors from 1950 and onwards played a role and shaped liver surgery, especially for hepatocellular carcinoma, as we know it today. Primarily the ability of bleeding control in liver trauma gave confidence to surgeons to proceed in large resections. Secondly, the control of blood supply and drainage of the liver to a more specific level rather than gross ligation of large vessels. The advance in supportive medicine such in fluid balance, adequate anesthesia, respiratory support, and hemodynamics played a key role in a successful operation. Following these, the advancement of imaging modalities and the multimodality team approach in treatment algorithm of HCC.

3. Multi-modality treatment of HCC

HCC remains the leading cause of cancer related mortality worldwide [16]. Hepatitis C is the most frequent risk factor for HCC in the Western world. On the other hand, chronic hepatitis B infection is the main risk factor in East Asia and sub-Saharan Africa, where incidence rates of HCC are the highest [17]. The MDT can establish patient access to well-established, as well as new multimodality therapies, consulting with all the involved specialists. These emerging therapeutic algorithms have led to review and updates of the treatment management in primary hepatobiliary cancers. Surgery remains the most-effective curative option for all primary hepatobiliary cancers; however, not all patients are good surgical candidates at the diagnosis, due to advanced disease. The Hepatobiliary MDT is crucial for ensuring that other treatment modalities are considered (palliation – best supportive care). This approach can optimize patient care, both on curative and palliative ways. HCC screening has undoubtedly helped earlier detection of tumors, allowing prompt commencement of treatment, positively impact on patients' outcomes [18].

4. Evolution of imaging modalities

Although current management guidelines for HCC do not require biopsy to prove the diagnosis, lesions greater than 2 cm on MRI or Computed Tomograph Angiography (CTA) scans, with elevated AFP (more than 400 ng/mL) or AFP incrising within sequential measurements, do not require pathologic confirmation according to the guidelines of the European Association for the Study of the Liver (EASL) [19].

According to American Assosiation of Liver Diseases (AASLD) guidelines, liver nodules detected on abdominal US, measuring less than 1 cm should be re-examined twice a year. If no radiological alteration of the hepatic lesion has occurred during a period of up to 2 consecutive years, routine surveillance should be considered.

Every suspicious lesion in high-risk population, with suggestive US-findings for HCC, should be further studied with additional imaging modalities. This radiology workup should include a 4-phase multidetector CT scan or dynamic contrast enhanced MRI. If the tumor has all the typical characteristics of HCC, it should be treated as HCC. If a liver nodule compatible with HCC is greater 2 cm at the initial diagnosis after one dynamic imaging study, biopsy is not mandatory. However, if the vascular profile of the lession on imaging studies of a non-cirrhotic patient is not compatible with HCC, a second imaging study or biopsy of the lesion should be performed to secure the correct diagnosis. If the biopsy is negative for HCC, patients should be further surveilled *via* an abdominal US every 3–6 months, until the lession presents enlarged or with altered imaging characteristics. According to the guidelines of the Asia-Pacific Association for the Study of the Liver 2010 [20], every liver lesion with non-typical vascular features should be further investigated with other modalities, such as endoscopic ultrasound (EUS).

It is well established that contrast-enhanced CT scans and MRI scans can be performed to examine, differentiate, and investigate a liver lesion. HCC has commonly a unique imaging array [21]. High arterial-phase contrast uptake followed by rapid washout in late phase are common in contrast-enhanced CT and MRI scans; these characteristics may not be present in earlier stages or in not well-differentiated tumors. Triphasic CTA can identify more lesions; however, in patients with nodular cirrhosis, contrast-enhanced MRI should be performed. Tumors sizing between 1 and 2 cm in cirrhotic patients, should be further studied with triphasic CTA and MRI to exclude HCC [22].

5. Anesthesiology management

During the last century, huge technological and medical advance aid surgeons to easier define their objective rather carefully and to overcome the shrieks and wails of their awake patients as in past times. Anesthesia of modern times came of age, so that the operating rooms became well-orchestrated exhibitions of joint expertise and support. We can now safely say that all matters are now a concern of the anesthetists; they furnished the hemodynamic support for complex operations, as liver surgery. Consequently, surgeons were allowed to focus on their meticulous procedures.

Matters of special interest are conditions that can cause an elevation of right-side cardiac and central venous pressure (CVP), which can significantly increase the risk of intra-operative bleeding. Invasive arterial and CVP monitoring allows for better hemodynamic control and regular blood sampling. All patients may benefit from cardiac output monitoring, enabling greater stability during the cardiovascular changes associated with vascular occlusion during hepatic resection. Core temperature should be monitored and normothermia maintained using warmed-fluids and forced warm-air blankets. Intra-operative coagulation profile should be monitored and corrected with fresh frozen plasma or/and coagulation factors, as indicated from laboratory results. Neuromuscular block should be also monitored [23].

6. Surgical approach

It well established that in patients without impaired underlying liver status (cirrhosis), an anatomical resection should be accomplished. Major hepatectomies can include up to two-thirds of the functional parenchyma. For cirrhotic patients, due to impaired liver regeneration process, resection is generally minimized to smaller hepatectomies, to maintain adequate liver function. Hypertrophy of the future liver remnant can be achieved with the use of pre-operative portal vein embolization (PVE).

One of the most important key factors during liver resection of HCC is the utilization of intra-operative ultrasound (IOUS), to identify tumor location, margins and its relation to the inflow and outflow vascular structures. The definition of a proper surgical strategy is important not only for achieving an adequate tumor-free margin, but also for avoiding inadvertent injuries to major intrahepatic vessels or bile duct pedicles during dissection or resection.

Management of hepatic inflow through the portal vein and/or vena cava, and hepatic outflow through the hepatic veins, can be routinely performed with control of this vessels. Controlling of the vascular inflow (Pringle maneuver) as an alternative to total vascular occlusion, has decrease deleterious effects of liver ischemia. Ischemic preconditioning of the liver has recently been proposed as a hepatoprotective measure, consisting of application of a brief period of ischemia (10 min) and reperfusion (10 min) after which, a prolonged-period of the liver inflow occlusion can be safely supported. In a prospective series, comparing major liver resections using the Pringle maneuver lasting 30–60 min, an advantage was found of ischemic preconditioning in young patients (<60 years), as well as in patients with steatosis or cirrhosis. Intermittent Pringle occlusion can be well tolerated by cirrhotic patients for up to 60 minutes, and is better tolerated than continuous clamping. The use of low CVP (less than 5 mm Hg) is also of great importance.

7. Techniques of liver parenchyma transection for HCC

7.1 Finger fracture technique

Hepatic transection remained a challenge for all surgeons, for more than a century. The first scheduled hepatectomy was performed in 1888 from Carl Langenbuch [24]. Liver surgery was minimal thus, up to the 20th century, when Pringle maneuver was first presented, for bleeding control during emergency hepatic resections [14]. Hepatectomy is particularly difficult in cirrhotic liver due to the fibrotic nature of liver tissue. The finger fracture technique, the liver tissue is fractured and crushed by the thumb and index finger followed by isolating and ligating the resistant intrahepatic vascular and ductal structures [15].

7.2 Crash-clamp (Kelly) technique

The finger fracture technique, in which the parenchymal transection is done by crushing the parenchyma between the thumb and another finger isolating vessels and bile ducts which were ligated and divided, after liver inflow occlusion, was afterward improved using a surgical instrument such as the Kelly clamp [25]. Using the Kelly clamp technique during hepatic resection of cirrhotic liver with HCC can be performed in less operative time, while help obtaining a clearer operative field [26].

7.3 Radiofrequency ablation (RFA) assisted technique

RF assisted hepatectomy, for the treatment of hepatocellular carcinoma amongst other liver malignancies, was first implemented by Habib's group at Hammersmith Hospital, London, UK [27]. Ever since, RFA has been widely used for the in-situ ablation of unresectable liver and other solid organ tumors [28], but it has now been incorporated into routine liver resection, being used to create a line of coagulative necrosis that can subsequently be divided with a scalpel with relatively little blood loss [29]. In recent years, the continuous use and development of RFA ablation in liver surgery have produced satisfactory results in the treatment of small HCC. It can also block small and medium-sized blood vessels in the liver through thermal coagulation, so it has been used in liver resection to reduce bleeding. However, the use of this technique remains controversial due to reported perioperative outcomes and complications; some studies have reported that radiofrequency-assisted liver resection causes severe postoperative liver dysfunction, and the incidence of postoperative complications is higher than that of simple hepatectomy [30].

7.4 Cavitron ultrasonic aspirator (CUSA) technique

Cavitron Ultrasonic Surgical Aspirator (CUSA), also known as Ultrasonic Dissector, was first popularized by Hodgson et al. in 1979 [31]. The ultrasonic waves generate energy to fragment and aspirate parenchymal tissue. Contact of the oscillating titanium tip instigate fragmentation of hepatocytes owing to the high-water content while, selectively sparing the blood vessels and bile ducts because of poor tissue water content. In the liver parenchyma, anatomically, both the Glissonean cords as the inflow system and the hepatic veins as the outflow system show branching, like a tree. Both systems rise from the dorsal side, where they are relatively close to each other, and branch towards the ventral side. Any liver resection can become simpler and safer by selectively dissecting in a plane, where no Glissonean cord runs, such as an intersegmental plane. When such planes are dissected with the CUSA, the hepatic veins, which are relatively thicker and can be more easily identified than those that appear when the other parts are divided, usually appear in the cutting plane. Further, some thinner branches, which cross the cutting plane and flow into the exposed thicker hepatic vein, should be cut at the confluence without incurring a split injury [32]. It has been proven that CUSA selectively destroys and aspirates parenchyma, leaving vessels and biliary ducts almost intact with larger vessels and large intrahepatic bile ducts amenable to ligation or clipping [33].

7.5 Sealing device-assisted technique

The LigaSure Vessel Sealing System (Valleylab, Boulder, CO, USA) is a hemostatic and dissecting tool, which is able seal blood vessels (up to 7 mm in diameter), by denaturing collagen and elastin within the vessel wall and in the surrounding connective tissue [34]. LigaSure can be safely applied in any type of liver and hepatectomy combined with the crush clamping method.

The Harmonic Scalpel (Ethicon Endo-Surgery, Cincinnati, OH, USA), utilizes ultrasonic vibration of two blades causing destruction of hydrogen bonds. This disturbance of hydrogen bonds causes protein denaturization coagulating small vessels of 3 mm diameter. The parenchyma is then transected with blade movement in a saw-like fashion [35].

7.6 Tools for resection

As mentioned above, the techniques used in liver transections were described in reports and were widely used. From the finger fracture technique described by Lin [15] to the use of the blunt end of a hemostat by Ogilvie [36] and the use of the blunt edge of a scalpel by Quattlebaum, a common goal can be perceived. The identification of different tissues, parenchyma vs. vessel, via the means of blunt dissection. Perseverance of great vessels and following appropriate ligation was the main aim of hepatic surgeons to avoid uncontrollable hemorrhage. Avoiding such complication could mean avoiding death.

In 1928 the first electrocautery device was invented. The Bovie knife, known from its inventors Bovie and Cushing, is the tool of choice up to this day by majority of centers when it comes to hemostasis and partial resection of the liver parenchyma [37]. A few years later, the need of new and perhaps more effective ways for liver surgery was explored.

Another technique that originates from compression characteristics of hemostasis is the hemostatic clamp. During the years, many surgeons have used such clamps. Back in 1960s the first clamp used in liver surgery was described by Stucke [38]. Variation of such were seen within the same decade. It needed the efforts of Nakayama to reach a newly designed clamp, specific to the liver [39].

8. Our technique

We have been performing liver resection routinely for the past 30 years. The first attempt towards a bloodless and uneventful hepatectomy was the formation of a proper HPB Unit, formed by specialist surgeons, dedicated anesthetists, ICU beds and experienced radiologists (invasive). Gradual implementation and enhancement of the new techniques followed. In the beginning, finger fracture/crash clamp technique was performed in all cases of liver resection, with the addition of electrocautery and argon beamer as adjuncts. Following that, from the beginning of 2000s, we adopted and evolved the RF-assisted liver resections, with favorable outcomes during numerous hepatectomies. However, we moved to the two surgeons' technique with newer abdominal retractors (Thompson Liver / Oncology System) since 2006; our transection tools have been standardized to implementation of CUSA for dissection of liver parenchyma and Aquamantis for hemostasis (**Figures 1** and **2**).

For major hepatectomies the ipsilateral major hepatic veins were encircled within vessel loops. When an anatomic resection was planned, hilar dissection was performed (**Figure 3**).

The ipsilateral branch of hepatic artery, portal vein, and common bile duct were encircled within vessel loops, but not divided, until the parenchymal dissection reached that point. Hilar dissection was not performed for non-anatomical hepatectomy. During major hepatectomies, the ipsilateral hepatic artery, portal vein branches and bile duct branches were ligated intra-hepatically during parenchymal transection. In addition, for major hepatectomies, the major hepatic veins were either suture-ligated and divided or divided using endovascular staplers at the end of parenchymal transection (**Figures 4–8**).

Drains are routinely placed in all patients.

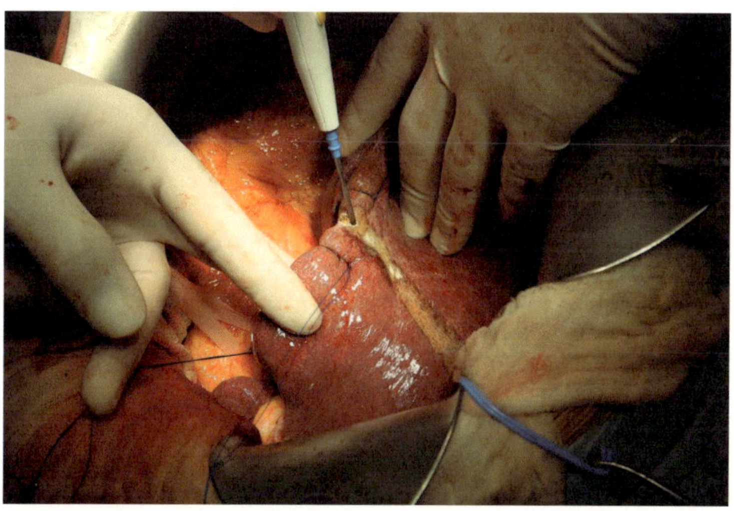

Figure 1.
Demarcation line using monopolar cautery.

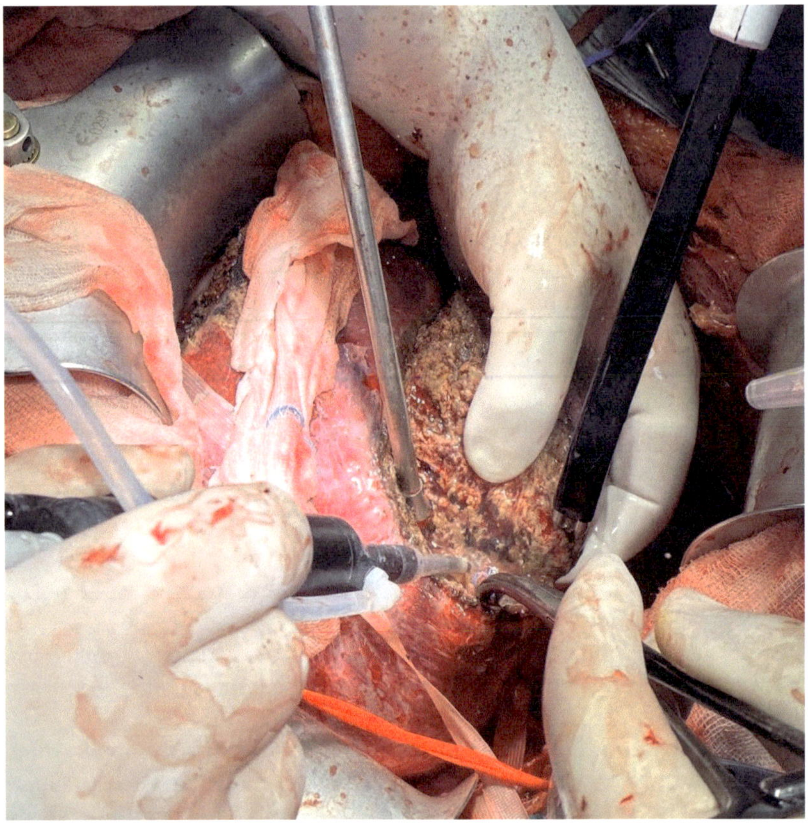

Figure 2.
Liver transection with CUSA and Aquamantis.

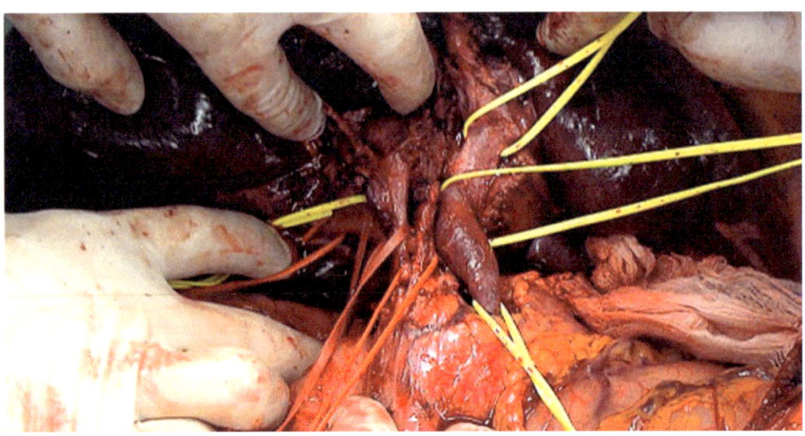

Figure 3.
Hilar dissection.

Anatomic and non-anatomic hepatectomies, wedge resections and liver ablations are routinely performed for the treatment of HCC from our team. Anatomic resections are selected in patients with unilobular disease and adequate liver function. Major hepatectomies include right and left hepatectomies, as well as extended right and extended left hepatectomies or trisectionectomies. Non-anatomic resections and liver ablation can be performed for smaller lesions, multilobular disease, in patients with previous hepatic resection (recurrence) or in cases with severely impaired liver function. Parenchymal sparing is crucial for maintaining adequate liver remnant post hepatectomy for these patients. In addition, vascular reconstructions in cases with vascular infiltration is possible in specific cases, as ex-vivo hepatectomy with auto-transplantation in cases of locally advanced/unresectable disease.

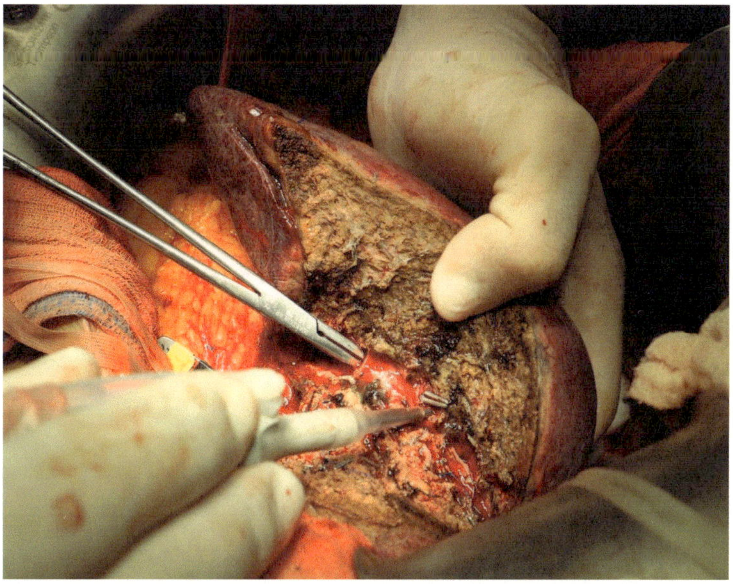

Figure 4.
Dissection of segmental branches.

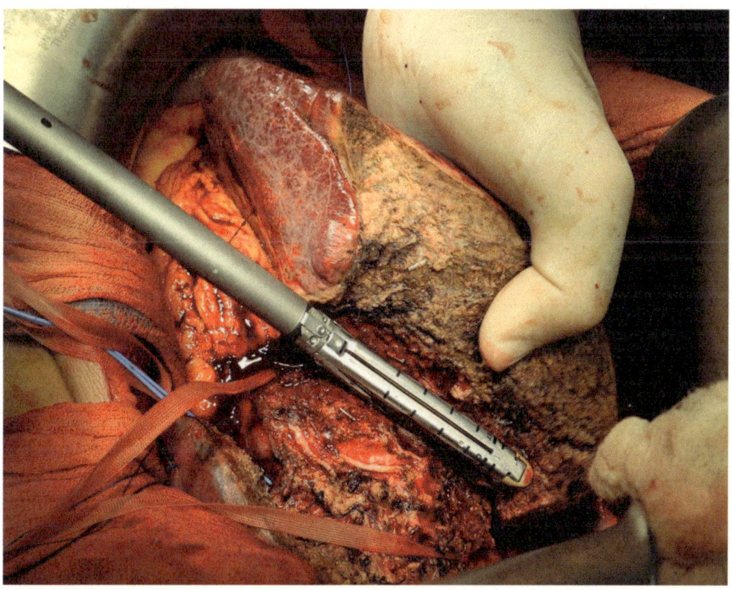

Figure 5.
Transection with vascular stapler.

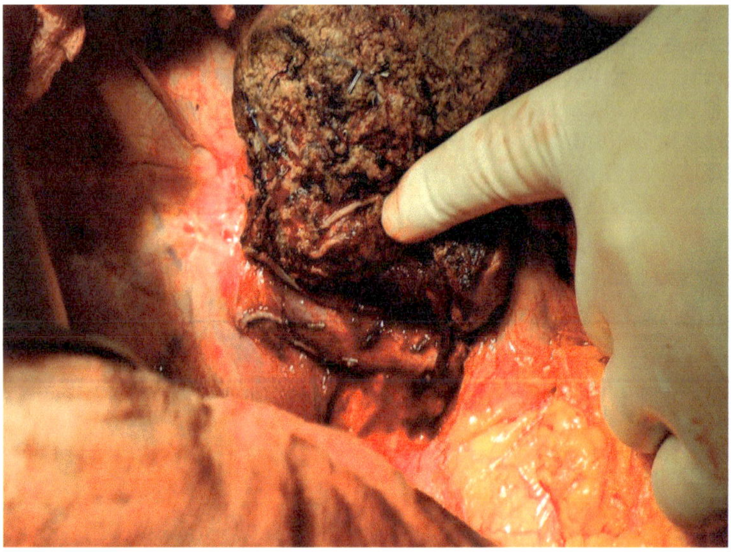

Figure 6.
Remaining liver parenchyma post right hepatectomy.

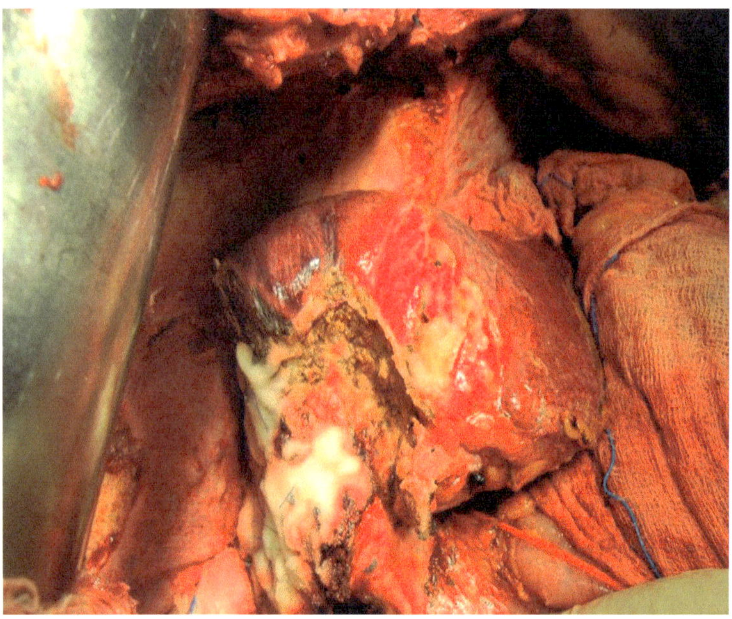

Figure 7.
Use of hemostatic-fibrin glue and final inspection.

9. Results

Between January 1st 2010 and January 1st 2021, more than n = 300 consecutive hepatectomies were performed in three referral hepatobiliary centers in Greece, from affiliated surgeons. Patients included in this study was treated for hepatocellular carcinoma and were treated with curative intent (hepatectomy). Adult patients that underwent elective operations were enrolled. All emergency operations or operations for other liver malignancies were excluded.

N = 170 patients underwent liver resection for HCC during the study period. Mean age was 75 years (Range: 20–85). There were 115 males and 55 female patients. Etiology of liver disease was liver cirrhosis in most cases, due to alcoholic liver disease (ALD) (23.5%), hepatitis B (HBV) infection (42.35%), hepatitis C (HBC) infection (17.64%) and hepatic steatosis (16.4%). Most of the patients (n = 99, 55%) were BCLC-A patients, while n = 71 (45%) patients were BCLC-B or BCLC-C staged. N = 89 patients (52.35%) passed away during the follow-up. Post-operative complications according to Clavien-Dindo classification, were grade I in 54.66%, grade II in 24% and III-IV in 17.33% of the cases, respectively. Thirty and 90-day mortality rates were 1.13%. Mean length of hospital stay was 17.5 days. Mean OS was 46.66 months, while mean PFS was 31.56 months. OS figures for 1, 3 and 5 years was 87.14%, 64% and 42% respectively.

This data indicates that liver resection for HCC with utilization of the combined technique of saline-linked radiofrequency ablation and ultrasonic aspiration, is safe and feasible, leading towards bloodless liver resection without the use of vascular occlusion, ensuring that surgical treatment for HCC becomes comparatively safer (**Figure 8**).

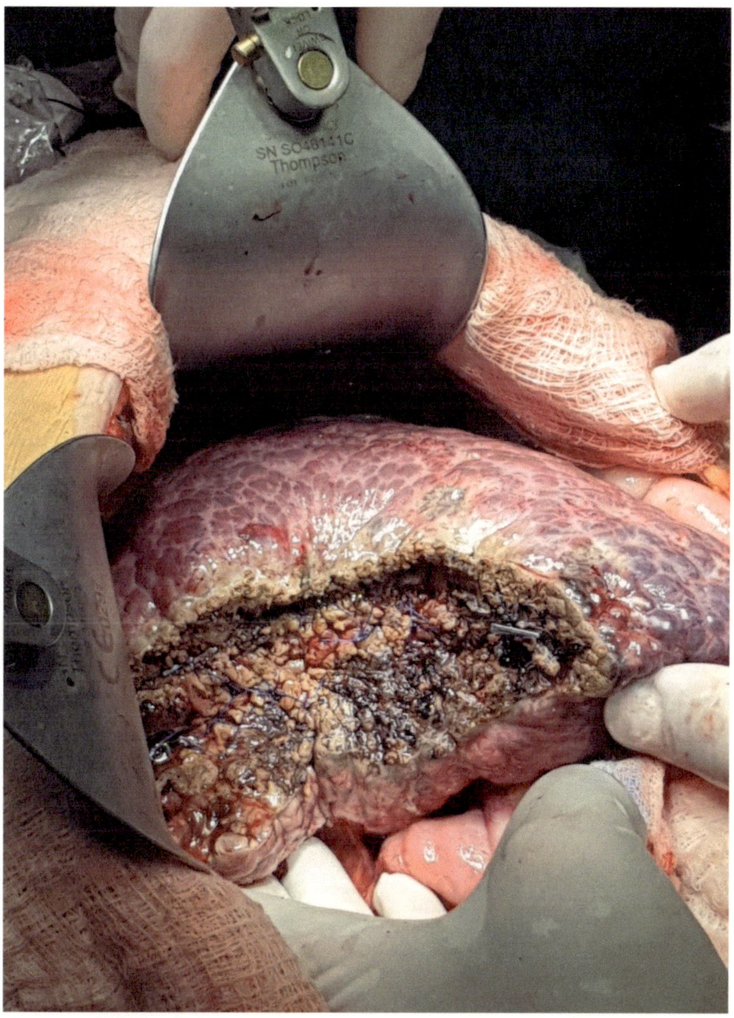

Figure 8.
Right hepatectomy for HCC in a cirrhotic patient.

9.1 Minimally invasive liver resection

Minimally invasive liver resection is on the rise. However, the majority of performed operations are minor or limited resections in highly selected patients, from experienced hepato-biliary surgeons. The first laparoscopic liver resection was reported in 1991 [40], was referred to excision of peripheral hepatic lesions. Anatomic resections such as left lateral hepatectomy were followed thereafter [41]. The first series of laparoscopic hepatectomies were published in 1998 by Hüscher et al. [42] using totally laparoscopic and hand-assisted (hybrid) approach for right-sided liver resections.

Although it has several theoretical advantages, only a small percentage of liver resections are performed by minimally invasive surgery. A French national database study, published in 2014, presented that only 15% of liver resections were performed through minimally invasive approach [43].

Minor laparoscopic resections in anterolateral segments, as well as left lateral sectionectomy are considered the gold-standard approach in the hands of experts nowadays [44]. On the other hand, excision of bilateral lesions or lesions in posterosuperior segments or in central locations of the liver (segments 1, 4a, 7, and 8), and mostly major hepatectomies are still considered rather challenging. Another key factor is the learning curve for minimally invasive liver resection, that can reach up to 75 operations [45].

Robot-assisted surgery has been gradually adopted as an alternative to laparoscopy, mainly in complex and major liver resections [46]. Despite all the potential advantages, most of the available evidence present no superiority of robotic assisted comparing to laparoscopic liver resections [47].

10. Conclusion

Hepatocellular Carcinoma (HCC) is the most frequent primary liver tumor. Well-established risk factors include chronic hepatitis B and C, non-alcoholic liver cirrhosis and liver steatosis amongst others, leading to impaired liver function in most cases. Surveillance programs and multi-disciplinary team approach aim to early diagnosis and effective therapy. Liver resection is the mainstay of treatment for HCC. All efforts are made towards bloodless hepatectomies, with adoption of newer techniques and evolvement of existing approaches. Laparoscopic or robotic liver resection can offer all the advantages of minimally invasive surgery in the hands of experts and for specific group of patients. Our technique of liver resection for HCC consists of saline-linked radiofrequency ablation and ultrasonic aspiration, is safe and feasible, leading towards bloodless liver resection without the use of vascular occlusion, ensuring that surgical treatment for HCC becomes comparatively safer in specialized hepatobiliary cancer centers.

Author details

Spyridon Davakis[1]*, Michail Vailas[1], Alexandros Kozadinos[1], Panagiotis Sakarellos[1], Anastasia Karampa[2], Dimitrios Korkolis[3], Georgios Glantzounis[2], Alexandros Papalampros[1] and Evangelos Felekouras[1]

1 First Department of Surgery, Laiko General Hospital, National and Kapodistrian University of Athens, Athens, Greece

2 Department of Surgery, Ioannina University Hospital, Ioannina, Greece

3 Department of Surgery, Saint Savvas Hospital, Hellenic Anticancer Institute, Athens, Greece

*Address all correspondence to: spdavakis@gmail.com

References

[1] Couinaud C. Liver anatomy: Portal (and suprahepatic) or biliary segmentation. Dig Surg 1999;16(6):459-467.

[2] Khatri VP, Schneider PD. Liver surgery: Modern concepts and techniques. Surg Clin North Am 2004;84(2):xv-xvi.

[3] Terblanche J, Krige JE, Bornman PC. Simplified hepatic resection with the use of prolonged vascular inflow occlusion. Arch Surg 1991;126(3): 298-301.

[4] Cescon M, Vetrone G, Grazi GL, Ramacciato G, Ercolani G, Ravaioli M, Del Gaudio M, Pinna AD. Trends in perioperative outcome after hepatic resection: analysis of 1500 consecutive unselected cases over 20 years. Ann Surg. 2009 Jun;249(6):995-1002. doi: 10.1097/SLA.0b013e3181a63c74. PMID: 19474679.

[5] Poon RT. Current techniques of liver transection. HPB (Oxford) 2007;9(3):166-173.

[6] Lesurtel M, Selzner M, Petrowsky H, McCormack L, Clavien PA. How should transection of the liver be performed? A prospective randomized study in 100 consecutive patients: Comparing four different transection strategies. Ann Surg 2005;242(6):814-822.

[7] Donadon M, Costa G, Torzilli G. State of the art of intraoperative ultrasound in liver surgery: current use for staging and resection guidance. Ultraschall Med. 2014 Dec;35(6):500-511; quiz 512-3. doi: 10.1055/s-0034-1385515. Epub 2014 Dec 4. PMID: 25474100.

[8] Moris D, Rahnemai-Azar AA, Tsilimigras DI, Ntanasis-Stathopoulos I, Marques HP, Spartalis E, Felekouras E, Pawlik TM. Updates and Critical Insights on Glissonian Approach in Liver Surgery. J Gastrointest Surg. 2018 Jan;22(1):154-163. doi: 10.1007/s11605-017-3613-9. Epub 2017 Nov 3. PMID: 29101722.

[9] Prassas E, Petrou A, Kontos M, Rizos D, Neofytou K, Pikoulis E, Diamantis T, Felekouras E. Radiofrequency ablation assisted resection for hepatocellular carcinoma: morbidity, mortality and long term survival. J BUON. 2014 Jan-Mar;19(1):256-262. PMID: 24659673.

[10] Felekouras E, Petrou A, Neofytou K, Giakoustidis A, Bagenal J, Cananzi F, Pikoulis E, Mudan S. Combined ultrasonic aspiration and saline-linked radiofrequency precoagulation: a step toward bloodless liver resection without the need of liver inflow occlusion: analysis of 313 consecutive patients. World J Surg Oncol. 2014 Nov 25;12:357. doi: 10.1186/1477-7819-12-357. PMID: 25424566; PMCID: PMC4256890.

[11] Blumgart LH, Belghiti J. Surgery of the liver, biliary tract, and pancreas. 4th ed. Philadelphia, PA: Saunders Elsevier, 2007.

[12] Keen WW IV. Report of a case of resection of the liver for the removal of a neoplasm, with a table of seventy-six cases of resection of the liver for hepatic tumors. Ann Surg. 1899;30:267-283.

[13] Lucke H. Zentralbl. Chir. 1891; 6:115.

[14] Pringle JH. V. Notes on the Arrest of Hepatic Hemorrhage Due to Trauma. Ann Surg. 1908 Oct;48(4):541-9. doi: 10.1097/00000658-190810000-00005. PMID: 17862242; PMCID: PMC1406963.

[15] Lin TY. A simplified technique for hepatic resection: the crush method. Ann Surg. 1974 Sep;180(3):285-90. doi: 10.1097/00000658-197409000-00005. PMID: 4368356; PMCID: PMC1343660.

[16] Siegel RL, Miller KD, Jemal A. Cancer statistics, 2016. CA: A Cancer Journal for Clinicians, 2016; 66: 7-30. https://doi.org/10.3322/caac.21332

[17] European Association For The Study Of The Liver; European Organisation For Research And Treatment Of Cancer. EASL-EORTC clinical practice guidelines: management of hepatocellular carcinoma. J Hepatol. 2012 Apr;56(4):908-43. doi: 10.1016/j.jhep.2011.12.001. Erratum in: J Hepatol. 2012 Jun;56(6):1430. PMID: 22424438.

[18] Alabraba E, Joshi H, Bird N, Griffin R, Sturgess R, Stern N, Sieberhagen C, Cross T, Camenzuli A, Davis R, Evans J, O'Grady E, Palmer D, Diaz-Nieto R, Fenwick S, Poston G, Malik H. Increased multimodality treatment options has improved survival for Hepatocellular carcinoma but poor survival for biliary tract cancers remains unchanged. Eur J Surg Oncol. 2019 Sep;45(9):1660-1667. doi: 10.1016/j.ejso.2019.04.002. Epub 2019 Apr 9. PMID: 31014988.

[19] Dimitroulis D, Damaskos C, Valsami S, Davakis S, Garmpis N, Spartalis E, Athanasiou A, Moris D, Sakellariou S, Kykalos S, Tsourouflis G, Garmpi A, Delladetsima I, Kontzoglou K, Kouraklis G. From diagnosis to treatment of hepatocellular carcinoma: An epidemic problem for both developed and developing world. World J Gastroenterol. 2017 Aug 7;23(29):5282-5294. doi: 10.3748/wjg.v23.i29.5282. PMID: 28839428; PMCID: PMC5550777.

[20] Omata M, Lesmana LA, Tateishi R, Chen PJ, Lin SM, Yoshida H, Kudo M, Lee JM, Choi BI, Poon RT, et al. Asian Pacific Association for the Study of the Liver consensus recommendations on hepatocellular carcinoma. Hepatol Int. 2010;4:439-474.

[21] Yu SC, Yeung DT, So NM. Imaging features of hepatocellular carcinoma. Clin Radiol. 2004;59:145-156.

[22] Hennedige T, Venkatesh SK. Imaging of hepatocellular carcinoma: diagnosis, staging and treatment monitoring. Cancer Imaging. 2013;12:530-547.

[23] Weiss E., Mantz J., Paugam-Burtz C. (2018) Liver Resection Surgery: Anesthetic Management, Monitoring, Fluids and Electrolytes. In: Wagener G. (eds) Liver Anesthesiology and Critical Care Medicine. Springer, Cham. https://doi.org/10.1007/978-3-319-64298-7_27

[24] Bismuth H, Eshkenazy R, Arish A. Milestones in the evolution of hepatic surgery. Rambam Maimonides Med J. 2011;2(1):e0021. Published 2011 Jan 31. doi:10.5041/RMMJ.10021.

[25] Kim KH, Lee SG. Usefulness of Kelly clamp crushing technique during hepatic resection. HPB (Oxford). 2008;10(4):281-284. doi:10.1080/13651820802167144.

[26] Weber JC, Navarra G, Jiao LR et al. New technique for liver resection using heat coagulative necrosis. Ann Surg 2002;236:560-563.

[27] Filippou DK, Avgerinos ED, Pavlakis E, Rizos S. Alternative interventional multimodality therapies for the management of liver malignancies. J BUON 2005;10:23-33.

[28] Delis S, Bakoyiannis A, Tassopoulos N et al. Clampcrush technique vs. radiofrequency-assisted liver resection for primary and metastatic liver neoplasms. HPB (Oxford) 2009;11: 339-344.

[29] Zhang F, Yan J, Feng XB, et al. Efficiency and safety of radiofrequency-assisted hepatectomy for hepatocellular carcinoma with cirrhosis: A single-center retrospective cohort study. World J Gastroenterol. 2015;21(35): 10159-10165. doi:10.3748/wjg.v21.i35.10159.

[30] Williams JW, Hodgson WJ. Histologic evaluation of tissues sectioned by ultrasonically powered instruments (a preliminary report). Mt Sinai J Med. 1979; 46:105-106.

[31] Honda G, Ome Y, Yoshida N, Kawamoto Y. How to dissect the liver parenchyma: Excavation with cavitron ultrasonic surgical aspirator. J Hepatobiliary Pancreat Sci. 2020 Nov;27(11):907-912. doi: 10.1002/jhbp.829. Epub 2020 Oct 4. PMID: 32897631.

[32] Saiura A, Yamamoto J, Koga R, Seki M, Yamaguchi T. Liver transection using the LigaSure sealing system. HPB (Oxford). 2008;10(4):239-43. doi: 10.1080/13651820802167714. PMID: 18773111; PMCID: PMC2518307.

[33] Poon RT. Current techniques of liver transection. HPB (Oxford). 2007;9(3):166-73. doi: 10.1080/13651820701216182. PMID: 18333217; PMCID: PMC2063596.

[34] Herman P, Perini MV, Coelho F, Saad W, D'Albuquerque LAC. Half-Pringle Maneuver: a useful tool in laparoscopic liver resection. J Laparoendosc Adv Surg Tech. 2010;20(1):35-37.

[35] Hüscher CG, Lirici MM, Chiodini S. Laparoscopic liver resections. Semin Laparosc Surg. 1998 Sep;5(3):204-210. doi: 10.1177/155335069800500308. PMID: 9787208.

[36] Ogilvie H. Partial hepatectomy. Br Med J. 1953; 2:1136.

[37] Tanabe KK. The past 60 years in liver surgery. Cancer 2008; 113:1888-1896.

[38] Stucke K. A new liver clamp. Chirurg. 1961;32:481-481.

[39] Nakayama K. Simplified hepatectomy. Br J Surg 1958; 45:645-649.

[40] Farges O, Goutte N, Dokmak S, Bendersky N, Falissard B. How surgical technology translates into practice: the model of laparoscopic liver resections performed in France. Ann Surg. 2014;260(5):916-921.

[41] Herman P, Perini MV, Coelho F, Saad W, D'Albuquerque LAC. Half-Pringle Maneuver: a useful tool in laparoscopic liver resection. J Laparoendosc Adv Surg Tech. 2010;20(1):35-37.

[42] Hüscher CG, Lirici MM, Chiodini S. Laparoscopic liver resections. Semin Laparosc Surg. 1998 Sep;5(3):204-210. doi: 10.1177/155335069800500308. PMID: 9787208.

[43] Wakabayashi G, Cherqui D, Geller DA, Buell JF, Kaneko H, Han HS, et al. Recommendations for laparoscopic liver resection: a report from the second international consensus conference held in Morioka. Ann Surg. 2015;261(4): 619-629.

[44] Coelho FF, Kruger JA, Fonseca GM, et al. Laparoscopic liver resection: Experience based guidelines. World J Gastrointest Surg. 2016;8(1):5-26. doi:10.4240/wjgs.v8.i1.5.

[45] Lee W, Woo JW, Lee JK, Park JH, Kim JY, Kwag SJ, et al. Comparison of learning curves for major and minor laparoscopic liver resection. J Laparoendosc Adv Surg Tech A. 2016;26(6):457-464.

[46] Fruscione M, Pickens R, Baker EH, Cochran A, Khan A, Ocuin L, et al. Robotic-assisted versus laparoscopic major liver resection: analysis of outcomes from a single center. HPB (Oxford). 2019;21(7):906-911.

[47] Montalti R, Berardi G, Patriti A, Vivarelli M, Troisi RI. Outcomes of robotic vs laparoscopic hepatectomy: a systematic review and meta-analysis. World J Gastroenterol.

2015;21(27):8441-51.) (Kim JK, Park JS, Han DH, Choi GH, Kim KS, Choi JS, et al. Robotic versus laparoscopic left lateral sectionectomy of liver. Surg Endosc. 2016;90:8.

Chapter 12

Systemic Therapy in Hepatocellular Carcinoma

Chanchai Charonpongsuntorn

Abstract

Systemic therapy of advanced stage hepatocellular carcinoma (HCC) was limited to the sorafenib in the past decade since 2007. Novel agents including multiple targeting agents, immune checkpoint inhibitors and anti-angiogenesis reported efficacy in treatment. This is the first time, the combination of atezolizumab and bevacizumab as first-line treatment is superior to sorafenib. Standard guideline in advanced HCC was changing. New novel drugs increase in available including multiple targeting agents and immune checkpoint blockade such as Lenvatinib, regorafenib, cabozantinib, ramucirumab and immunotherapy as first line or second line therapy will benefit in term of survival benefit and quality of life in advanced stage or unresectable hepatocellular carcinoma.

Keywords: hepatocellular carcinoma, immunotherapy, targeted therapy, systemic therapy, advanced stage

1. Introduction

During the many years, numerous randomized control clinical studies have been performed for testing treatments for advanced hepatocellular carcinoma (HCC) [1]. Historical studies performed to prove efficacy of cancer chemotherapy as single agent or in combination. However, this class of cancer therapy have had no proven benefits on overall survival in advanced stage HCC. Sorafenib a multi-tyrosine kinase inhibitor with antiangiogenesic effects showed a survival benefit and it was established as first-line systemic therapy for advanced stage HCC patients or progression form locoregional therapy since 2007. In recent years, there are new agents has been approved for advanced stage HCC as first line and second line options. Exploratory analyses of these drugs indicate that a cumulative median overall survival more than 20 months with good liver function and quality of life.

2. Systemic chemotherapy

Historically, systemic chemotherapy has not shown survival efficacy in treatment of HCC when used in advance stage HCC. This result comes from single-arm, open label studies evaluating the use of some traditionally chemotherapeutic, that did not lead in the past years and limiting their use in palliative setting or some situations. Single agent anthracyclines and fluoropyrimidines have been most widely used in clinical practice in the past. Unfortunately, that result reported poor response rates and short timing in tumor progression [2]. New chemotherapeutic agents, such as oxaliplatin, have shown clinical benefit in cancers of gastrointestinal tract (stomach cancer, colorectal cancer, or pancreatic cancer). These drugs have also been evaluated for the treatment of advanced stage setting with some benefit findings. As previously said, rational of combination use of chemotherapy might be a valuable option for advance stage HCC. FOLFOX4 regimen (Fluorouracil, leucovorin, oxaliplatin) was evaluated efficacy in comparison with single agent of doxorubicin for advanced stage HCC patients whom ineligible for locoregional therapies or surgery in Phase III EACH study [3]. FOLFOX4 had better results in term of progression free survival (PFS) (2.93 mons vs. 1.77 mons, $P < 0.001$) and in response rate and disease control rate. Although, these positive results and good safety profile in adverse effect but do not necessarily translate to better overall survival that is primary endpoint of the study (6.40 mons vs. 4.97 mons, $P = 0.07$), leading to a negatively result of study. Still, an unplanned subsequent analysis performed at 7 months after the end of the previous study has shown an improvement of survival outcomes (6.46 mons vs. 4.90 mons, $P = 0.04$) but progression free survival, response rate and disease rate control in the Chinese populations [4], leading to FOLFOX4 approval in Chines FDA for advanced HCC. Others, combination drug, GEMOX regimen (Gemcitabine, oxaliplatin) was evaluated in a large, multicenter retrospective study (AGEO) [5]. Results of the study had high response rate with 22%, 66% disease control rate and 4.5 months with 11.0 months in term of progression free survival and overall survival. This interesting result should be considered, response to GEMOX led to better overall survival in comparison with lack of response but possible serious side effects of this regimen (Neurotoxicity, thrombocytopenia, neutropenia, and diarrhea). Furthermore, studies are therefore required in phase III trial to assess the role of this regimen in treatment of advanced stage HCC. Some other oxaliplatin-based regimens have been studies in phase II studies, showing interesting results, such as XELOX (oxaliplatin plus capecitabine) or GP (Gemcitabine plus cisplatin) [6, 7]. Meta-analysis study defined the efficacy of oxaliplatin-based regimens but it as an important limitation having evaluated only small single arm studies [8].

All this result suggests that better efficacy in some situation could be obtained with oxaliplatin-base regimen and GEMOX combination in some setting. But current trials are emerging and focusing on targeted therapies and immunotherapy that have significantly improve survival outcome.

3. Targeted therapies

The vascular nature of HCC and that vascular endothelial growth factor (VEGF) play role of HCC development and metastasis, anti-angiogenesis agents have been studies extensively in the setting of advanced HCC. All, this knowledge dramatically leaded changing of systemic therapies form chemotherapy to molecular targeted agent. Since sorafenib was established as standard first line therapy in advanced HCC.

3.1 Targeted first line therapies

3.1.1 Sorafenib

Sorafenib, a multi-tyrosine kinase inhibitor with antiangiogenic effects is thought to be mediated by the blockade of VEGFR 2–3, platelet-derived growth factor receptor (PDGFR)-B, and other receptor tyrosine kinases. Sorafenib was approved in 2007 by the FDA as first-line therapy for unresectable HCC with BCLC stage C,

Child-Pugh class A or BCLC stage B that progressing after locoregional therapy. It was recommended in patient with well performance status (Eastern cooperative oncology group or ECOG PS 0–2) and preserve liver function test. The efficacy of this drug was demonstrated in two phase III, randomized, placebo-controlled clinical trials: the SHARP study [9] and the Asia-Pacific study (ORIENTAL) [10]. The patient population was mainly recruited form Europe and North America in SHARP study and Asian population in Asia-Pacific study. In the SHARP phase III studies, Sorafenib treatment with dose 400 mg twice a day compared to placebo. Among 602 patients, sorafenib significantly improved overall survival compared with placebo (HR 0.69; 10.7 mons vs. 7.9 mons, $P < 0.001$), DCR (disease control rate) about 43% in sorafenib arm compared to 32% in placebo arm ($P = 0.002$). Sorafenib study arm had significantly prolong time to radiologic progression in 5.5 mons compared with 2.8 mons in placebo arm ($P < 0.001$), Even though sorafenib prolong time to radiologic progression but there is no significant difference in term of time to symptomatic progression. Population of this trial was mostly patients with advanced stage HCC including 35% with macrovascular invasion and 50% with extrahepatic disease. The observed side effects were diarrhea, weight loss, hand-foot syndrome and hypophosphatemia. The result of the SHARP trial was subsequently confirmed in Asia-Pacific study and in 10 subsequent trials with and median overall survival in the range of 10–12 months. Efficacy of sorafenib was conducted in Asia-Pacific region population (The ORIENTAL study). The study was performed with the same design study to the SHARP trial. The Sorafenib arm group had significantly increase overall survival with 6.5 mons compared to 4.2 mons in placebo arm ($P = 0.014$). The overall survival-time and progression free survival time was lower compared to the SHARP study. Unfortunately, objective responses rate is poor with 2% by Response Evaluation Criteria in Solid Tumors (RECIST) and 10% by modified RECIST (mRECIST) [11] and no predictive biomarkers of responsiveness to sorafenib have been identified.

From the positively result, Sorafenib was approved with patient who has well Child-Pugh score (CTP A only); however, result for the GIDEON (Global investigation of therapeutic decision in Hepatocellular Carcinoma and its Treatment with Sorafenib) study, a large observational study assessing the safety profile and efficacy in patients with poor liver dysfunction, the result had a similar safety profile irrespective of Child-Pugh scoring [12]. However, Clinical practice guideline recommended that sorafenib in patient with underlying liver dysfunction is not recommended based on these data alone. The risks and benefits of sorafenib should be carefully consideration prior to start.

The recommended dose of sorafenib is 800 mg. Median treatment duration is estimated 5–6 months, but early recognition and prevention of toxicities can enhance tolerability. Sorafenib toxicities can be manageable. Common toxicities are diarrhea, hand-foot skin reaction (HFS), fatigue and hypertension. 35% of the patient in the study needed dose reduction and 15% of patients need to withdraw from the study due to adverse side effect sorafenib. Liver failure that related to sorafenib complications are marginal. Considering the restrictive indication of sorafenib in Child-Pugh A class only. However, because of its poor antitumor effect and relatively toxicity, developing a new targeted agent with superior efficacy and/or lower toxicity has been a critical issue.

3.1.2 Lenvatinib

After sorafenib has been approved for advanced HCC then several studies have been conducted to compare sorafenib in front line therapy such as sunitinib [13], brivatinib [14], erlotinib [15], linifanib [16] or everolimus [17] without showing superiority (or at least non-inferiority) to sorafenib. Lenvatinib has only recently shown non-inferior clinical benefit in REFLECT study [18]. Lenvatinib is an oral multi-kinase inhibitor that targets VEGFR 1–3 and fibroblast growth factor receptor (FGFR) 1–4, among others. REFLECT study is an open-label, Phase III, multicenter, non-inferiority study demonstrated efficacy in Lenvatinib compared with sorafenib in patients with advanced HCC (excluding main portal vein invasion, clear bile duct invasion and > 50% of tumor to total liver volume occupancy). Lenvatinib was adjusted to body weight of patient. The study was evaluated in the first line therapy. The study met the primary endpoint of non-inferiority in overall survival (HR = 0.92, 13.6 mons, Lenvatinib compared 12.3 mons, sorafenib, 95% CI = 0.79–1.06). Secondary outcomes in PFS and time to progression were better for Lenvatinib. Overall response rate (ORR) by mRECIST had significant better response (24% versus 9.2% for sorafenib, $P < 0.001$). This drug has shown a higher response rate compared with other tyrosine kinase inhibitors (TKIs) and sorafenib. Most common adverse effects compared with sorafenib were as follows: hypertension (42% versus 30%), diarrhea (39% versus 45%) and HFS (27% versus 52%). These results, Lenvatinib was approved as an option in first line therapy for advanced HCC.

Arguing for a use of Lenvatinib when rapid tumor shrinkage is warranted. Further subgroup analyses showed that Asian populations, patients with hepatitis B infection and high serum AFP > 200 ng/mL demonstrated a particular benefit form treatment with Lenvatinib. Comparing in term of side effects Lenvatinib was associated with more frequent side effects than sorafenib but manageable. More important high side effects were hypertension and weight loss for Lenvatinib. Based on these documents, current clinical practice guidelines recommended both Lenvatinib and sorafenib as frontline therapy for unresectable or advance stage HCC that are not amendable to surgery or locoregional therapies [19].

3.2 Targeted second-line therapies

In the SHARP/ASIAN-Pacific and REFLECT studies, it was shown that administration of TKIs only leads to relatively short periods of tumor control. The recent data evaluated the efficacy of targeted therapies in second-line therapy that shown clinical benefit in patients with advanced HCC that progressed on prior sorafenib therapy in front-line treatment, drugs that considered in this setting was regorafenib, carbozantinib and ramucirumab.

3.2.1 Regorafenib

Regorafenib, a multi-kinase inhibitor targeting similar kinases as sorafenib. Phase III study (RESOUCE) study [20] was conducted to comparing regorafenib with placebo in advanced HCC patients progressing despite sorafenib. The starting dose of regorafenib is 160 mg/day (3 weeks on and 1 week off). The primary endpoint of this study is overall survival. The study was positive for its primary end points (HR = 0.62, $P < 0.001$, 10.6 months in the regorafenib group vs. 7.8 months in the placebo). The secondary endpoints were PFS, ORR and safety profile. Regorafenib had significantly prolonged time to disease progression (3.1 versus 1.5 months). The efficacy of treatment improved survival in all subgroups of patients. Population in this trial, 88% were BCLC stage C and 12% were BCLC stage B, with all of them tolerant to sorafenib but progression on treatment. 70% of patients had extrahepatic spread and 30% had macrovascular invasion. Around half of patients has high AFP more than 400 ng/dL. The response rate was only 10%, based on mRECIST. Median time on treatment was 3.5 months. Hypertension was the most common adverse effect, occurring in 15% of patients on regorafenib, followed by HFS. Adverse effects led to 51% dose reductions and 10% treatment discontinuation. Sequential administration of sorafenib and regorafenib resulted in an OS of 26 months compared with 19 months in patients receiving only sorafenib as first-line and placebo as second line treatment [21].

Regorafenib is the standard of care for patients with advanced HCC who have tolerated sorafenib but progressed and recommended in patients with well-preserved liver function test (Child-Pugh A class) and good ECOG PS 0–1.

3.2.2 Cabozantinib

Cabozantinib is another TKI targeting VEGFR 1–3, MET, RET and AXL [22]. Carbozantinib was approved for thyroid and renal cancer. Phase III study (CELESTIAL) [23] compared the efficacy of carbozantinib as second- and third-line therapy in advanced HCC patients after failure of a sorafenib compared with placebo. In contrast to regorafenib, this study allowed the inclusion of patients that were intolerant to sorafenib and who had progressive disease on one or two systemic therapies. Carbozantinib led to a significant improvement in overall survival (HR = 0.76, 95% CI = 0.63–0.92, P = 0.0049, 10.2 mons versus 8.0 mons). Other secondary end points such as PFS and ORR were also positive. It is worth noting that 27% of the patients had received 2 previous systemic agents. 30% of populations in this study presented with macrovascular invasion, 78% with extra-hepatic spreading and 45% with AFP > 400 ng/dL. Response rate was only 4% with carbozantinib based upon RECIST criteria. The most common adverse effects are HFS, hypertension, increased level of aspartate aminotransferase (AST), fatigue and diarrhea. These adverse effects led to 62% dose reduction and 16% treatment discontinuation.

Carbozantinib can be considered for patients who had progressive disease on one or two systemic therapies with well-preserve liver function and good ECOG PS 0–1.

Because RESORCE and CELESTIAL compared with a placebo arm, it is no data shown that which is superior or inferior in term of efficacy to the other. Biomarkers have not yet been identified. The RESORCE study recently identified a total of five proteins (angiopoietin 1, cystatin B, the latency-associated peptide of TGF-β1, oxidized low-density lipoprotein receptor 1 and C-C motif chemokine ligand 3) that were associated with prolonged survival with regorafenib [24]. In addition, nine plasma miRNAs (MIR30A, MIR122, MIR125B, MIR200A, MIR374B, MIR15B, MIR107, MIR320 and MIR645) were correlated with an improved survival. To what extent these findings will become clinically relevant remains to be seen.

3.2.3 Ramucirumab

Ramucirumab is a human immunoglobulin G1 (IgG1) monoclonal antibody (mAb) that inhibits ligand activation of VEGFR2. Phase III study (REACH) [25] conducted for tested efficacy of ramucirumab in term of overall survival in advanced HCC after the failure of sorafenib. The primary end point of the study is OS was not statistically significant, but a meaningful improvement was observed in subgroup patients with baseline AFP > 400 ng/mL. Based on these data, the REACH-2 phase III study [26] analyzed the efficacy of ramucirumab in patients with baseline AFP > 400 ng/mL after failure with sorafenib. Result of this study shown ramucirumab significantly improved overall survival from 7.3 mons to 8.5 mons (HR = 0.71, 95% CI = 0.53–0.95) and median PFS from 1.6 mons to 2.8 mons (HR = 0.45, 95% CI = 0.34–0.60) compared with placebo. Overall response rate was 4.6%. The safety profile observed in this study was consistent with previously study, only grade III adverse effects occurring were hypertension (12.2%) and hyponatremia (5.6%)

Ramucirumab can be considered for patients in second-line therapy with baseline AFP > 400 ng/mL with well-preserved liver function and good ECOG PS 0–1, thus, the AFP may serve as a marker for the benefit of ramucirumab in the second line setting for advanced hepatocellular carcinoma. Ramucirumab remains the only systemic agent that demonstrated clinical benefit in biomarker selected population in HCC.

3.3 Immunotherapy

The most promising immunotherapeutic approach has been the use of immune checkpoint inhibitors in vary of cancer type including gastrointestinal malignancies. Immune checkpoint inhibitor can change paradigm of treatment and improve survival and quality of life in many type of cancer. Tumor-infiltrating lymphocytes (TILs) in the tumor microenvironment was demonstrated in hepatocellular carcinoma cell, which shown that HCC is also immunogenic cancer [27]. Some studies have also shown the presence of an immunosuppressive intratumoral milieu driven by constant exposure of the liver to antigens via the portal system and immune dysfunction related to cirrhosis [28]. These results of a phenomenon of immune escape might predict that HCC could be response to immunotherapy and immune checkpoint inhibitor drugs.

3.4 First-line immunotherapy

Single agent of Immunotherapy has been conducted in two phase III studies as first line therapy. The Checkmate 459 trial, Nivolumab compared to standard of care as sorafenib, failed to meet the primary endpoint as overall survival [29]. Also, with, The KEYNOTE-240 trial of pembrolizumab as second line treatment of advance HCC after failure to sorafenib compared with placebo, failed to meet endpoints of OS and progression free survival [30]. They are not recommended as monotherapy for the treatment of advanced HCC.

To date, new combination immunotherapy with Atezolizumab plus bevacizumab were change paradigm of treatment in advanced HCC. This combination therapy is the first treatment to demonstrate a significant OS benefit compared with sorafenib in Phase III international, open label of patients with locally advanced or metastatic and/or unresectable HCC (IMbrave 150 study) [31]. Patients were allocated randomization with 2:1 ratio to compare efficacy of Atezolizumab plus bevacizumab to sorafenib. The coprimary endpoints were overall survival and progression free survival. The combination therapy demonstrated a significant overall survival benefit (HR = 0.66, 95% CI = 0.52–0.85). The median overall survival was not reached (Not estimate or NE) in the Atezolizumab plus bevacizumab arm, whereas sorafenib arm had median overall survival at 13.2 months. The study reported a significantly PFS of combination therapy compared to sorafenib (6.8 mons vs. 4.3 mons, HR = 0.59, 95% CI = 0.47–0.76, P < 0.0001). The difference in overall response rate was significant (stratified $P < 0.0001$): Atezolizumab plus Bevacizumab arm = 27%, and sorafenib arm = 12%. Complete response was achieved in 18 patients (6%), which is quite promising. The median duration of response of NE and the proportion (80%) of responders with a DOR of >6 months by Atezolizumab plus Bevacizumab arm therapy indicate a considerable durable response to this treatment. Successful benefit both the OS and PFS endpoints at first analysis was surprising and coming to a new era of systemic therapy for HCC as standard of care in first-line therapy due to meet primary endpoint of overall survival benefit.

Treatment related adverse effects especially grades III or IV were found more in sorafenib arm (46%) compared to Atezolizumab plus Bevacizumab arm (36%). Immune-related adverse effects were rarely observed in the Atezolizumab plus Bevacizumab arm (expect for infusion reaction in 10.9%, AIHA in 0.3% and adrenal insufficiency in 0.3%). Bleeding events form bevacizumab was minimal occurring at 6.4%. The data suggest that the acceptable safety profile in Atezolizumab plus Bevacizumab.

However, the median progression free survival is only 6.8 months and only 20% of patients do not response to atezolizumab plus bevacizumab, experimental studies need to define options for second-line therapy after progression on immunotherapy. Most of drugs only been tested after sorafenib intolerance or progression and there are currently no phase III study to inform the choice of therapy in this setting. However, a clear rationale for offering a targeted therapy given the existing evidence for efficacy in first- and second-line therapy.

3.5 Other combination immunotherapies

To current knowledge of combination immune checkpoint blockade plus anti-angiogenesis translate to new combination therapy that need to find out the clinical benefit. Basic research studies show that lenvatinib and anti-PD-1 antibodies have synergistic effects [32]. Immunotherapy and Molecular targeting agents as combination therapy might have a role in the treatment of HCC in the future. A phase Ib trial of combination use of lenvatinib plus pembrolizumab reported promising results [33]. This combination had a median progression free survival and overall survival of 9.3 months (95% CI: 5.6–9.7) and 22.0 months (95% CI: 20.4–NE), respectively. Overall response rate was higher in 46% (95% CI: 36.0–56.3). A phase III trial (LEAP002) of this combination is currently ongoing. On the other hand, rationale of dual combination immune checkpoint blockade (PD-L1 plus CTLA-4 inhibitor) might have a clinical response too. The results of combination therapy with the durvalumab (PD-L1 antibody) and the tremelimumab (CTLA-4 antibody). The study revealed a median PFS and OS of 2.17 months (95% CI: 1.91–5.42) and 18.73 months (95% CI: 10.78–27.27), respectively. ORR this combination therapy was 24.0% (95% CI, 14.9–35.3). Therefore, this combination therapy is promising, and the phase III HIMALAYA trial of this combination is ongoing too.

3.6 Second-line immunotherapy

Second-line therapy after the failure of sorafenib apart from molecular targeting agents. Data of immunotherapy both pembrolizumab (an anti-PD-1 monoclonal antibody) and nivolumab (a fully humanized monoclonal antibody against PD-1) shown efficacy in Phase Ib studies (CheckMate-040 [34] and Keynote-224 [35]). Unfortunately, for pembrolizumab, these results were negative in the Phase III study, randomized double-blind keynote-240 study, which included a total of 413 patients with pretreated advanced HCC. The study was comparable with pembrolizumab or placebo. The median OS was 13.9 months in the pembrolizumab arm versus 10.6 months in the control arm (HR: 0.78; P = 0.024), the median PFS was 3.0 mons versus 2.8 mons (HR: 0.72; P = 0.002). However, since the prespecified alpha level was significantly lower, the study must be considered statistically negative. CTLA-4 antibodies were also tested in second-line therapy of advance stage HCC; The study reported results (response rate was 17.6% and a median time to progression was 6.48 months) from patients treated with tremelimumab [36]. Nivolumab as single agent in advance HCC treated with sorafenib reported an ORR of 14% and median OS of 16 months. Due to the promising results the study was conducted the efficacy and safety of the combination of nivolumab and ipilimumab [37]. The study was randomized into three different dose and time arms of nivolumab and ipilimumab. Of note, the first arm (Nivolumab 1 mg/kg + ipilimumab 3 mg/kg every 3 weeks (Q3W) followed by n 240 mg Q2W) demonstrated the most promising efficacy in term of OS (23 months). ORR and disease control rate were 31% and 49%, respectively. Interestingly, the different combinations were well tolerated, potentially offering a novel treatment option for patients with pretreated HCC.

4. Conclusion

Current data of systemic therapy in advanced stage/unresectable or failure to locoregional therapy HCC shown efficacy and safety profile of multiple targeting agents such as Lenvatinib, regorafenib, cabozantinib and ramucirumab in addition to standard treatment with sorafenib. New emerging current standard of care in advanced HCC is change to combination therapy with Bevacizumab plus atezolizumab as first line therapy due to improvement of progression free survival and with overall survival. The increase in available multiple targeting agents and immune checkpoint blockade will benefit in many patients. Sequential therapy and drug selection will become more challenging as **Figure 1**. New strategies of systemic therapy with new combination therapy are needed to explore.

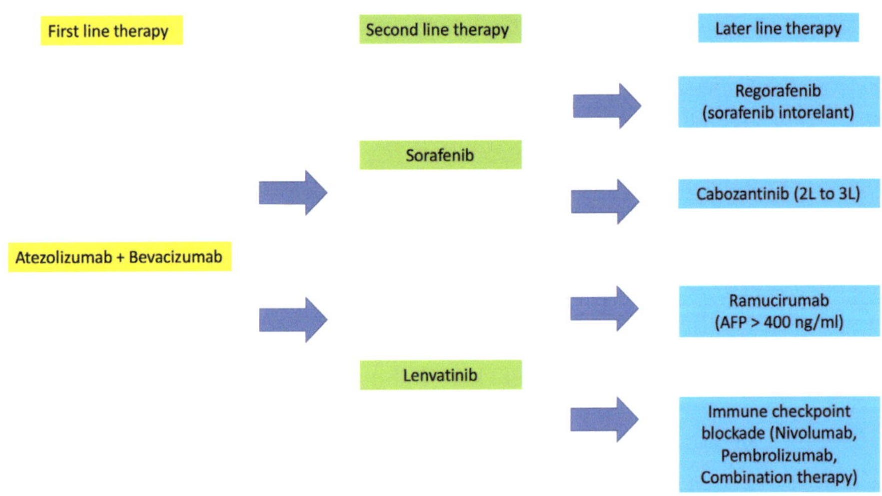

Figure 1.
Possible sequential systemic therapy for advanced stage/unresectable or failure to locoregional treatment HCC, hepatocellular carcinoma; 2 L, second line; 3 L, third line; AFP, alpha-fetoprotein.

Acknowledgements

The authors would like to thank all colleagues in the Department of Internal Medicine, Faculty of Medicine, Srinakharinwirot University especially the Hepatocellular excellent center team for their invaluable help and encouragement throughout the course of this work.

Conflict of interest

The authors declare no conflict of interest.

Author details

Chanchai Charonpongsuntorn
Department of Internal Medicine, Faculty of Medicine, Srinakharinwirot University, Bangkok, Thailand

*Address all correspondence to: chanchaic@g.swu.ac.th

References

[1] Llovet JM, Villanueva A, Lachenmayer A, Finn RS. Advances in targeted therapies for hepatocellular carcinoma in the genomic era. Nat Rev Clin Oncol 2015; 12: 436.

[2] Llovet JM, Bruix J. Novel advancements in the management of hepatocellular carcinoma in 2008. J Hepatol. 2008;48 Suppl 1:S20-S37.

[3] Qin S, Bai Y, Lim HY, et al. Randomized, multicenter, open-label study of oxaliplatin plus fluorouracil/leucovorin versus doxorubicin as palliative chemotherapy in patients with advanced hepatocellular carcinoma from Asia. J Clin Oncol. 2013;31:3501-3508. PMID: 23980077.

[4] Qin S, Cheng Y, Liang J, Shen L, Bai Y, Li J, Fan J, Liang L, Zhang Y, Wu G, et al. Efficacy and safety of the FOLFOX4 regimen versus doxorubicin in Chinese patients with advanced hepatocellular carcinoma: a subgroup analysis of the EACH study. Oncologist. 2014;19:1169-1178

[5] Zaanan A, Williet N, Hebbar M, Dabakuyo TS, Fartoux L, Mansourbakht T, Dubreuil O, Rosmorduc O, Cattan S, Bonnetain F, et al. Gemcitabine plus oxaliplatin in advanced hepatocellular carcinoma: a large multicenter AGEO study. J Hepatol. 2013;58:81-88

[6] Boige V, Raoul JL, Pignon JP, Bouché O, Blanc JF, Dahan L, Jouve JL, Dupouy N, Ducreux M. Multicentre phase II trial of capecitabine plus oxaliplatin (XELOX) in patients with advanced hepatocellular carcinoma: FFCD 03-03 trial. Br J Cancer. 2007;97: 862-867.

[7] Chia WK, Ong S, Toh HC, Hee SW, Choo SP, Poon DY, Tay MH, Tan CK, Koo WH, Foo KF. Phase II trial of gemcitabine in combination with cisplatin in inoperable or advanced hepatocellular carcinoma. Ann Acad Med Singapore. 2008;37:554-558.

[8] Petrelli F, Coinu A, Borgonovo K, Cabiddu M, Ghilardi M, Lonati V, Barni S. Oxaliplatin-based chemotherapy: a new option in advanced hepatocellular carcinoma. a systematic review and pooled analysis. Clin Oncol (R Coll Radiol) 2014;26: 488-496.

[9] Llovet JM, Ricci S, Mazzaferro V et al. Sorafenib in advanced hepatocellular carcinoma. N Engl J Med 2008; 359: 378-390.

[10] Cheng AL, Kang YK, Chen Z, Tsao CJ, Qin S, Kim JS, Luo R, Feng J, Ye S, Yang TS, et al. Efficacy and safety of sorafenib in patients in the Asia-Pacific region with advanced hepatocellular carcinoma: a phase III randomised, double-blind, placebo-controlled trial. Lancet Oncol. 2009;10:25-34.

[11] Lencioni R, Llovet JM. Modified RECIST (mRECIST) assessment for hepatocellular carcinoma. Semin Liver Dis 2010; 30: 52-60.

[12] Marrero JA, Kudo M, Venook AP, et al. Observational registry of sorafenib use in clinical practice across Child-Pugh subgroups: the GIDEON study. J Hepatol. 2016;65(6):1140-1147.

[13] Cheng AL, Kang YK, Lin DY et al. Sunitinib versus sorafenib in advanced hepatocellular cancer: results of a randomized Phase III trial. J. Clin. Oncol. 31(32), 4067-4075 (2013).

[14] Johnson PJ, Qin S, Park JW et al. Brivanib versus sorafenib as first-line therapy in patients with unresectable, advanced hepatocellular carcinoma: results from the randomized Phase III BRISK-FL study. J. Clin. Oncol. 31(28), 3517-3524

[15] Zhu AX, Rosmorduc O, Evans TR et al. SEARCH: a Phase III, randomized, double-blind, placebo-controlled trial of sorafenib plus erlotinib in patients with advanced hepatocellular carcinoma. J. Clin. Oncol. 33(6), 559-566 (2015).

[16] Cainap C, Qin S, Huang WT et al. Linifanib versus sorafenib in patients with advanced hepatocellular carcinoma: results of a randomized Phase III trial. J. Clin. Oncol. 33(2), 172-179 (2015)

[17] Zhu AX, Kudo M, Assenat E et al. Effect of everolimus on survival in advanced hepatocellular carcinoma after failure of sorafenib: the EVOLVE-1 randomized clinical trial. JAMA 312(1), 57-67 (2014).

[18] Kudo M, Finn RS, Qin S et al. Lenvatinib versus sorafenib in first-line treatment of patients with unresectable hepatocellular carcinoma: a randomised phase 3 non-inferiority trial. Lancet 2018; 391: 1163-1173.

[19] EASL clinical practice guidelines: management of hepatocellular carcinoma. J. Hepatol. 69(1), 182-236 (2018).

[20] Bruix J, Qin S, Merle P et al. Regorafenib for patients with hepatocellular carcinoma who progressed on sorafenib treatment (RESORCE): a randomised, double-blind, placebo-controlled, Phase III trial. Lancet 389(10064), 56-66 (2017).

[21] Finn RS, Merle P, Granito A et al. Outcomes of sequential treatment with sorafenib followed by regorafenib for HCC: additional analyses from the Phase III RESORCE trial. J. Hepatol. 69(2), 353-358 (2018).

[22] Durante C, Russo D, Verrienti A, Filetti S. XL184 (cabozantinib) for medullary thyroid carcinoma. Expert Opin. Investig. Drugs 20(3), 407-413 (2011).

[23] Abou-Alfa GK, Meyer T, Cheng AL et al. Cabozantinib in patients with advanced and progressing hepatocellular carcinoma. N. Engl. J. Med. 379(1), 54-63 (2018).

[24] Teufel M, Seidel H, Kochert K et al. Biomarkers associated with response to regorafenib in patients with hepatocellular carcinoma. Gastroenterology156(6), 1731 1741 (2019)

[25] Zhu AX, Park JO, Ryoo BY et al. Ramucirumab versus placebo as second-line treatment in patients with advanced hepatocellular carcinoma following first-line therapy with sorafenib (REACH): a randomised, double-blind, multicentre, Phase III trial. Lancet Oncol. 16(7), 859-870 (2015)

[26] Zhu AX, Kang Y-K, Yen C-J et al. REACH-2: a randomized, double- blind, placebo-controlled phase 3 study of ramucirumab versus placebo as second-line treatment in patients with advanced hepatocellular car- cinoma (HCC) and elevated baseline alpha-fetoprotein (AFP) following first-line sorafenib. J Clin Oncol 2018; 36: 4003-4003.

[27] Yoong KF, McNab G, Hübscher SG, Adams DH. Vascular adhesion protein-1 and ICAM-1 support the adhesion of tumor-infiltrating lymphocytes to tumor endothelium in human hepatocellular carcinoma. J Immunol. 1998;160(8): 3978-3988.

[28] Thomson AW, Knolle PA. Antigen-presenting cell function in the tolerogenic liver environment. Nat Rev Immunol. 2010;10(11):753-766.

[29] Yau T, Park JW, Finn RS, et al. CheckMate 459: a randomized, multi-center phase III study of nivolumab (NIVO) vs sorafenib (SOR) as first-line (1L) treatment in patients (pts) with advanced hepatocellular carcinoma (aHCC). Ann Oncol. 2019;30(5): v874-v875.

[30] Finn RS, Ryoo BY, Merle P, et al. Pembrolizumab as second-line therapy in patients with advanced Hepato cellular carcinoma in KEYNOTE-240: a randomized, double-blind, phase III Trial. J Clin Oncol. 2020;38(3):193- 202.

[31] Finn RS, Qin S, Ikeda M, et al. Atezolizumab plus bevacizumab in unre- sectable hepatocellular carcinoma. N Engl J Med. 2020;382(20):1894- 1905.

[32] Kudo M. Immune checkpoint inhibition in hepatocellular carcinoma: basics and ongoing clinical trials. Oncology. 2017;92(Suppl1):50-62.

[33] Finn RS, Ikeda M, Zhu AX, Sung MW, Baron AD, Kudo M, et al. Phase Ib study of lenvatinib plus pembrolizumab in patients with unresectable hepatocellular carcinoma. J Clin Oncol. 2020;38(26):2960-2970.

[34] El-Khoueiry AB, Sangro B, Yau T et al. Nivolumab in patients with advanced hepatocellular carcinoma (CheckMate 040): an open-label, non-comparative, Phase I/II dose escalation and expansion trial. **Lancet** 389(10088), 2492-2502 (2017).

[35] Zhu AX, Finn RS, Edeline J et al. Pembrolizumab in patients with advanced hepatocellular carcinoma previously treated with sorafenib (KEYNOTE-224): a non-randomised, open-label Phase II trial. **Lancet Oncol.** 19(7), 940-952 (2018).

[36] Sangro B, Gomez-Martin C, de la Mata M et al. A clinical trial of CTLA-4 blockade with tremelimumab in patients with hepatocellular carcinoma and chronic hepatitis C. **J. Hepatol.** 59(1), 81-88

[37] Yau T, Zagonel V, Santoro A et al. Nivolumab (NIVO) + ipilimumab (IPI) + cabozantinib (CABO) combination therapy in patients (pts) with advanced hepatocellular carcinoma (aHCC): results from CheckMate 040. Presented at: **GI Cancers Symposium**. San Francisco, CA, USA (2020)